AF101378

Advances in Marine Natural Product Characterisation and Separation Methodologies

Advances in Marine Natural Product Characterisation and Separation Methodologies

Editor

Sylvia Urban

MDPI • Basel • Beijing • Wuhan • Barcelona • Belgrade • Manchester • Tokyo • Cluj • Tianjin

Editor
Sylvia Urban
RMIT University (City Campus)
Australia

Editorial Office
MDPI
St. Alban-Anlage 66
4052 Basel, Switzerland

This is a reprint of articles from the Special Issue published online in the open access journal *Marine Drugs* (ISSN 1660-3397) (available at: https://www.mdpi.com/journal/marinedrugs/special_issues/Advances_Characterisation_Separation_Methodologies).

For citation purposes, cite each article independently as indicated on the article page online and as indicated below:

LastName, A.A.; LastName, B.B.; LastName, C.C. Article Title. *Journal Name* **Year**, *Article Number*, Page Range.

ISBN 978-3-03943-128-1 (Hbk)
ISBN 978-3-03943-129-8 (PDF)

© 2020 by the authors. Articles in this book are Open Access and distributed under the Creative Commons Attribution (CC BY) license, which allows users to download, copy and build upon published articles, as long as the author and publisher are properly credited, which ensures maximum dissemination and a wider impact of our publications.
The book as a whole is distributed by MDPI under the terms and conditions of the Creative Commons license CC BY-NC-ND.

Contents

About the Editor vii

Preface to "Advances in Marine Natural Product Characterisation and Separation Methodologies" ix

Gennaro Pescitelli
For a Correct Application of the CD Exciton Chirality Method: The Case of Laucysteinamide A
Reprinted from: *Mar. Drugs* **2018**, *16*, 388, doi:10.3390/md16100388 1

José Antonio Vázquez, Javier Fraguas, Ramón Novoa-Carvallal, Rui L. Reis, Luis T. Antelo, Ricardo I. Pérez-Martín and Jesus Valcarcel
Isolation and Chemical Characterization of Chondroitin Sulfate from Cartilage By-Products of Blackmouth Catshark (*Galeus melastomus*)
Reprinted from: *Mar. Drugs* **2018**, *16*, 344, doi:10.3390/md16100344 13

Giuseppe Di Sanzo, Sanjeet Mehariya, Maria Martino, Vincenzo Larocca, Patrizia Casella, Simeone Chianese, Dino Musmarra, Roberto Balducchi and Antonio Molino
Supercritical Carbon Dioxide Extraction of Astaxanthin, Lutein, and Fatty Acids from *Haematococcus pluvialis* Microalgae
Reprinted from: *Mar. Drugs* **2018**, *16*, 334, doi:10.3390/md16090334 29

Yingqi Mi, Wenqiang Tan, Jingjing Zhang, Lijie Wei, Yuan Chen, Qing Li, Fang Dong and Zhanyong Guo
Synthesis, Characterization, and Antifungal Property of Hydroxypropyltrimethyl Ammonium Chitosan Halogenated Acetates
Reprinted from: *Mar. Drugs* **2018**, *16*, 315, doi:10.3390/md16090315 47

Takeshi Yamada, Tetsuya Kajimoto, Takashi Kikuchi and Reiko Tanaka
Elucidation of the Relationship between CD Cotton Effects and the Absolute Configuration of Sixteen Stereoisomers of Spiroheterocyclic-Lactams
Reprinted from: *Mar. Drugs* **2018**, *16*, 223, doi:10.3390/md16070223 61

Caleb Singleton, Robert Brkljača and Sylvia Urban
Absolute Configuration Determination of Retroflexanone Using the Advanced Mosher Method and Application of HPLC-NMR
Reprinted from: *Mar. Drugs* **2018**, *16*, 205, doi:10.3390/md16060205 73

Feifei Wang, Luodong Huang, Baoyan Gao and Chengwu Zhang
Optimum Production Conditions, Purification, Identification, and Antioxidant Activity of Violaxanthin from Microalga *Eustigmatos* cf. *polyphem* (Eustigmatophyceae)
Reprinted from: *Mar. Drugs* **2018**, *16*, 190, doi:10.3390/md16060190 83

Yong Liu, Xuezhen Zhou, C. Benjamin Naman, Yanbin Lu, Lijian Ding and Shan He
Preparative Separation and Purification of Trichothecene Mycotoxins from the Marine Fungus *Fusarium* sp. LS68 by High-Speed Countercurrent Chromatography in Stepwise Elution Mode
Reprinted from: *Mar. Drugs* **2018**, *16*, 73, doi:10.3390/md16020073 97

Sara Kildgaard, Karolina Subko, Emma Phillips, Violaine Goidts, Mercedes de la Cruz, Caridad Díaz, Charlotte H. Gotfredsen, Birgitte Andersen, Jens C. Frisvad, Kristian F. Nielsen and Thomas O. Larsen
A Dereplication and Bioguided Discovery Approach to Reveal New Compounds from a Marine-Derived Fungus *Stilbella fimetaria*
Reprinted from: *Mar. Drugs* **2017**, *15*, 253, doi:10.3390/md15080253 . . . . **107**

Amanda Lawrence, Shadaesha Green and Jum Sook Chung
Isolation and Tissue Distribution of an Insulin-Like Androgenic Gland Hormone (IAG) of the Male Red Deep-Sea Crab, *Chaceon quinquedens*
Reprinted from: *Mar. Drugs* **2017**, *15*, 241, doi:10.3390/md15080241 . . . . **127**

About the Editor

Sylvia Urban Sylvia is an associate professor at the School of Science, RMIT University, and a fellow of the Royal Australian Chemical Society (FRACI). She completed her Ph.D. at The University of Melbourne and has held research appointments in the field of natural product drug discovery (with AstraZeneca and PharmaMar SA) at Griffith University and at the University of Canterbury, Christchurch, New Zealand, respectively. She was awarded an ASP Research Starter grant from the American Society of Pharmacognosy and the Gerald Blunden Award for her activities in natural product chemistry research. Her research interests include marine and terrestrial natural products chemistry; isolation and structural characterisation; NMR spectroscopy and analytical separation and profiling methodologies for natural product discovery. Sylvia leads the Marine and Terrestrial Natural Product research group at RMIT University. Sylvia is also Program Manager of the Bachelor of Science degree at RMIT University, and is a passionate chemistry educator and a leader in transforming education in STEM. In 2019, she was awarded an Australian Award for University Teaching (AAUT) Citation for Outstanding Contribution to Student Learning, and was elected as a Senior Fellow of the Higher Education Academy (SFHEA) in 2018. Sylvia has served as Deputy Chair and a committee member of the Women Researchers Network (WRN) at RMIT University, and is a committee member of the Royal Australian Chemical Society (RACI) Women in Chemistry group (WinC). Her goal is to promote better opportunities for women in science, technology, engineering and mathematics (STEM), and she has been selected for some key leadership programs that provide leadership training and support to women in the university sector. Finally, Sylvia is Reconcilation Facilitator and Ingidenous Coordinator for the School of Science at RMIT University, a role that she is passionate about, especially as it entails better understanding how we can embed indigenous knowledge into the STEM education sector.

Preface to "Advances in Marine Natural Product Characterisation and Separation Methodologies"

The search for bioactive marine natural products calls for the need for efficient chemical profiling strategies, together with the need for advances in separation and characterization methodologies, in order to expedite their discovery. This Special Issue of Marine Drugs highlights some advances in extraction, isolation, purification and dereplication methodologies in the quest for bioactive marine natural products. In total, ten articles have been published, covering applications such as the application of the CD Exciton Chirality method, Super critical carbon dioxide extraction, dereplication approaches, synthesis and preparative separation, as well as various approaches to deducing the absolute configuration of a range of marine natural products.

Sylvia Urban
Editor

marine drugs

MDPI

Article

For a Correct Application of the CD Exciton Chirality Method: The Case of Laucysteinamide A

Gennaro Pescitelli

Department of Chemistry and Industrial Chemistry, University of Pisa, Via G. Moruzzi 13, 56124 Pisa, Italy; gennaro.pescitelli@unipi.it; Tel.: +39-050-2219-339

Received: 21 September 2018; Accepted: 15 October 2018; Published: 16 October 2018

Abstract: The circular dichroism (CD) exciton chirality method (ECM) is a very popular approach for assigning the absolute configuration (AC) of natural products, thanks to its immediacy and ease of application. The sign of an exciton couplet (two electronic CD bands with opposite sign and similar intensity) can be directly correlated with the molecular stereochemistry, including the AC. However, a correct application of the ECM necessitates several prerequisites: knowledge of the molecular conformation; knowledge of transition moment direction; and preeminence of the exciton coupling mechanism with respect to other sources of CD signals. In recent years, by using quantum-chemical CD calculations, we have demonstrated that some previous applications of ECM were wrong or based on incorrect assumptions. In a recent publication of this journal (*Mar. Drugs*, **2017**, *15*(4), 121), the ECM was employed to assign the AC of a marine metabolite, laucysteinamide A. This is a further case of incorrect application of the method, where none of the aforementioned prerequisites is fully met. Using this example, we will discuss the criteria required for a correct application of the ECM.

Keywords: electronic circular dichroism; absolute configuration; molecular conformation; electric transition dipole moment; exciton coupling; TDDFT calculations

1. Introduction

The very large majority of known natural products is chiral and contains multiple centers of chirality [1]. The two enantiomers of a chiral substance most often display different biological and pharmaceutical properties [2]. As a consequence, a complete stereochemical elucidation is a common requirement in natural products discovery. A novel chiral natural compound cannot be said to be fully characterized until its absolute configuration (AC) is determined. Marine natural products are, of course, not an exception [3]. The most important method for assigning ACs is X-ray structure determination [4]. Unfortunately, it is restricted to crystalline materials of compounds exhibiting enough strong anomalous dispersion. Alternatively, a wide family of chiroptical techniques exists specifically designed to analyze chiral nonracemic substances [5,6]. Of these, electronic circular dichroism (ECD, or simply CD) remains the most popular one in the field of natural products discovery [7], although vibrational CD (VCD) and Raman optical activity are gaining progressive interest [8,9]. Currently, the most common approach to assign AC by ECD or VCD analysis consists in the comparison between experimental and quantum-chemical calculated spectra [10]. However, there are several other means for interpreting ECD spectra to be used for AC determination [7,11].

The exciton chirality method (ECM) has been for a long time the most employed approach for assigning the AC of natural products by ECD spectra [12]. First developed for compounds containing a diol moiety convertible into a bis(benzoate) [13], it has then been applied to hundreds of natural compounds with very diverse skeletons and functionalities [14,15]. In a nutshell, the essence of the method is the following: a chiral molecule containing two separate chromophores with electric-dipole-allowed electronic transitions—if properly arranged with respect to each other—displays a CD spectrum containing a so-called exciton couplet, that is, two bands of opposite sign and similar intensity, centered around the chromophores UV maxima. The couplet sign (defined as that of the long-wavelength component) correlates with the absolute angle of twist defined by the two transition dipoles: a positive couplet indicates that the two transition dipoles define a positive chirality, that is, when viewed along the line connecting the dipoles, one would need a clockwise rotation to move from the dipole in the front onto that in the back. Obviously, the dipole chirality is dictated by the AC, but it also depends on the molecular conformation. In many favorable cases, just looking at the CD spectrum will yield the AC assignment, provided that a good molecular model is utilized. The most important quality of the ECM is its ease of application; it is also very robust, because it is based on a well-established theoretical basis [6,12]. These two facts render the ECM still popular, in the present computational era, to assign the AC of natural products including marine-derived ones, as demonstrated by a few recent references selected from this journal [16–21]. The method is so useful that when a compound lacks the necessary chromophores, it may be convenient to introduce them covalently or noncovalently to apply the ECM [15,22], rather than resorting to a different approach.

Any method for structural determination, however robust and efficient it may be, relies upon a correct application which meets all necessary prerequisites and hypotheses. For the ECM, the latter includes the knowledge of the molecular conformation and of transition moment directions, and confidence that the ECM dominates the CD spectrum. Strictly speaking, the ECM should not be applied unless all these pieces of information are safely known; otherwise, its application is not justified and may lead to incorrect AC assignments. We have demonstrated that incautious applications of the ECM still happen to appear in recent literature reports [23–25]. In this contribution, we will examine a recent example of AC assignment of a marine product published in this journal, laucysteinamide A (**1**) [17]. We will first present an independent interpretation of the CD spectrum of **1** by means of density functional theory (DFT) calculations. Based on our analysis, we will then criticize the previous assignment to emphasize which are, and how to meet, the necessary criteria for a safe and accurate application of the ECM.

2. Results

Laucysteinamide A (**1**, Scheme 1) is a cytotoxic compound isolated from *Caldora penicillate* [17]. During its structural elucidation, the AC at the C-2 chirality center was established by recording the CD spectrum and applying the ECM. The CD spectrum of **1** contains a single negative band above 200 nm (Figure 1). Although the quality of the experimental spectrum is poor (see legend of Figure 1), we can confidently assume the presence of a negative CD band above 210 nm or at least a tail due to the same band above 220 nm. This band was assigned by the authors to the long-wavelength component of a "couplet" emerging from the nondegenerate exciton coupling between the C-3/C-4 alkene (absorbing below 200 nm) and the thiazoline chromophore (absorbing above 200 nm).

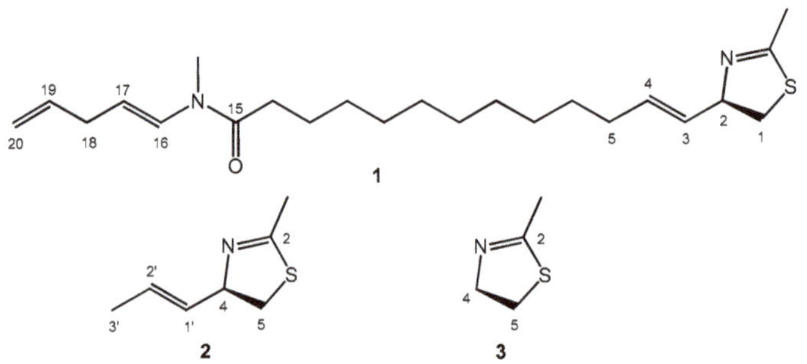

Scheme 1. Molecular diagram of (2*R*)-laucysteinamide A (**1**), of its truncated analog (2*R*)-2-methyl-4-(prop-1-en-1-yl)-4,5-dihydrothiazole (**2**), and the model chromophore 2-methyl-4,5-dihydrothiazole (**3**).

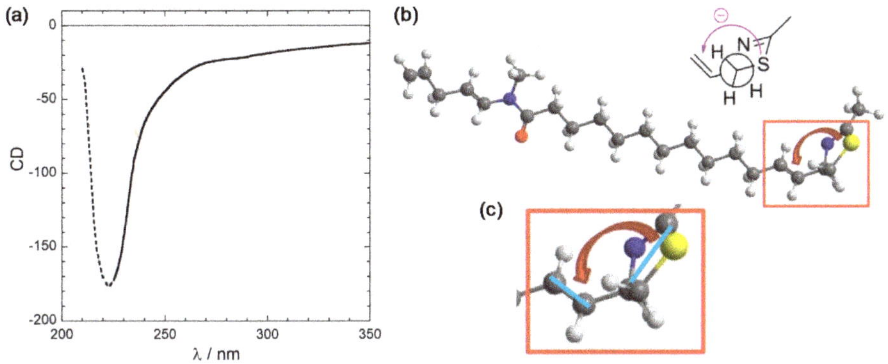

Figure 1. (**a**) CD spectrum of laucysteinamide A (**1**) recorded in CH_2Cl_2. Measurement conditions (concentration and path length) were not given, thus the *y*-axis units are undetermined. The trend below 225 nm (dotted part) is probably an artifact because of the solvent cutoff. (**b**) Exciton chirality reported in the original publication. Notice the absence of transition dipole moment directions as well as the unclear perspective. (**c**) Zoom of the relevant molecular portion where we added the most likely transition dipole moment directions (light blue bars) as suggested by the curved arrows. Panel (**a**) is adapted and (**b**,**c**) are reproduced from ref. [17].

Exciton coupling is said to be degenerate (DEC) when it occurs between equivalent transitions of two identical chromophores. Conversely, nondegenerate exciton coupling (NDEC) arises between different chromophores [6,12,26]. While DEC generates a couplet centered around the single chromophore transition, NDEC generates two distant CD bands, still with opposite signs and similar intensity, each centered in correspondence with one chromophore transition. In the extreme situation, one of the two transitions involved in NDEC may occur at too high energy (or short wavelengths, <200 nm) to be observed. This is the case of the alkene π–π^* transition, which is polarized along the double-bond direction and normally occurs at 195 nm. For instance, in the so-called allylic benzoate method [12,27], the alkene π–π^* transition is excitonically coupled to the benzoate π–π^* transition occurring around 230 nm. The long-wavelength component of the "couplet" will then appear at 230 nm, while the short-wavelength component will be often masked by the solvent cutoff.

Although not openly stated by the authors [17], the ECM analysis of laucysteinamide A (**1**) was possibly inspired by the similarity with allylic benzoates, with the thiazoline ring replacing the benzoate. As a matter of fact, the CD section in the original paper is very concise and many details were uncovered. For example, the authors apparently neglected the presence of the other two chromophoric moieties, the enamide from C-15 to C-17, and the further alkene at C-19/C-20 (Scheme 1). Though not explicitly justified, this is in fact a correct procedure because these chromophores are separated from the C-2 chirality center by a long flexible chain, therefore their contribution to the CD spectrum is negligible. In other words, one can safely consider, instead of the whole molecule of **1**, its truncated analog **2** (Scheme 1). This truncation approach has been successfully employed in CD analyses [28], and we will use it again here.

Apart from the missing details and poor experimental spectrum, the reported application of the ECM to laucysteinamide A (**1**) is flawed by many mistakes and oversights, and must be considered incorrect. As we shall see below, the assigned absolute configuration (2*R*)-**1** is the right one, although its correct assignment [17] must be consider fortuitous. A list of the most important issues, which will be analyzed more in detail in the Discussion section, is the following:

1. The nature and polarization of the transition of the thiazoline chromophore responsible for the CD band above 220 nm were not discussed; it was not clear whether this is a π–π^* transition, namely, the kind of transition which is expected to be involved in exciton coupling;

2. In the drawing of **1** used to establish the chirality associated with the NDEC, the direction of the transition moment allied with the thiazoline chromophore was not shown, and an ambiguous viewpoint was assumed;
3. No conformational analysis of **1** was run, or at least it is not reported; ECM was applied to a single conformer whose relative population is unclear.

These inconsistencies prompted us to run an independent analysis of the CD spectrum of **1**, by means of a well-established computational procedure based on DFT and time-dependent DFT (TDDFT) calculations [7,29]. The procedure was run on the truncated analog (*R*)-**2** and the model for the thiazoline chromophore **3** (Scheme 1), and the results of the various steps are reported in the following sections.

2.1. Electronic Transitions of the Model Thiazoline Chromophore 3

The ECM applied to laucysteinamide A (**1**) invoked the exciton coupling between an alkene and a thiazoline chromophore [17]. While the former is well known and its participation to exciton coupling mechanism well documented, like in the allylic benzoate method mentioned above [12,27], no previous application of ECM to the thiazoline chromophore is described in the literature, to the best of our knowledge. CD analyses of chiral thiazoline-2-thiones have been reported in several instances [30,31], but this is indeed a totally different chromophore. Also different are chromophores like luciferins, subject to much attention [32], where the thiazoline ring is part of an extended chromophoric system. On the contrary, little is known on the simpler thiazoline chromophore which is of interest for the current ECM application.

To fill the gap, we first investigated compound **3** as model chromophore of the thiazoline ring in **1**. Its geometry was optimized at ωB97X-D/6-311+G(d,p) level and TDDFT calculations were run at CAM-B3LYP/ def2-TZVP level, yielding the data shown in Table 1 and summarized below:

- the first calculated transition is a magnetic-dipole-allowed sulfur-centered n–σ*;
- the second calculated transition is a magnetic-dipole-allowed nitrogen-centered n–π*;
- the third calculated transition is a π–π* transition; this is an electric-dipole-allowed transition associated with a rather weak electric transition dipole (oscillator strength *f* ~0.05).

Table 1. Main parameters for the first three electronic transitions of **3** calculated at CAM-B3LYP/def2-TZVP level.

State	Energy (eV)	Wavelength (nm)	Oscillator Strength
1	5.208	238.1	0.0018
2	5.697	217.6	0.0040
3	5.775	214.7	0.0495

In Figure 2, the natural transition orbitals (NTO) [33] for the three transitions are depicted. This approach offers a compact representation of the electronic transition densities associated with the various transitions. The main character of each transition is described as a single excitation from an occupied to a virtual NTO. Notice how, for the first two transitions, the occupied → virtual excitation describes a rotation of the transition density, which is typical of magnetic-dipole-allowed transitions. The third excitation describes instead a translation of the transition density, which is typical of electric-dipole-allowed transitions like π–π* ones. The direction of the transition dipole for the π–π* transition is drawn in Figure 2; it is oriented approximately as the C-5/S bond of **3**.

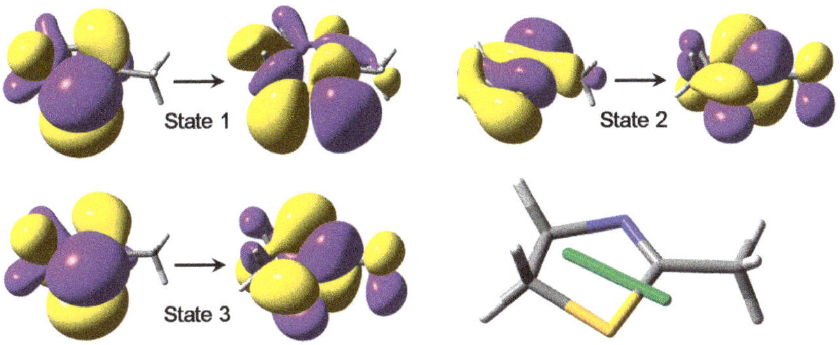

Figure 2. NTO plots of the first three transitions of **3** calculated at CAM-B3LYP/def2-TZVP level. The molecular orientation is shown in the lower right panel, also displaying the electric transition dipole for the 3rd transition (π–π*).

2.2. Conformational Analysis and Geometry Optimizations of Truncated Model **2**

The conformation of the model compound **2** was investigated by molecular mechanics conformational analysis and DFT geometry optimizations. All possible conformers of (*R*)-**2** were generated by a systematic conformational search using the Merck molecular force field (MMFF). The structures were then optimized with DFT at ωB97X-D/6-311+G(d,p) level. Six low-energy conformers were obtained due to the rotamerism around the C-4/C-1′ bond and the five-membered ring puckering. They can be described using the anti/gauche notation for the reciprocal orientation of H-4 and H-1′, and the pseudo-equatorial/axial position of the propenyl group attached at C-4. The structures and relative energies are displayed in Figure 3; notice the small energy differences between the various conformers.

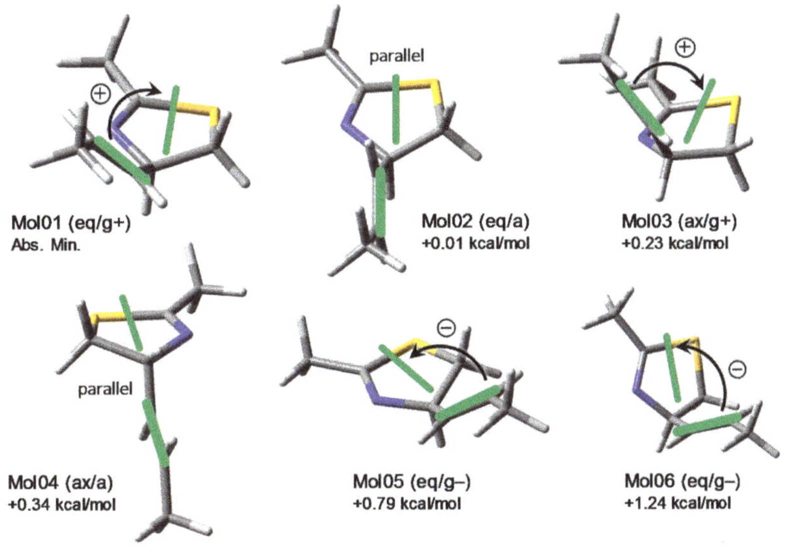

Figure 3. Conformers and relative energies of model compound **2** obtained after ωB97X-D/6-311+G(d,p) geometry optimization, and exciton chirality defined by the two transition dipole moments (green bars, for alkene and thiazoline π–π* transition, see text). Legend for the notation: ax/eq, pseudo-axial/equatorial position of the propenyl group; a/g+/g−, anti/gauche+/gauche− relation between H-4 and H-1′.

These results suggest that laucysteinamide A (**1**) may also exhibit a pronounced flexibility around the C-2/C-3 bond and in the thiazoline ring, although the relative populations between the various conformers may differ from those of its truncated model **2**. Such a flexibility is crucial for the exciton coupling mechanism because the noticed motions affect directly the relative orientation of the two chromophores supposed to be involved in the ECM. This fact can be appreciated by looking at the green bars shown in Figure 3 representing the transition dipole directions for the alkene π–π* (polarized along the C=C bond) and the thiazoline π–π* transition. This latter corresponds to the third calculated excited state for model chromophore **3** discussed above. It can be seen that, for a given axial/equatorial conformer of **2**, the three rotamers around the C-4/C-1′ bond exhibit variable chirality defined by the transition dipoles, either positive, negative, or negligible (when the two dipoles are approximately parallel). It is impossible to establish with certainty the resulting sign of the exciton chirality on a qualitative ground (i.e., without quantitative exciton coupling calculations) [34], though one might expect a dominant positive chirality. Regrettably, in the original publication, a negative chirality was inferred (see Figure 1 and Section 3.3 below).

2.3. CD Calculations on Truncated Model **2** and Transition Analysis

To simulate the CD spectrum of model compound (*R*)-**2**, which retains the same chromophoric portion as (*R*)-**1**, TDDFT calculations were run on the six conformers described above using B3LYP and CAM-B3LYP functionals and def2-TZVP basis sets, including the IEF-PCM solvent model for dichloromethane. CAM-B3LYP/def2-TZVP results are described below; B3LYP functional led to consistent results. The six calculated spectra were averaged using internal energies estimated at ωB97X-D/6-311+G(d,p) level. The final weighted-average-calculated CD spectrum for (*R*)-**2** is shown in Figure 4. In the wavelength region >230 nm, it displays a negative CD band which corresponds to the experimental band >220 nm. A second positive band appears between 200 and 230 nm, which is impossible to compare with the experimental spectrum because of the solvent cutoff. Therefore, we must limit our discussion to the first band. We can confirm, at least on the basis of this limited spectral comparison, that the absolute configuration of laucysteinamide A (**1**) is (2*R*). It must, however, be stressed that AC assignments based only on a single band are discouraged [11], and the present case is especially critical because the experimental band is poorly defined (Section 2.1).

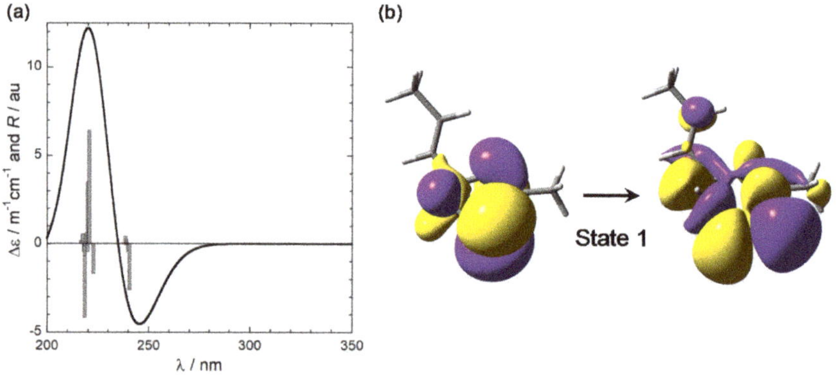

Figure 4. (**a**) Calculated CD spectrum of truncated model **2** at CAM-B3LYP/def2-TZVP level. The vertical bars represent the rotational strengths *R* calculated for the various conformers. (**b**) NTO plot of the first transition of **2** for the lowest-energy conformer (Mol01 in Figure 3).

In all relevant conformers of **2**, the first calculated transition around 240 nm, responsible for the "diagnostic" CD band, is essentially a magnetic-dipole-allowed sulfur-centered n–σ* transition, like in the model chromophore **3**; in addition, some character of charge transfer from the thiazoline to the alkene can be recognized. The NTOs calculated for the lowest-energy conformer of **2** (Mol01 in Figure 3) are depicted in Figure 4. In conclusion, TDDFT calculations on model compounds **2** and **3** demonstrate that the negative band (or tail) appearing in the CD spectrum of laucysteinamide A (**1**) is not a component of a "couplet" arising from nondegenerate exciton coupling. Though centered on the thiazoline ring, it is not an electric-dipole-allowed π–π^* transition but a magnetic-dipole-allowed sulfur-centered n–σ^* transition.

3. Discussion

Having analyzed the conformation, CD spectrum, and electronic properties of the truncated model **2** in detail, we shall now examine the major pitfalls and inconsistencies found in the reported application of the ECM to laucysteinamide A (**1**). This exercise will help in recapitulating the criteria for a safe and accurate application of the ECM.

3.1. Missing Conformational Analysis

The published report on the AC assignment of laucysteinamide A (**1**) contains no detail on its conformation [17]. Apparently, no conformational analysis of **1** was run. The procedure used to obtain the molecular model used to establish the transition moment chirality is briefly described: «Computational molecular models […] were subjected to energy minimization with MOPAC software»; then, a single structure was considered for the ECM application (Figure 1). One must conclude that only a single conformer was taken into account, with unspecified relative population. The validity of this approximation is contradicted by experimental and computational data. Among the few available NMR data of **1**, we noticed the following $^3J_{HH}$ coupling constants relative to H-1, H-2, and H-3: $^3J_{H1a,H2}$ = $^3J_{H1a,H2}$ = 8.4 Hz; $^3J_{H2,H3}$ = 6.6 Hz. The single conformer used for the ECM (Figure 1) has a pseudo-axial H-2, which would lead to substantially different couplings with the pseudo-axial/equatorial H-1a and H-1b. Moreover, the expected $^3J_{H2,H3}$ vinylic coupling constant would be 11–12 Hz for anti-oriented and 3–4 Hz for gauche-oriented H-2 and H-3, respectively [35]. Thus, the experimental values of the diagnostic $^3J_{HH}$'s indicate an average situation allied with a large conformational freedom in the ring conformation and around the C-2/C-3 bond. The results of our conformational study on truncated model **2** (Section 2.2) also confirm the existence of multiple conformers. More importantly, we have demonstrated that the exciton coupling may vary sizably in intensity and even in sign from conformer to conformer. Any exciton-coupled CD, if observed at all, would be the weighted average of all possible situations, yielding an overall couplet difficult to predict.

The impact of conformation on exciton-coupled CD spectra has been demonstrated in several instances [36–38], and it is just a specific case of the well-known sensitivity and dependence of CD spectra on molecular conformation [39]. The first criterion for a correct ECM application is then: *run a thorough conformational analysis and estimate the exciton coupling for the various conformers.* The *ECM can be safely applied only if a dominant sign of the exciton chirality is apparent* among the most populated conformers. As a corollary, we recommend that the *conformational analysis is run by a combination of experimental and computational methods* [39,40].

3.2. Nature of the Transition Involved

In the published report on the AC assignment of laucysteinamide A (**1**), the NDEC between the alkene and thiazoline chromophores was invoked [17]. The authors noticed that the «CD spectrum of compound **1** showed a negative local maximum at 223 nm, corresponding to the thiazoline chromophore», while «the maximum expected from the C-3/C-4 alkene would be around 190 nm, but was not observed in the spectrum due to solvent absorptions». This is analogous to the allylic benzoate method recalled above (Section 2.1). As a matter of fact, the nature of the specific transition of the thiazoline chromophore involved in the NDEC was not discussed [17]. Since π–π^* transitions are normally considered in ECM, because of their electric-dipole-allowed character, one might expect that the authors assumed the existence of a π–π^* transition around 220 nm. In addition, the direction of the electric dipole moments should be known prior to ECM applications, because it is the reciprocal arrangement between the transition dipoles which dictates the sign of the CD spectrum. Most of the aromatic or π-conjugated chromophores usually encountered in ECM, for example, *p*-substituted benzoates [12,13], naphthalene [41,42], enones [43], etc., have a well-known electronic structure and the direction of the relevant transition dipoles is certain. In many other cases, the transition dipole polarization may be inferred from the symmetry properties of the chromophores. For example, an all-*trans* polyene chain, or a polyenone, has an effective cylindrical symmetry for which the relevant π–π^* transitions are necessary polarized along the chain direction; ECM applications are therefore straightforward [16]. On the contrary, the thiazoline ring lacks any element of axial symmetry, therefore π–π^* transitions can be, in principle, oriented in any direction in the plane. It appears that this chromophore is not ideal at all for ECM applications. Still, in this situation, one may resort to running excited-state calculations to study the chromophore and to assess the direction of the transition moments. Apparently, such necessity was overlooked by the authors [17].

As a result of our TDDFT calculations on **2** and **3**, we already demonstrated that the transition responsible for the CD band >220 nm is not an electric-dipole-allowed π–π^* transition, which could give exciton coupling with the alkene π–π^* transition. The first calculated transition is instead a magnetic-dipole-allowed sulfur-centered n–σ^* transition. This means that the diagnostic band in the CD spectrum of **1** is not due to the exciton coupling mechanism but to other mechanisms capable of generating CD signals, in this case, those typically associated with sulfur n–σ^* transitions [44].

In summary, the *ECM should be applied to well-known chromophores* for which *the direction of the transition dipole moment is established*. "New" chromophores require their electronic structure to be studied independently. *ECM can be invoked only for electric-dipole-allowed transitions*, in most cases, π–π^* transitions of aromatic chromophores or extended π-conjugated chromophores. In all cases, moreover, one must be confident that the *ECM is truly responsible for the observed CD spectrum*, and interference from other sources of CD signals may be excluded. This is especially important for NDEC, which is intrinsically weaker than DEC and generates weak CD "couplets" easily overruled by other sources of CD signals [24]. Polavarapu provided a useful formula to estimate the strength of CD signals associated with NDEC; see p. 360 in Ref. [6].

3.3. Viewpoint Used to Establish the Transition Moment Chirality

When assessing the exciton chirality defined by the two transition dipole moments, one must follow a few steps: (a) generate one (or more) meaningful molecular model representative of the most relevant conformer(s), see Section 2.2; (b) depict it in an intelligible way with one chromophore clearly placed in the front and the other in the back; (c) draw the transition dipole moments with their correct direction in the middle of the respective chromophores, see Section 2.1; (d) establish the sense of rotation (clockwise or anticlockwise), which is conceptually necessary to move the dipole in the front onto that in the back. Figure 3 was conceived according to these prescriptions. This is instead not the case for the drawing used to establish the exciton chirality in laucysteinamide A (**1**) [17], reproduced in Figure 1. We have already noticed the missing transition moment directions (Section 3.2). More importantly, even admitting the most plausible directions, the viewpoint adopted by the authors remains ambiguous, as one cannot safely establish which chromophore lies in front and which in back. This problem can be appreciated using our molecular model for the lowest-energy DFT conformer of (*R*)-**2** (Mol01 in Figure 3), which corresponds to the conformation used by the authors for (*R*)-**1**. In Figure 5a, we plot this molecular model, on which the correct transition moments are projected, using the same viewpoint of the original drawing: it is impossible to establish the exciton chirality unambiguously. This is instead possible by plotting the same molecular model more meaningfully as in Figure 5b: once the correct viewpoint is assumed, the chirality defined by the transition dipole moments turns out to be positive. Regrettably enough, this is opposite to the negative chirality inferred in the original publication for (*R*)-**1** (Figure 1) [17].

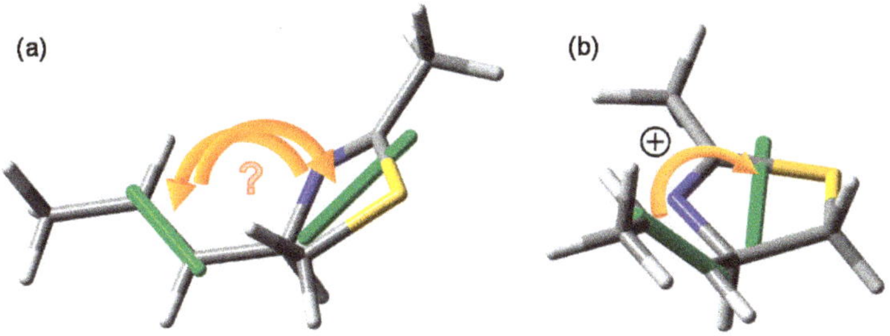

Figure 5. Lowest-energy conformer of model compound (*R*)-**2** seen in two different perspectives. Viewpoint (**a**) is the same assumed in the original publication (see Figure 1c), where a negative chirality was seen for (*R*)-**1** [17]. The chirality defined by the transition moments is in fact ambiguous. Viewpoint (**b**) offers a better perspective of the actual positive chirality.

One can expect that such a trivial error is unique; unfortunately, this is not unprecedented [23]. The take-home message is that *the molecular model used to establish the transition moment chirality must be drawn in an unambiguous way*, that is, with one chromophore clearly placed in the front and the other in the back. The *less ambiguous viewpoint is along the line connecting the middle of the two chromophores*, although often this does not offer a good perspective of the molecule. A more extensive treatment of this latest issue may be found elsewhere [23].

4. Materials and Methods

Molecular mechanics and preliminary Density Functional Theory (DFT) calculations were run with Spartan'16 (Wavenfunction, Irvine, CA, USA, 2016) with default parameters, default grids, and convergence criteria; DFT and Time-Dependent DFT (TDDFT) calculations were run with Gaussian16 (Gaussian. Inc., Wallingford, CT, USA) [45] with default grids and convergence criteria. Conformational analyses were run with the Monte Carlo procedure implemented in Spartan'16 using Merck molecular force field (MMFF). All structures obtained thereof were optimized with DFT at the ωB97X-D/6-311+G(d,p) level in vacuo. TDDFT calculations were run with B3LYP and CAM-B3LYP functionals and def2-TZVP basis set, and included the polarizable continuum model (PCM) for CH_2Cl_2 in its Integral Equation Formalism (IEF) formulation. Average ECD spectra were computed by weighting ECD spectra (calculated for each conformer) with Boltzmann factors at 300K estimated from DFT internal energies. CD spectra were plotted using the program SpecDis [46,47], applying the dipole-length formalism for rotational strengths; the difference with dipole-velocity values was negligible. Natural transition orbitals were plotted with GaussView6 (Semichem, Inc., Shawnee Mission, KS, USA).

5. Conclusions

The exciton chirality method (ECM) is a powerful, robust, and rapid method for assigning the absolute configuration (AC) of natural products, provided that they contain two or more chromophores giving rise to electric-dipole-allowed electronic transitions. The two chromophores need to be (relatively) close in space but not directly conjugated with each other or mutually involved in charge-transfer transitions. To apply the method, the CD spectrum should display a *diagnostic CD couplet*, or at least its long-wavelength component should be clearly identified. Henceforth, by looking at the *molecular structure*, one must establish the chirality defined by the two *transition dipoles*, and correlate it with the experimental CD sign.

At first sight, one may expect that the above facts can be simply assessed by looking at the molecular diagram and spectra. In fact, crucial details are hidden within the italicized words. Looking at the *molecular structure* means that this latter must be known, that is, the molecular conformation must have been safely determined and all the important conformers identified—namely, those most contributing to the experimental CD spectrum. Establishing the chirality defined by the two *transition dipoles* means that their exact direction within each chromophore must be known in advance, or must be established before applying the ECM. Finally, identifying a *diagnostic CD couplet* implies that the CD spectrum is dominated by the exciton coupling mechanism, while other sources of CD signals are absent or negligible. None of these pieces of information is trivial and their importance is easily overlooked by nonexperts. Not surprisingly, then, they are the main sources of incorrect applications of the ECM. Laucysteinamide A (**1**) seems to be a very unfortunate case where none of the above prescriptions was met. It lends itself as a negative but instructive example of the major traps which can be encountered on the way to assigning ACs by the ECM. The present critical analysis was mainly intended to stress the necessary prerequisites and criteria for a safe application of the ECM, and to guide on how to achieve them.

Funding: This research received no external funding.

Acknowledgments: We acknowledge the CINECA award under the ISCRA initiative for the availability of high-performance computing resources and support.

Conflicts of Interest: The author declares no conflict of interest.

References

1. Krastel, P.; Petersen, F.; Roggo, S.; Schmitt, E.; Schuffenhauer, A. Aspects of Chirality in Natural Products Drug Discovery. In *Chirality in Drug Research*; Francotte, E., Lindner, W., Eds.; Wiley-VCH: Weinheim, Germany, 2006; pp. 67–94.
2. Lin, G.-Q.; You, Q.-D.; Cheng, J.-F. (Eds.) *Chiral Drugs: Chemistry and Biological Action*; Wiley: Hoboken, NJ, USA, 2011.
3. Blunt, J.W.; Carroll, A.R.; Copp, B.R.; Davis, R.A.; Keyzers, R.A.; Prinsep, M.R. Marine natural products. *Nat. Prod. Rep.* **2018**, *35*, 8–53. [CrossRef] [PubMed]
4. Albright, A.L.; White, J.M. Determination of Absolute Configuration Using Single Crystal X-Ray Diffraction. In *Metabolomics Tools for Natural Product Discovery: Methods and Protocols*; Roessner, U., Dias, A.D., Eds.; Humana Press: Totowa, NJ, USA, 2013; pp. 149–162.
5. Berova, N.; Polavarapu, P.L.; Nakanishi, K.; Woody, R.W. (Eds.) *Comprehensive Chiroptical Spectroscopy*; John Wiley & Sons, Inc.: Hoboken, NJ, USA, 2012.
6. Polavarapu, P.L. *Chiroptical Spectroscopy: Fundamentals and Applications*; CRC Press: Boca Raton, FL, USA, 2016.
7. Superchi, S.; Scafato, P.; Górecki, M.; Pescitelli, G. Absolute Configuration Determination by Quantum Mechanical Calculation of Chiroptical Spectra: Basics and Applications to Fungal Metabolites. *Curr. Med. Chem.* **2018**, *25*, 287–320. [CrossRef] [PubMed]
8. Hopmann, K.H.; Šebestík, J.; Novotná, J.; Stensen, W.; Urbanová, M.; Svenson, J.; Svendsen, J.S.; Bouř, P.; Ruud, K. Determining the Absolute Configuration of Two Marine Compounds Using Vibrational Chiroptical Spectroscopy. *J. Org. Chem.* **2012**, *77*, 858–869. [CrossRef] [PubMed]
9. Joseph-Nathan, P.; Gordillo-Román, B. Vibrational Circular Dichroism Absolute Configuration Determination of Natural Products. In *Progress in the Chemistry of Organic Natural Products*; Kinghorn, A.D., Falk, H., Kobayashi, J., Eds.; Springer: Cham, Switzerland, 2015; Volume 100, pp. 311–452.
10. Srebro-Hooper, M.; Autschbach, J. Calculating Natural Optical Activity of Molecules from First Principles. *Annu. Rev. Phys. Chem.* **2017**, *68*, 399–420. [CrossRef] [PubMed]
11. Berova, N.; Di Bari, L.; Pescitelli, G. Application of electronic circular dichroism in configurational and conformational analysis of organic compounds. *Chem. Soc. Rev.* **2007**, *36*, 914–931. [CrossRef] [PubMed]
12. Harada, N.; Nakanishi, K. *Circular Dichroic Spectroscopy—Exciton Coupling in Organic Stereochemistry*; University Science Books: Mill Valley, CA, USA, 1983.
13. Harada, N.; Nakanishi, K. Exciton chirality method and its application to configurational and conformational studies of natural products. *Acc. Chem. Res.* **1972**, *5*, 257–263. [CrossRef]
14. Berova, N.; Ellestad, G.A.; Harada, N. Characterization by Circular Dichroism Spectroscopy. In *Comprehensive Natural Products II*; Mander, L., Liu, H.-W., Eds.; Elsevier: Oxford, UK, 2010; Volume 9, pp. 91–146.

15. Harada, N.; Nakanishi, K.; Berova, N. Electronic CD Exciton Chirality Method: Principles and Applications. In *Comprehensive Chiroptical Spectroscopy*; Berova, N., Polavarapu, P.L., Nakanishi, K., Woody, R.W., Eds.; John Wiley & Sons, Inc.: Hoboken, NJ, USA, 2012; pp. 115–166.
16. Meng, J.; Cheng, W.; Heydari, H.; Wang, B.; Zhu, K.; Konuklugil, B.; Lin, W. Sorbicillinoid-Based Metabolites from a Sponge-Derived Fungus Trichoderma saturnisporum. *Mar. Drugs* **2018**, *16*, 226. [CrossRef] [PubMed]
17. Zhang, C.; Naman, C.; Engene, N.; Gerwick, W. Laucysteinamide A, a Hybrid PKS/NRPS Metabolite from a Saipan Cyanobacterium, cf. Caldora penicillata. *Mar. Drugs* **2017**, *15*, 121. [CrossRef] [PubMed]
18. Yang, F.; Zou, Y.; Wang, R.-P.; Hamann, M.; Zhang, H.-J.; Jiao, W.-H.; Han, B.-N.; Song, S.-J.; Lin, H.-W. Relative and Absolute Stereochemistry of Diacarperoxides: Antimalarial Norditerpene Endoperoxides from Marine Sponge Diacarnus megaspinorhabdosa. *Mar. Drugs* **2014**, *12*, 4399–4416. [CrossRef] [PubMed]
19. Wang, Y.; Wang, L.; Zhuang, Y.; Kong, F.; Zhang, C.; Zhu, W. Phenolic Polyketides from the Co-Cultivation of Marine-Derived Penicillium sp. WC-29-5 and Streptomyces fradiae 007. *Mar. Drugs* **2014**, *12*, 2079–2088. [CrossRef] [PubMed]
20. Zhu, G.; Kong, F.; Wang, Y.; Fu, P.; Zhu, W. Cladodionen, a Cytotoxic Hybrid Polyketide from the Marine-Derived Cladosporium sp. OUCMDZ-1635. *Mar. Drugs* **2018**, *16*, 71. [CrossRef] [PubMed]
21. Wang, P.; Xi, L.; Liu, P.; Wang, Y.; Wang, W.; Huang, Y.; Zhu, W. Diketopiperazine Derivatives from the Marine-Derived Actinomycete Streptomyces sp. FXJ7.328. *Mar. Drugs* **2013**, *11*, 1035–1049. [CrossRef] [PubMed]
22. Berova, N.; Pescitelli, G.; Petrovic, A.G.; Proni, G. Probing molecular chirality by CD-sensitive dimeric metalloporphyrin hosts. *Chem. Commun.* **2009**, 5958–5980. [CrossRef] [PubMed]
23. Pescitelli, G.; Di Bari, L. Revision of the Absolute Configuration of Preussilides A-F Established by the Exciton Chirality Method. *J. Nat. Prod.* **2017**, *80*, 2855–2859. [CrossRef] [PubMed]
24. Pescitelli, G.; Di Bari, L. Exciton coupling between enones: Quassinoids revisited. *Chirality* **2017**, *29*, 476–485. [CrossRef] [PubMed]
25. Shi, X.-W.; Lu, Q.-Q.; Pescitelli, G.; Ivšić, T.; Zhou, J.-H.; Gao, J.-M. Three Sesquiterpenoid Dimers from Chloranthus japonicus: Absolute Configuration of Chlorahololide A and Related Compounds. *Chirality* **2016**, *28*, 158–163. [CrossRef] [PubMed]
26. Pescitelli, G.; Bari, L.D. Comment on "Breakdown of Exciton Splitting through Electron Donor–Acceptor Interaction: A Caveat for the Application of Exciton Chirality Method in Macromolecules". *J. Phys. Chem. C* **2014**, *118*, 24197–24198. [CrossRef]
27. Harada, N.; Iwabuchi, J.; Yokota, Y.; Uda, H.; Nakanishi, K. A chiroptical method for determining the absolute configuration of allylic alcohols. *J. Am. Chem. Soc.* **1981**, *103*, 5590–5591. [CrossRef]
28. Iwahana, S.; Iida, H.; Yashima, E.; Pescitelli, G.; Di Bari, L.; Petrovic, A.G.; Berova, N. Absolute Stereochemistry of a 4a-Hydroxyriboflavin Analogue of the Key Intermediate of the FAD-Monooxygenase Cycle. *Chem. Eur. J.* **2014**, *20*, 4386–4395. [CrossRef] [PubMed]
29. Pescitelli, G.; Bruhn, T. Good Computational Practice in the Assignment of Absolute Configurations by TDDFT Calculations of ECD Spectra. *Chirality* **2016**, *28*, 466–474. [CrossRef] [PubMed]
30. Roschester, J.; Berg, U.; Pierrot, M.; Sandström, J. Conformational analysis of *N*-(1-phenylethyl)-Δ4-thiazoline-2-thiones and analogs. A proton NMR, circular dichroism, x-ray crystallographic, and molecular mechanics study. *J. Am. Chem. Soc.* **1987**, *109*, 492–507. [CrossRef]
31. Roschester, J.; Sandström, J. Conformational analysis of *N*-(1-methoxycarbonylethyl)-Δ4-thiazoline-2-thiones by temperature-dependent circular dichroism and NMR spectroscopy and by molecular mechanics calculations. *Tetrahedron* **1989**, *45*, 5081–5100. [CrossRef]
32. Orlova, G.; Goddard, J.D.; Brovko, L.Y. Theoretical Study of the Amazing Firefly Bioluminescence: The Formation and Structures of the Light Emitters. *J. Am. Chem. Soc.* **2003**, *125*, 6962–6971. [CrossRef] [PubMed]
33. Martin, R.L. Natural transition orbitals. *J. Chem. Phys.* **2003**, *118*, 4775–4777. [CrossRef]
34. Superchi, S.; Giorgio, E.; Rosini, C. Structural determinations by circular dichroism spectra analysis using coupled oscillator methods: An update of the applications of the DeVoe polarizability model. *Chirality* **2004**, *16*, 422–451. [CrossRef] [PubMed]
35. Garbisch, E.W. Conformations. VI. Vinyl-Allylic Proton Spin Couplings. *J. Am. Chem. Soc.* **1964**, *86*, 5561–5564. [CrossRef]

36. Chisholm, J.D.; Golik, J.; Krishnan, B.; Matson, J.A.; Van Vranken, D.L. A Caveat in the Application of the Exciton Chirality Method to N,N-Dialkyl Amides. Synthesis and Structural Revision of AT2433-B1. *J. Am. Chem. Soc.* **1999**, *121*, 3801–3802. [CrossRef]
37. Matile, S.; Berova, N.; Nakanishi, K. Intramolecular Porphyrin π,π-Stacking: Absolute Configurational Assignment of Acyclic Compounds with Single Chiral Centers by Exciton Coupled Circular Dichroism. *Enantiomer* **1996**, *1*, 1–12. [PubMed]
38. Gargiulo, D.; Derguini, F.; Berova, N.; Nakanishi, K.; Harada, N. Unique ultraviolet-visible and circular dichroism behavior due to exciton coupling in a biscyanine dye. *J. Am. Chem. Soc.* **1991**, *113*, 7046–7047. [CrossRef]
39. Pescitelli, G.; Di Bari, L.; Berova, N. Conformational Aspects in the Studies of Organic Compounds by Electronic Circular Dichroism. *Chem. Soc. Rev.* **2011**, *40*, 4603–4625. [CrossRef] [PubMed]
40. Mazzanti, A.; Casarini, D. Recent trends in conformational analysis. *WIREs Comput. Mol. Sci.* **2012**, *2*, 613–641. [CrossRef]
41. Mason, S.F.; Seal, R.H.; Roberts, D.R. Optical activity in the biaryl series. *Tetrahedron* **1974**, *30*, 1671–1682. [CrossRef]
42. Di Bari, L.; Pescitelli, G.; Salvadori, P. Conformational study of 2,2′-homosubstituted 1,1′-binaphthyls by means of UV and CD spectroscopy. *J. Am. Chem. Soc.* **1999**, *121*, 7998–8004. [CrossRef]
43. Koreeda, M.; Harada, N.; Nakanishi, K. Exciton chirality methods as applied to conjugated enones, esters, and lactones. *J. Am. Chem. Soc.* **1974**, *96*, 266–268. [CrossRef]
44. Rosenfield, J.S.; Moscowitz, A. Optical activity data as an aid in the assignment of electronic transitions: Application to dialkyl sulphides. In *Fundamental Aspects and Recent Developments in ORD and CD*; Ciardelli, F., Salvadori, P., Eds.; Heyden: London, UK, 1967; pp. 41–49.
45. Frisch, M.J.; Trucks, G.W.; Schlegel, H.B.; Scuseria, G.E.; Robb, M.A.; Cheeseman, J.R.; Scalmani, G.; Barone, V.; Petersson, G.A.; Nakatsuji, H.; et al. *Gaussian 16, Revision A.03*, Gaussian, Inc.: Wallingford, CT, USA, 2016.
46. Bruhn, T.; Schaumlöffel, A.; Hemberger, Y.; Bringmann, G. SpecDis: Quantifying the Comparison of Calculated and Experimental Electronic Circular Dichroism Spectra. *Chirality* **2013**, *25*, 243–249. [CrossRef] [PubMed]
47. Bruhn, T.; Schaumlöffel, A.; Hemberger, Y.; Pescitelli, G. *SpecDis Version 1.71*; SpecDis: Berlin, Germany.

© 2018 by the author. Licensee MDPI, Basel, Switzerland. This article is an open access article distributed under the terms and conditions of the Creative Commons Attribution (CC BY) license (http://creativecommons.org/licenses/by/4.0/).

marine drugs

MDPI

Article

Isolation and Chemical Characterization of Chondroitin Sulfate from Cartilage By-Products of Blackmouth Catshark (*Galeus melastomus*)

José Antonio Vázquez [1,*], Javier Fraguas [1,2], Ramón Novoa-Carvallal [3,4], Rui L. Reis [3,4,5], Luis T. Antelo [6], Ricardo I. Pérez-Martín [2] and Jesus Valcarcel [1,*]

1 Group of Recycling and Valorisation of Waste Materials (REVAL), Marine Research Institute (IIM-CSIC), Eduardo Cabello, 6. Vigo, 36208 Galicia, Spain; xavi@iim.csic.es

2 Group of Food Biochemistry, Marine Research Institute (IIM-CSIC), Eduardo Cabello, 6. Vigo, 36208 Galicia, Spain; ricardo@iim.csic.es

3 3B's Research Group—Biomaterials, Biodegradables and Biomimetics, University of Minho, Headquarters of the European Institute of Excellence on Tissue Engineering and Regenerative Medicine, AvePark, Barco, 4805-017 Guimarães, Portugal; ramon.novoa@i3bs.uminho.pt (R.N.-C.); rgreis@i3bs.uminho.pt (R.L.R.)

4 ICVS/3B's—PT Government Associate Laboratory, 4805-017 Braga/Guimarães, Portugal

5 The Discoveries Centre for Regenerative and Precision Medicine, Headquarters at University of Minho, Avepark, Barco, 4805-017 Guimarães, Portugal

6 Group of Bioprocess Engineering, Marine Research Institute (IIM-CSIC), Eduardo Cabello, 6. Vigo, 36208 Galicia, Spain; ltaboada@iim.csic.es

* Correspondence: jvazquez@iim.csic.es (J.A.V.); jvalcarcel@iim.csic.es (J.V.); Tel.: +34-986-231-930 (J.A.V. & J.V.); Fax: +34-986-292-762 (J.A.V. & J.V.)

Received: 5 September 2018; Accepted: 18 September 2018; Published: 20 September 2018

Abstract: Chondroitin sulfate (CS) is a glycosaminoglycan actively researched for pharmaceutical, nutraceutical and tissue engineering applications. CS extracted from marine animals displays different features from common terrestrial sources, resulting in distinct properties, such as anti-viral and anti-metastatic. Therefore, exploration of undescribed marine species holds potential to expand the possibilities of currently-known CS. Accordingly, we have studied for the first time the production and characterization of CS from blackmouth catshark (*Galeus melastomus*), a shark species commonly discarded as by-catch. The process of CS purification consists of cartilage hydrolysis with alcalase, followed by two different chemical treatments and ending with membrane purification. All steps were optimized by response surface methodology. According to this, the best conditions for cartilage proteolysis were established at 52.9 °C and *pH* = 7.31. Subsequent purification by either alkaline treatment or hydroalcoholic alkaline precipitation yielded CS with purities of 81.2%, 82.3% and 97.4% respectively, after 30-kDa membrane separation. The molecular weight of CS obtained ranges 53–66 kDa, depending on the conditions. Sulfation profiles were similar for all materials, with dominant CS-C (GlcA-GalNAc6S) units (55%), followed by 23–24% of CS-A (GlcA-GalNAc4S), a substantial amount (15–16%) of CS-D (GlcA2S-GalNAc6S) and less than 7% of other disulfated and unsulfated disaccharides.

Keywords: chondroitin sulfate production; cartilage *Galeus melastomus* by-products; sulfation patterns; process optimization; molecular weight glycosaminoglycans determination; bycatch waste management

1. Introduction

Glycosaminoglycans (GAGs) are linear polymers consisting of repeating *O*-linked disaccharide units present in the extracellular matrix or at the cell surface of most animal tissues. GAGs' ability to interact with proteins is behind their involvement in important cellular events such as cell proliferation, differentiation and migration [1]. As a consequence, GAGs have shown a range of biological activities and are actively explored in the pharmaceutical and tissue engineering fields [2–4].

Most GAGs are commercially produced from terrestrial animals, but can also be isolated from marine organisms. Because of the different evolutionary pathways followed by each group of organism, marine and terrestrial GAGs are different, mainly in terms of molecular weight and sulfation [5,6]. Both chemical characteristics are particularly important for the biological functionality of GAGs. In some cases, a specific sequence of saccharides is required for biological activity, for example a pentasaccharide in heparin is responsible for its anticoagulant properties. However, interactions between GAGs and proteins are generally not so specific and seem to be rather influenced by charge density and the presence of particular sulfated units [7]. Thus, sulfated marine GAGs probably represent the most interesting molecules from a therapeutic perspective, chondroitin sulfate (CS) in particular [5].

CS is composed of glucuronic acid (GlcA) and *N*-acetyl galactosamine (GalNAc) linked via alternating β-(1→4) and β-(1→3) glycosidic bonds, and each disaccharide unit can be sulfated at different positions. Marine CS were reported to have different activities such as antiviral, anti-metastatic, anticoagulant and anti-inflammatory activities [1,8,9], to provide signaling properties to cartilage engineering constructs and to improve their mechanical performance [10,11] and to promote neurite outgrowth when hybridized with dermatan sulfate [12]. These biological activities are associated in many cases to the abundance and kind of sulfation pattern, and both are characteristic of each organism [13]. Accordingly, exploration of new sources of CS holds potential to expand the possibilities of different sulfation configurations that may have improved therapeutic properties.

Because of the current overexploitation of marine resources and associated challenges for the fishing industry, new marine sources should be evaluated from the point of view of sustainability. In this regard, valorization of fish by-catch represents an interesting alternative to current discard practices. Within the wide scope of this approach, CS from fish cartilage has been identified as one of the most suitable products for valorization due to its high price and relatively low environmental impact [14]. A number of species of cartilaginous fish have little economic value; however, under current European Union legislation, fishing vessels must keep on board these non-target species if they are subject to quota regulations [15]. This is the case of the blackmouth catshark (*Galeus melastomus*), a shark common in the Northeastern Atlantic Ocean and the Mediterranean Sea. Being abundant, *G. melastomus* is incidentally caught by commercial trawl fisheries [16,17].

Blackmouth catshark appears therefore as a sustainable source of CS, a valorization product that could increase the economic value of this species and serve as an incentive to abandon discard practices. Furthermore, the characteristics of CS extracted from *G. melastomus* are largely unknown, since only one previous report has described some structural features and properties of this material [18]. Important characteristics of CS such as molecular weight and disaccharide composition have not been quantitatively evaluated and, to the best of our knowledge, remain unknown.

In the present work, we aim to fully characterize CS isolated from blackmouth catshark under optimal conditions, defined by response surface methodology. In line with the sustainability principles that guide this study, hydrolysis of cartilage is carried out by enzymatic methods, instead of conventional chemical treatments with toxic guanidine hydrochloride and concentrated alkali [19]. Finally, time-consuming chromatographic separations for CS purification are replaced with more straightforward ultrafiltration-diafiltration techniques.

2. Results and Discussion

The average (±confidence interval) proportion of cartilage in the analyzed individuals amounted to 6.80 ± 0.40% (percentage of total weight) with a moisture content of 67.9 ± 3.7%. Chemical composition of cartilage, as % of dry weight, results in 55.0 ± 0.9% protein, 37.0 ± 1.8% ash, 2.0 ± 0.5% fat and 6.0 ± 0.3% carbohydrates. These values are in agreement with the proximal composition found for *Scyliorhinus canicula* cartilage [20].

2.1. Hydrolysis of Cartilage by Enzyme Proteolysis

The first step for the isolation of glycosaminoglycans was the enzymatic digestion of cartilage from heads, central skeletons and fins of *G. melastomus* by-products. The enzyme selected was alcalase, a well-known endoprotease with excellent capacity to hydrolyze several marine substrates [21–24], including cartilage from other fish species [25,26]. The kinetics of enzyme hydrolysis were performed under the experimental conditions defined in Table 1 and the Materials and Methods Section.

Table 1. Experimental domains and codification of the independent variables in the factorial rotatable designs performed to optimize the enzyme hydrolysis of cartilage and the chemical treatments of the hydrolysates using alkaline or alkaline-hydroalcoholic solutions.

Coded Values	Natural Values					
	Enzyme Hydrolysis		NaOH Treatment		NaOH-EtOH Treatment	
	pH	*T* (°C)	*NaOH* (M)	Time (h): *t*	*NaOH* (M)	Ethanol (*v*)
−1.41	6.0	30.0	0.20	1.0	0.10	0.30
−1	6.6	37.3	0.39	4.4	0.20	0.46
0	8.0	55.0	0.85	12.5	0.45	0.85
+1	9.4	72.7	1.31	20.6	0.70	1.24
+1.41	10.0	80.0	1.50	24.0	0.80	1.40

Codification: $V_c = (V_n - V_0)/\Delta V_n$; decodification: $V_n = V_0 + (\Delta V_n \times V_c)$; V_c = codified value of the variable; ΔV_n = increment of V_n per unit of V_c; V_n = natural value of the variable to codify; V_0 = natural value in the center of the domain.

The kinetic data of hydrolysis, with hyperbolic trends, were perfectly modelled by the Weibull equation [23], achieving determination coefficients ranging from 0.980–0.998 and complete statistical significance of kinetic parameters (data not shown). One of those parameters, maximum hydrolysis (H_m), was chosen as the response variable to study the joint influence of *pH* and temperature (*T*) on alcalase hydrolysis. The concentration of chondroitin sulfate (*CS*) from samples of the hydrolysates extracted at 0.5 M NaOH/1 *v* EtOH and the index of CS purity (I_p) were also determined. In all cases, the predicted response surfaces were very similar with clear convex shapes (Figure 1). The second order equations that calculated those theoretical surfaces are summarized in Table 2.

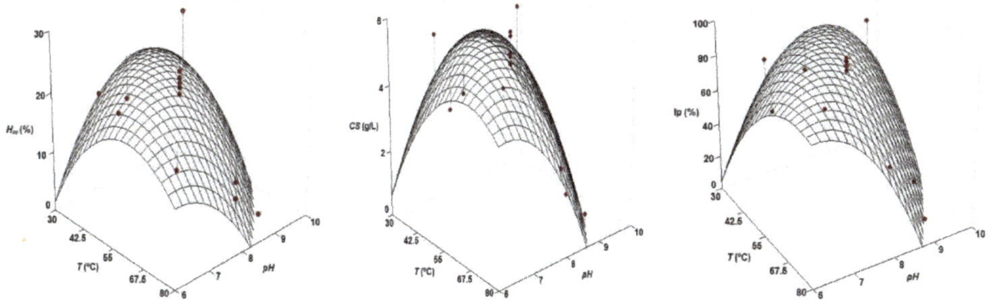

Figure 1. Experimental data and theoretical surfaces obtained from the equations shown in Table 1 describing the joint effect of *pH* and T on the maximum hydrolysis (H_m), chondroitin sulfate (*CS*) concentration and CS purity (I_p) generated by alcalase hydrolysis of cartilage by-products of *G. melastomus*.

Table 2. Polynomial equations modelling NaOH and time influence in alkaline treatment and NaOH and EtOH in an alkaline-alcoholic precipitation applied to cartilage hydrolysates. Optima values of the independent variables ($NaOH_{opt}$, t_{opt} and $EtOH_{opt}$) are also calculated.

Treatment	Second Order Equations	R^2_{adj}	$NaOH_{opt}$ (M)	t_{opt} (h)
Alkaline	CS (g/L) = 6.42 + 1.34 t $NaOH$ − 0.88 $NaOH^2$ + 1.68 t^2	0.687	0.85	1 or 24
	I_p (%) = 19.05 + 3.03 t $NaOH$ − 2.61 $NaOH^2$ + 4.37 t^2	0.709	0.85	1 or 24
		R^2_{adj}	$NaOH_{opt}$ (M)	$EtOH_{opt}$ (v)
Alkaline-alcoholic	CS (g/L) = 6.56 + 1.91 $EtOH$ − 2.39 $NaOH^2$ − 1.28 $EtOH^2$	0.742	0.45	1.14
	I_p (%) = 67.0 + 20.90 $EtOH$ − 20.06 $NaOH^2$ − 13.03 $EtOH^2$	0.710	0.45	1.16

Statistically, the consistency of models was always validated after overcoming the $F1$ and $F2$ ratios from F-Fisher tests (data not shown). The numerical derivation of equations to obtain the optimal values of both variables, maximizing the response studied, led to the results indicated in Table 3. pH_{opt} and T_{opt} ranged from 7.06–7.61 and from 47.5–57.8, respectively. In this context, the best conditions to hydrolyze cartilage from *G. melastomus* with alcalase (compromise option as the average of the mentioned intervals) were established at T = 52.9 °C and pH = 7.31.

Table 3. Polynomial equations modelling pH and T effects on alcalase hydrolysis of *G. melastomus* cartilage. Adjusted determination coefficients (R^2_{adj}) and optimal values of T and pH (T_{opt} and pH_{opt}) that maximized the dependent variables are also shown.

Second Order Equations	R^2_{adj}	T_{opt} (°C)	pH_{opt}
H_m (%) = 22.02 − 5.18 T − 4.82 pH − 5.56 T pH − 4.26 T^2 − 4.44 pH^2	0.801	47.5	7.61
CS (g/L) = 5.25 − 0.80 T − 1.36 pH − 1.20 T pH − 0.80 T^2 − 1.16 pH^2	0.796	53.3	7.25
I_p (%) = 85.06 − 11.81 T − 23.06 pH − 22.76 T pH − 10.59 T^2 − 20.02 pH^2	0.890	57.8	7.06

2.2. Isolation of CS by Chemical Treatments

For the present step, two strategies for improving chondroitin sulfate isolation were evaluated: (1) alkaline hydrolysis to produce CS useful for nutraceutical formulations and (2) selective precipitation of CS in alkaline-alcoholic solutions to yield purer CS useful for medical applications. Initially, hydrolysates of cartilage were produced under the optimal conditions previously defined (t_h = 8 h, T = 53 °C, pH = 7.3, [alcalase] = 0.5% (v/w), solid:liquid ratio (1:1), agitation = 200 rpm), in enough amount to perform the two factorial designs of the chemical processing (Table 1). CS concentration and I_p responses (both experimental points and predicted surfaces) from such treatments of the hydrolysates are depicted in Figure 2, and the second order equations are given in Table 2.

ALKALINE HYDROLYSIS

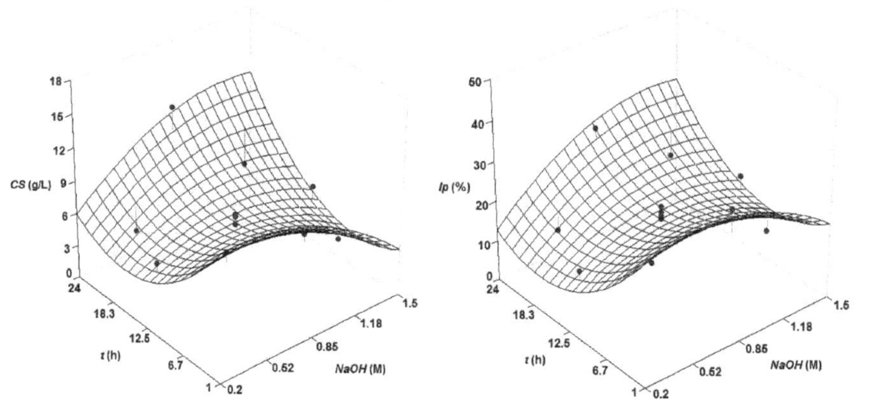

Figure 2. *Cont.*

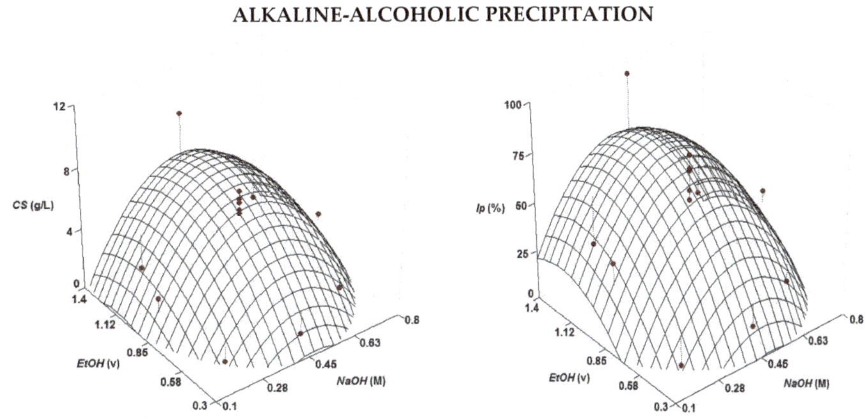

Figure 2. Experimental data and predicted response surfaces by empirical equations summarized in Table 2 corresponding to the combined effect of NaOH and EtOH on the selective treatment of CS from cartilage hydrolysates of *S. canicula*. Responses were *CS* concentration (**left**) and purity index, I_p (**right**).

The correlation between experimental and predicted was is relatively good with values greater than 0.69, but a lack of fit could be observed in some experimental data (Figure 2). Nevertheless, the consistency of the four cases was confirmed by the values of the F1 and F2 ratios and their comparison to the values from the Fisher F-test (data not shown). In the alkaline hydrolysis, the surfaces showed a heterogeneous concave shape with higher values of CS recovered and purity at short and long times of processing (1 h and 24 h). In both situations, the best concentration of alkalis to maximize the responses was 0.85 M (Table 2). These outcomes were certainly surprising since the expected pattern for the hydrolysis time would be an asymptotic curve (e.g., sigmoid or hyperbolic) rather than the present concave surface observed. No clear assumption could be set to explain this behavior, but a similar parabolic trend for the time of hydrolysis was found in the extraction of antioxidants from surplus tomato crop assisted by microwave [27], the solubilization of collagen from croaker skin by pepsin hydrolysis [28], enzyme hydrolysis of fish processing waste [29] and the production of fish protein hydrolysates [30]. For the NaOH-EtOH treatment, the surfaces were convex domes, with a clear maximum response, in agreement with the results obtained in the precipitation of CS from other cartilaginous fish species [26,31].

Optimal levels of alkalis and ethanol Table 2 were similar, in the case of alcohol, and lower, for NaOH, to those achieved in *Prionace glauca* [26] and *S. canicula* [20]. The purity of CS isolated after enzyme digestion and chemical processing, in the best conditions of operation, were 30% and 75% for alkaline and alkaline-ethanolic treatments, respectively.

2.3. Diafiltration for CS Purification

The most common protocols for the final purification of glycosaminoglycans are based on chromatography [32,33] or membrane technologies [34,35]. In the present work, we studied the recovery of CS by the ultrafiltration (UF) and diafiltration (DF) steps. Thus, samples obtained by enzyme hydrolysis and subsequent chemical treatments (in all cases, employing optimal conditions) were passed through a membrane of 30 kDa operating in total recirculation. Figure 3 shows the results of the UF-DF stages for the samples generated by selective precipitation (EtOH) and alkaline hydrolysis (NaOH at 1 h and 24 h).

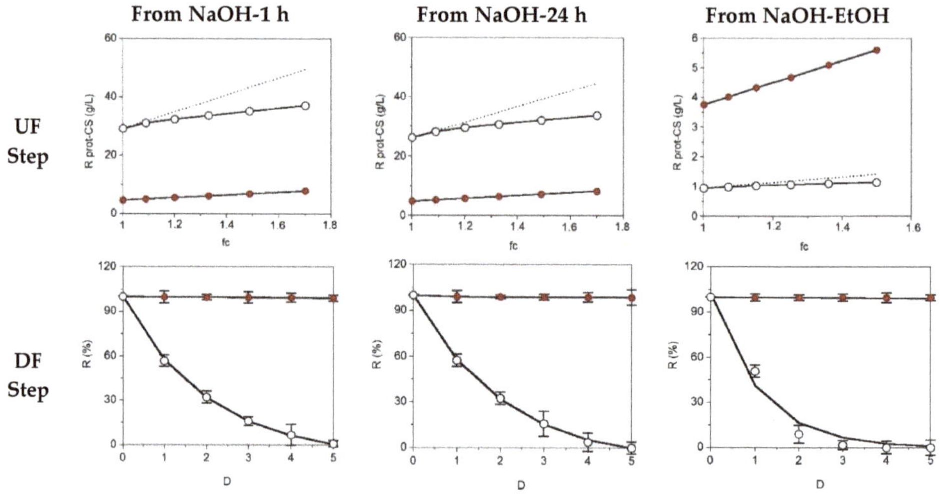

Figure 3. Ultrafiltration (UF) and diafiltration (DF) progress for samples obtained from NaOH (1 h and 24 h of hydrolysis) and NaOH-EtOH treatment. Top: concentration of retained protein (o) and CS (●) in linear relation with the factor of volumetric concentration (fc) depicting experimental data (points) and theoretical profiles corresponding to a fully-retained solute (discontinuous line). Bottom: progress of protein (o) and CS (●) retention with the increase of diavolume from DF step (D). Error bars are the confidence intervals (α = 0.05; n = 2).

For the case of CS, complete correlation between the experimental and predicted concentration factor was observed, but for the protein fraction, a remarkable amount of this material permeated at the 30-kDa molecular weight cut-off. The DF data were perfectly modelled by the exponential equation [3], obtaining determination coefficients higher than 0.980. The values of the specific retention (s), the parameter derived from that equation, indicated the high and low retention of CS and protein, respectively: 0.992 $\pm$ 0.017 for CS-NaOH/EtOH, 0.980 $\pm$ 0.025 for CS-NaOH-1 h, 0.971 $\pm$ 0.023 for CS-NaOH-24 h, 0.090 $\pm$ 0.009 for CS-NaOH/EtOH, 0.505 $\pm$ 0.021 for CS-NaOH-1 h and 0.523 $\pm$ 0.016 for CS-NaOH-24 h. The transmembrane flows during the concentration stage (UF) were maintained, working at 0.8–0.9 bar, at the following levels: 114 $\pm$ 21 mL/min, 175 $\pm$ 10 mL/min and 182 $\pm$ 11 mL/min for the NaOH-1 h, NaOH-24 h and NaOH/EtOH samples, respectively. After drying of retentates, the purities of CS (I_p-values) stood at 81.2%, 82.3% (samples from NaOH treatment) and 97.4% (sample from NaOH/EtOH precipitation). Finally, the yield of CS ranged between 3.5% and 3.7% of wet weight cartilage.

2.4. Molecular Weight of CS

The number average molecular weight (Mn) of CS treated with NaOH for 1 h was estimated at 66 kDa; increasing hydrolysis time to 24 h reduced Mn to 53 kDa, comparable to the 55 kDa obtained for hydroalcoholic alkaline precipitation (Table 4). GPC eluograms depicted in Figure 4 show a second peak at low retention times in all samples, which can be observed in the light scattering signals, but is barely visible in the refractive index (RI) trace. This indicates high molecular weight species at a very low concentration. Proteinaceous composition seems unlikely, since additional on-line UV detection from 240–310 nm did not produce any signals. The peak might corresponded to CS aggregates, which have been described in other polyelectrolytes such as chitosan [36,37] or heparin [38], but also other high molecular GAGs occurring in cartilage such as hyaluronan. Unfortunately, hyaluronan presence could not be confirmed by ^{1}H NMR because of signal overlap, as discussed in the next section.

Regardless of its nature, the low species concentration makes its contribution to CS composition relatively unimportant.

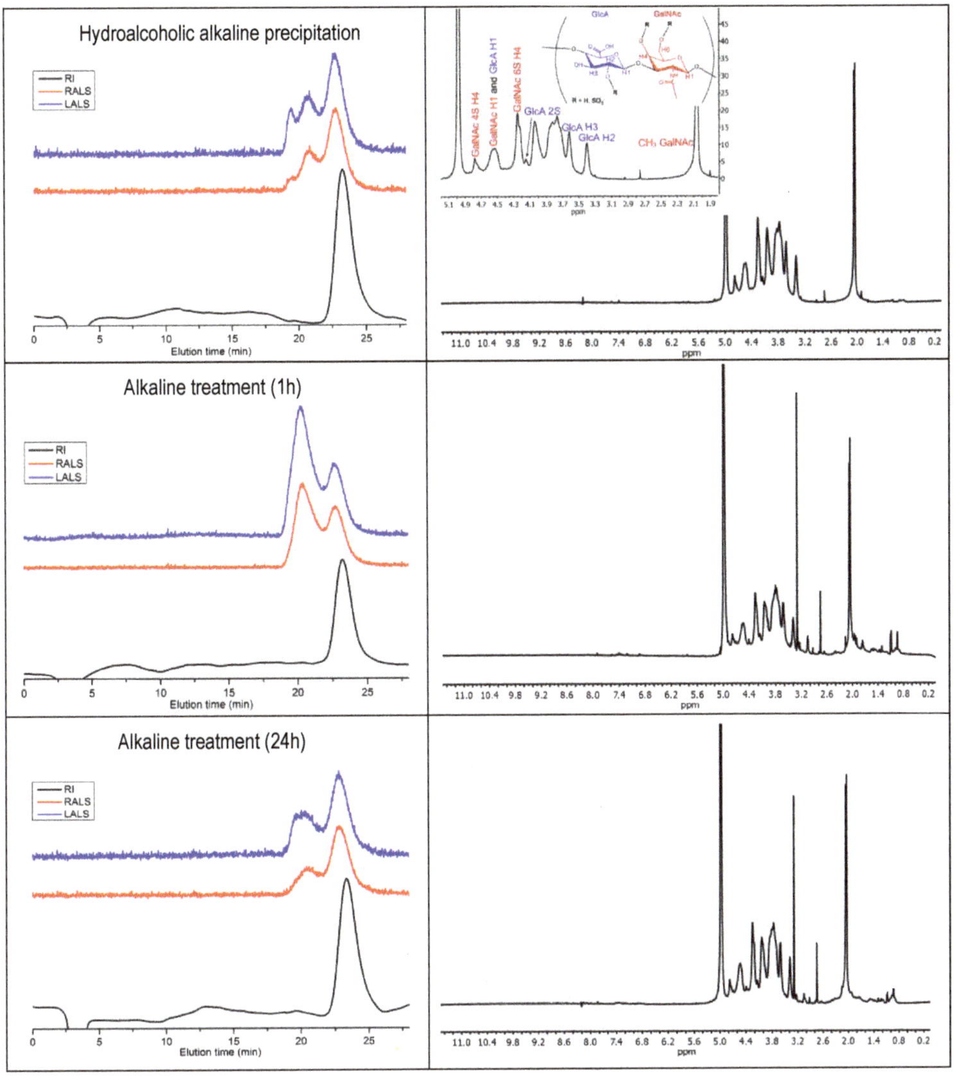

Figure 4. Gel permeation chromatography (GPC) eluograms (**left**) and ^{1}H NMR spectra (**right**) of CS extracted from *Galeus melastomus*. Red line: right angle light scattering signal (RALS); blue line: low angle light scattering signal (LALS); black line: refractive index (RI) signal.

A previous report tentatively estimated the chain length of CS extracted from *G. melastomus* at 27 disaccharide units [18]. This value was calculated from the relative intensities of ^{1}H NMR signals of terminal and non-terminal GlcA residues. As the authors recognize, the approximation was only qualitative since other polysaccharide moieties may have contributed to the signal assigned to terminal GlcA, therefore leading to molecular weight underestimation. Indeed, 27 disaccharide units correspond to around 10 kDa (assuming 80% of units mono-sulfated and 15% disulfated), 5–6-times lower than the Mn values reported herein. In other shark species, molecular weight ranges from 31 kDa (unidentified species) [39] to 60 kDa in blue shark (*Prionace glauca*) [40]. In comparison, the molecular weight of CS from *G. melastomus* was relatively high.

Table 4. Molecular weight and disaccharide composition of CS isolated from *G. melastomus* following alkaline hydrolysis (1 h and 24 h) and hydroalcoholic-alkaline precipitation. Mn: number average molecular weight, PDI: polydispersity index; disaccharide composition expressed as the mean% ± the standard deviation; ^{1}H NMR, strong anion exchange (^{2}SAX)-HPLC.

	Alkaline Hydrolysis 1 h	Alkaline Hydrolysis 24 h	Hydroalcoholic Alkaline Precipitation
Mn	66 kDa	53 kDa	55 kDa
PDI	1.14	1.25	1.26
CS-A (GlcA-GalNAc 4S)^1	23.9	22.78	23.01
CS-A (GlcA-GalNAc 4S)^2	23.43 ± 0.23	23.52 ± 0.11	23.77 ± 0.13
CS-C (GlcA-GalNAc 6S)^2	54.78 ± 0.02	55.11 ± 0.16	54.93 ± 0.36
CS-0 (GlcA-GalNAc 0S)^2	3.96 ± 0.03	3.92 ± 0.27	4.23 ± 0.55
CS-D (GlcA 2S-GalNAc 6S)^2	15.75 ± 0.19	15.37 ± 0.00	15.00 ± 0.05
CS-E (GlcA-GalNAc 4,6S)^2	1.46 ± 0.05	1.46 ± 0.00	1.48 ± 0.01
CS-B (GlcA 2S-GalNAc 4S)^2	0.61 ± 0.00	0.62 ± 0.01	0.59 ± 0.01

2.5. Composition of CS

^{1}H NMR spectra shown in Figure 4 provide an overview of CS composition. Characteristic CS signals appeared at 2.05 ppm, corresponding to the acetyl group in GalNAc, and in the region from to 3.5–5 ppm. Additional signals outside this range probably correspond to impurities. Amino acids in particular typically appeared between 0.5 and 1.5 ppm (aliphatic) and 7.0–8.5 (aromatic). The number and intensity of these signals were higher for alkaline treatment after 1 h than after 24 h and decreased to its minimum after hydroalcoholic precipitation. This is in line with CS purity index (I_p) values of 81–82% for alkaline treatment and 97.4% for hydroalcoholic alkaline precipitation.

Additional GAGs present in cartilage could also remain as impurities in the final product, specifically hyaluronan, keratan sulfate (KS) and dermatan sulfate (DS). CS and DS both contain GalNAc in their structure, but GlcA in CS is replaced by its epimer iduronic acid (IdoA) in DS. Characteristic signals of DS at 4.87 ppm (H1 of IdoA) and 3.52 ppm (H2 of IdoA) [41] were barely visible in the alkaline-treated samples, implying possible DS presence in minute amounts. Unlike CS and DS, KS and HA share N-acetyl glucosamine (GlcNAc) in their constitutive disaccharides, instead of GalNAc. Anomeric carbons of GlcNAc (H1) present signals at 4.54 ppm in HA and 4.7 ppm in KS [41]. Small amounts of KS can be seen in alkaline-treated samples (Figure 4). The absence of DS and KS signals in the hydroalcoholic precipitated samples indicates that 1.4–1.16 volumes of ethanol used here were capable of separating these GAGs from CS. This agrees with previous reports, which found that DS and KS precipitation occurred below one and above 1.2 volumes of ethanol, respectively, while CS precipitated above one volume of ethanol [42,43]. In the case of HA, it is not possible to assert its presence because the signal at 4.54 ppm overlapped with those of GalNAc and GlcA (H1).

Beyond contaminating compounds, NMR profiles in Figure 4 appear similar for all samples, indicating that differences in treatments did not impact disaccharide composition. Quantification in NMR is difficult because of signal overlap; however, the percentage of units sulfated in position 4 of GalNAc (CS-A) could be estimated by comparing the signal intensities of the acetyl group in GalNAc (2.05–2.07 ppm) with the singlet at 4.78 (H4 of four sulfated GalNAc) [44]. This resulted in 23–24% of CS-A (Table 4), in agreement with the values obtained by strong anion exchange (SAX)-HPLC. Qualitatively, the strong signal at 4.25 denoted a high percentage of CS-C and the singlet at 4.15 the presence of some two sulfated glucuronic acid.

Chromatographic analysis after enzymatic treatment was carried out to complement the information provided by NMR (Figure 5). However, it must be noted that a previous report had shown that treatment with chondroitinase ABC led to 70% hydrolysis after 2.5 h. Even extensive digestion with lyases ABC and C for seven days can only convert 80–85% of the initial polymer to disaccharides [45]. Although this work used an enzyme to substrate ratio 100-times lower than in the present work, it is possible that the hydrolysis performed in the current study was not complete, and disaccharide composition may not fully reflect the proportion in the original polymer. Bearing this in mind, quantitative analysis from chromatography shows that in all cases, the majority of CS disaccharides consisted of CS-C (55%), followed by CS-A (23–24%), with unsulfated CS accounting for only 4% of total CS. Disulfated disaccharides represented 17–18% of total CS, mainly GlcA 2S-GalNAc 6S (CS-D), with only minor quantities of GlcA-GalNAc 4,6S (CS-E) and GlcA 2S-GalNAc 4S (CS-B).

These data showed that CS from *G. melastomus* represents a good source of CS-A and CS-D. Compared to other shark species, CS-C proportion (55%) lied at the high end of the range, typically from 30–60% [40,44,46]. In the case of CS-D, this disaccharide unit is quite uncommon. Cartilaginous fish are its main source, despite the fact that it is not the main disaccharide in fish cartilage. In *G. melastomus*, CS-D accounts for 15–16% of total CS, close to up to 20% reported in *Chimaera phantasma* [46].

While particular applications lie beyond the scope of the current report, CS rich in C units have shown positive results for cartilage regeneration. In vitro, the presence of CS-C appears to enhance chondrocyte proliferation [47–49]; favor differentiation of mesenchymal stem cells to chondrocytes and increase extracellular matrix secretion [50,51]. In vivo studies seem to confirm that CS-C improves the ability of hydrogels and scaffolds to repair cartilage lesions [10,52]. Furthermore, CS-C also appears to modulate inflammation to a greater extent than CS-A by reducing NO production and pro-inflammatory cytokines, while increasing the anti-inflammatory cytokine interleukin-10 [53]. These examples serve to illustrate the potential of CS rich in C-units, such as CS from *G. melastomus*.

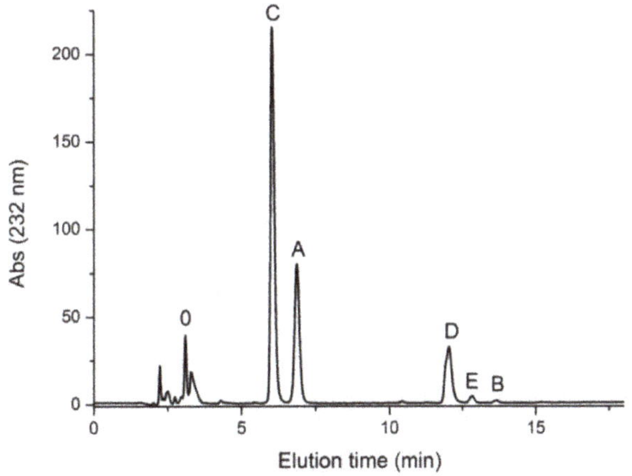

Figure 5. SAX-HPLC chromatogram (UV detection at 232 nm) of CS from *G. melastomus* purified by hydroalcoholic alkaline precipitation after enzymatic digestion with chondroitinase ABC. 0: ΔUA-GalNAc (CS-0); A: ΔUA-GalNAc4S (CS-A); C: ΔUA-GalNAc6S (CS-C); D: ΔUA(2S)-GalNAc6S (CS-D); E: ΔUA-GalNAc4,6S (CS-E); B: ΔUA2S-GalNAc4S (CS-B).

3. Experimental Section

3.1. Preparation of Cartilage and Proximal and Analytical Determinations

Cartilage from blackmouth catshark (*Galeus melastomus*) individuals, kindly supplied by Opromar (Marín, Spain), was isolated from the heads, fins and skeletons by treatment with water at 90 °C for 30 min and subsequent manual cleaning. These substrates were crushed and homogenized to ≈1–4 mm and stored at −20 °C until use. The proximal composition of cartilage was determined in triplicate, including moisture, ash, fat, total nitrogen and total protein according to the AOAC protocols [54]. Total carbohydrate content was estimated by subtracting protein, fat, ash and moisture to total sample weight. In CS solutions, total soluble protein (Pr) was determined by the method of

Lowry et al. [55]; CS, as glucuronic acid, was quantified by the method of Van den Hoogen et al. [56], according to the modifications of Murado et al. [57]. The CS purity index (I_p), defined as I_p (%) = CS × 100/(CS + Pr), was also calculated in all purification stages.

3.2. Factorial Designs and Statistical Analysis

Three experimental designs were performed in the present work to study and optimize: (1) the simultaneous effect of temperature (T) and pH on the hydrolysis degree of blackmouth catshark cartilage catalyzed by alcalase; (2) the influence of the concentration of NaOH and the time of alkaline hydrolysis on the hydrolysates of cartilage obtained under previous optimal conditions; (3) the effect of NaOH concentration and ethanol volume needed for the selective isolation of CS from cartilage hydrolysates obtained under optimal conditions of hydrolysis. In all cases, the factorial experiments were rotatable second order designs with five replicates in the center of the experimental domains [58]. Codified and natural values for all experimental conditions tested in the factorial designs are summarized in Table 1.

Orthogonal least-squares calculation on factorial design data was used to obtain empirical equations describing the different dependent variables studied (Y), each one related to T and pH for enzymatic hydrolysis and $NaOH$ and $EtOH$ for CS production. The general form of the polynomial equations is:

$$Y = \mathrm{b}_0 + \sum_{i=1}^{n} \mathrm{b}_i X_i + \sum_{\substack{i=1 \\ j>i}}^{n-1} \sum_{j=2}^{n} \mathrm{b}_{ij} X_i X_j + \sum_{i=1}^{n} \mathrm{b}_{ii} X_i^2 \quad (1)$$

where Y is the dependent variable evaluated, b_0 the constant coefficient, b_i the coefficient of the linear effect, b_{ij} the coefficient of the combined effect, b_{ii} the coefficient of the quadratic effect, n the number of variables and X_i and X_j the independent variables studied in each case. Student's t-test ($\alpha = 0.05$) was employed to determine the statistical significance of coefficients. The coefficient of adjusted coefficients of determination (R^2_{adj}) was used to establish goodness-of-fit, and the following mean squares ratios from the Fisher F-test ($\alpha = 0.05$) were calculated to define model consistency: $F1$ = model/total error, the model being acceptable when $F1 \geq F^{\mathrm{num}}_{\mathrm{den}}$; and $F2$ = (Model + lack of fitting)/model, the model being acceptable when $F2 \leq F^{\mathrm{num}}_{\mathrm{den}}$. $F^{\mathrm{num}}_{\mathrm{den}}$ are the theoretical values for $\alpha = 0.05$ with corresponding degrees of freedom for the numerator (num) and denominator (den).

3.3. Cartilage Enzymatic Digestion

Cartilage was digested with 2.4 L of alcalase from *Bacillus licheniformis* (Novozyme Nordisk, Bagsvaerd, Denmark). The enzyme/substrate ratio was 24 U/kg (1% v/w of fresh cartilage); the solid:liquid ratio was (1:1); and T and pH conditions are defined in Table 1. Hydrolysis was performed in a thermostated reactor as indicated in previous work [20,26]. The progress of enzymatic hydrolysis was determined by the pH-Stat method [59], and the non-linear kinetics of hydrolysis degree (H, in %) were modelled by the Weibull equation [23]. The maximum degree of hydrolysis (H_m) was the parameter selected from such an equation as the dependent variable for the optimization study.

3.4. Chemical Processing of the Hydrolysates

Two kinds of chemical treatments were applied in parallel to the hydrolysates of cartilage obtained by alcalase digestion: (a) alkaline hydrolysis and (b) selective precipitation using hydroalcoholic solutions of NaOH. In the former, NaOH was added to the enzymatic hydrolysates until the concentrations defined in Table 1. The corresponding mixtures were maintained in continuous agitation at 200 rpm and room temperature for the different times studied. At the end of hydrolysis, mixtures were centrifuged at 6000× g for 20 min and supernatants neutralized with 6 M HCl. In the second treatment, CS present in the hydrolysates was precipitated by slowly adding NaOH solutions in hydroalcoholic media with different ethanol volumes (Table 1) under medium agitation at room temperature. A concentration of 2.5 g/L NaCl was also present in the mixtures. Suspensions formed were centrifuged (6000× *g*/20 min) after 2 h in agitation and the sediments resuspended in water and neutralized with 6 M HCl.

3.5. Purification of CS by UF-DF

A UF membrane of 30 kDa (spiral polyethersulfone, 0.56 m^2, Prep/Scale-TFF, Millipore Corporation, Burlington, MA, USA) was used to concentrate, desalinate and purify CS solutions obtained in chemical processing. The configuration and operation mode of the membrane system, initial concentration by the UF and then the DF step, were performed according to the description reported by [20]. DF data were modeled by a first-order equation [60], and the specific retention (*s*) parameter from that was calculated for comparative reasons.

3.6. Molecular Weight of CS

Absolute molecular weight of CS was determined on a GPC/SEC system (Agilent 1260, Agilent, Waldbronn, Germany) equipped with quaternary pump (G1311B), injector (G1329B), column oven (G1316A), refractive index (G1362A) and dual angle static light scattering (G7800A) detectors. Sample separation was achieved with a set of four columns (PSS, Mainz, Germany): Suprema precolumn (5 µm, 8 × 50 mm), Suprema 30 Å (5 µm, 8 × 300 mm), Suprema 100 Å (5 µm, 8 × 300 mm) and Suprema ultrahigh (10 µm, 8 × 300 mm). A sample volume of 100 µL was injected onto the above system and eluted at 1 mL/min with a solution composed of 0.1 M NaN_3 and 0.01 M NaH_2PO_4 at *pH* 6.6. The column oven and light scattering detector were kept at 30 °C, while the refractive index detector was kept at 40 °C. Both detectors were calibrated with a polyethylene oxide standard (PSS, Mainz, Germany) of 106 kDa (Mp) and a polydispersity index (PDI) of 1.05. Samples and standards were dissolved in the mobile phase solution. Refractive index increments (dn/dc) of 0.110 were calculated from the RI detector response.

3.7. CS Composition by ^{1}H NMR and SAX-HPLC

Chemical composition of CS was assessed by the combination of NMR and chromatographic techniques.

NMR spectra were recorded on a Bruker DPX 600 (Bruker, Rheinstetten, Germany) operating at 600 Mhz. The temperature was set to 10 °C to avoid overlapping with residual HOD. Samples were dissolved in D_2O at 1 g/L for ^{1}H experiments. Spectral processing was carried out with MestReNova 10.0.2 software (Mestrelab Research, Santiago de Compostela, Spain). Spectra were referenced from the solvent signal.

Disaccharide composition of CS was determined by strong anion exchange (SAX) chromatography after enzymatic digestion with chondroitinase ABC from *Proteus vulgaris* (EC 4.2.2.4., 1.66 U mg^{-1}, Product number C2905, Sigma-Aldrich, Saint Louis, MO, USA) at 0.2 U mg^{-1} of CS. The reaction was carried out in 0.05 M Tris-HCl/0.15 M sodium acetate buffer at *pH* 8 and 37 °C. After 24 h, the enzyme was inactivated by heating at 70 °C for 25 min, followed by centrifugation at 12,857× *g*. Supernatants were collected and filtered through 0.2-µm polyethersulfone (PES) syringe filters. Unsaturated disaccharide standards were purchased from Grampenz (Aberdeen, UK) and dissolved in water. Samples and standards were manually injected onto an HPLC system (Agilent 1200) consisting of a binary pump (G1312A), column oven (G1316A) and UV-visible detector (G1314B). Separation was carried out with a Waters Spherisorb SAX column (5 µm, 4.6 × 250 mm, Prod. No. PSS832715, Waters Corp, Milford, MA, USA) fitted with a guard cartridge (Waters Spherisorb, 5 µm, 4.6 × 10 mm) based on a previously reported method [61]. Elution was performed in isocratic mode from 0–5 min with 50 mM NaCl at *pH* 4. The linear gradient was applied from 5–20 min starting with 50 mM NaCl at *pH* 4 and ending with 76% 50 mM NaCl at *pH* 4 and 24% 1.2 M NaCl at *pH* 4. A sample volume of 20 µL was injected onto the system with a flow rate of 1.5 mL min^{-1}. Detection was made at 232 nm. An external calibration curve was built with each standard to calculate the amount of disaccharide units in the sample and reported as percentage of weight.

4. Conclusions

In the present work, we study CS isolation from *G. melastomus* by initial enzymatic cartilage proteolysis, followed by two different chemical treatments and ending in membrane purification. All steps are mathematically optimized by response surface methodologies. The conditions to maximize CS recovery are established as: 52.9 °C and *pH* 7.31 for enzyme digestion of cartilaginous material; 0.85 M NaOH for alkaline treatment of the EH and 0.45 M NaOH, 1.14–1.16 *v* EtOH for alkaline hydroalcoholic precipitation of the EH; and UF at 30 kDa using at least five diavolumes of water to obtain CS with more than 81–82% of purity (97.4% with NaOH-EtOH solutions). Molecular weights were estimated at 53–66 kDa, relatively high compared to other cartilaginous fish. Sulfation profiles were similar for both chemical treatments, revealing dominant CS-C units (55%), followed by 23–24% CS-A, a substantial amount of CS-D (15–16%) and less than 7% of other disulfated and unsulfated disaccharides.

Author Contributions: J.A.V. and J.V. conceived and designed the experiments. J.A.V., J.F. and J.V. performed the experiments. J.A.V., R.N.C. and J.V. analyzed the data. J.A.V., R.N.C. and J.V. wrote the paper. R.I.P.-M., L.T.A. and R.L.R. participated in the interpretation of the data and also critically revised the manuscript.

Funding: Acknowledgments for financial support to projects iSEAS LIFE13 ENV/ES/000131 (LIFE+Programme, EU), IBEROS (0245_IBEROS_1_E, POCTEP 2015), CVMar+I (0302_CVMAR_I_1_P, POCTEP 2015) and BLUEHUMAN (EAPA_151/2016, UE-INTERREG Atlantic Area Programme) and support of the publication fee by the CSIC Open Access Publication Support Initiative through its Unit of Information Resources for Research (URICI). RNC thanks the Portuguese Foundation for Science and Technology (IF/00373/2014).

Conflicts of Interest: The authors declare no conflict of interest.

References

1. Yamada, S.; Sugahara, K. Potential therapeutic application of chondroitin sulfate/dermatan sulfate. *Curr. Drug Discov. Technol.* **2008**, *5*, 289–301. [CrossRef] [PubMed]
2. Celikkin, N.; Rinoldi, C.; Costantini, M.; Trombetta, M.; Rainer, A.; Święszkowski, W. Naturally derived proteins and glycosaminoglycan scaffolds for tissue engineering applications. *Mater. Sci. Eng. C* **2017**, *78*, 1277–1299. [CrossRef] [PubMed]
3. Lima, M.; Rudd, T.; Yates, E. New applications of heparin and other glycosaminoglycans. *Molecules* **2017**, *22*, 749. [CrossRef] [PubMed]
4. Pomin, V.H. A dilemma in the glycosaminoglycan-based therapy: Synthetic or naturally unique molecules? *Med. Res. Rev.* **2015**, *35*, 1195–1219. [CrossRef] [PubMed]
5. Valcarcel, J.; Novoa-Carballal, R.; Pérez-Martín, R.I.; Reis, R.L.; Vázquez, J.A. Glycosaminoglycans from marine sources as therapeutic agents. *Biotechnol. Adv.* **2017**, *35*, 711–725. [CrossRef] [PubMed]
6. Yamada, S.; Sugahara, K.; Özbek, S. Evolution of glycosaminoglycans: Comparative biochemical study. *Commun. Integr. Biol.* **2011**, *4*, 150–158. [CrossRef] [PubMed]
7. Soares da Costa, D.; Reis, R.L.; Pashkuleva, I. Sulfation of glycosaminoglycans and its implications in human health and disorders. *Annu. Rev. Biomed. Eng.* **2017**, *19*, 1–26. [CrossRef] [PubMed]
8. Basappa; Murugan, S.; Sugahara, K.N.; Lee, C.M.; ten Dam, G.B.; van Kuppevelt, T.H.; Miyasaka, M.; Yamada, S.; Sugahara, K. Involvement of chondroitin sulfate E in the liver tumor focal formation of murine osteosarcoma cells. *Glycobiology* **2009**, *19*, 735–742. [CrossRef] [PubMed]
9. Pomin, V.H. Holothurian fucosylated chondroitin sulfate. *Mar. Drugs* **2014**, *12*, 232–254. [CrossRef] [PubMed]
10. Chen, W.-C.; Wei, Y.-H.; Chu, I.M.; Yao, C.-L. Effect of chondroitin sulphate C on the in vitro and in vivo chondrogenesis of mesenchymal stem cells in crosslinked type II collagen scaffolds. *J. Tissue Eng. Regen. Med.* **2013**, *7*, 665–672. [CrossRef] [PubMed]
11. Zhao, Y.; Nakajima, T.; Yang, J.J.; Kurokawa, T.; Liu, J.; Lu, J.; Mizumoto, S.; Sugahara, K.; Kitamura, N.; Yasuda, K.; et al. Proteoglycans and glycosaminoglycans improve toughness of biocompatible double network hydrogels. *Adv. Mater.* **2014**, *26*, 436–442. [CrossRef] [PubMed]

12. Nandini, C.D.; Mikami, T.; Ohta, M.; Itoh, N.; Akiyama-Nambu, F.; Sugahara, K. Structural and functional characterization of oversulfated chondroitin sulfate/dermatan sulfate hybrid chains from the notochord of hagfish: Neuritogenic and binding activities for growth factors and neurotrophic factors. *J. Biol. Chem.* **2004**, *279*, 50799–50809. [CrossRef] [PubMed]
13. Kozlowski, E.O.; Gomes, A.M.; Silva, C.S.; Pereira, M.S.; de Vilela Silva, A.C.E.S.; Pavão, M.S.G. Structure and biological activities of glycosaminoglycan analogs from marine invertebrates: New therapeutic agents? In *Glycans in Diseases and Therapeutics*; Pavão, S.G.M., Ed.; Springer: Berlin/Heidelberg, Germany, 2011; pp. 159–184.
14. Antelo, L.T.; de Hijas-Liste, G.M.; Franco-Uría, A.; Alonso, A.A.; Pérez-Martín, R.I. Optimisation of processing routes for a marine biorefinery. *J. Clean. Prod.* **2015**, *104*, 489–501. [CrossRef]
15. EC (European Commission). Regulation (EU) No 1380/2013 of the European Parliament and of the Council of 11 December 2013 on the Common Fisheries Policy, Amending Council Regulations (EC) No 1954/2003 and (EC) No 1224/2009 and Repealing Council Regulations (EC) No 2371/2002 and (EC) No 639/2004 and Council Decision 2004/585/EC, 2013. Available online: http://data.europa.eu/eli/reg/2013/1380/oj (accessed on 5 September 2018).
16. Ordóñez-Del Pazo, T.; Antelo, L.T.; Franco-Uría, A.; Pérez-Martín, R.I.; Sotelo, C.G.; Alonso, A.A. Fish discards management in selected Spanish and Portuguese métiers: Identification and potential valorisation. *Trends Food Sci. Technol.* **2014**, *36*, 29–43. [CrossRef]
17. Berrow, S. Incidental capture of elasmobranchs in the bottom-set gill-net fishery off the south coast of Ireland. *J. Mar. Biol. Assoc. UK* **1994**, *74*, 837–848.
18. Krylov, V.B.; Grachev, A.A.; Ustyuzhanina, N.E.; Ushakova, N.A.; Preobrazhenskaya, M.E.; Kozlova, N.I.; Portsel, M.N.; Konovalova, I.N.; Novikov, V.Y.; Siebert, H.-C.; et al. Preliminary structural characterization, anti-inflammatory and anticoagulant activities of chondroitin sulfates from marine fish cartilage. *Russ. Chem. Bull.* **2011**, *60*, 746. [CrossRef]
19. Vázquez, J.A.; Rodríguez-Amado, I.; Montemayor, M.; Fraguas, J.; González, M.; Murado, M.Á. Chondroitin sulfate, hyaluronic acid and chitin/chitosan production using marine waste sources: Characteristics, applications and eco-friendly processes: A review. *Mar. Drugs* **2013**, *11*, 747–774. [CrossRef] [PubMed]
20. Blanco, M.; Fraguas, J.; Sotelo, C.G.; Pérez-Martín, R.I.; Vázquez, J.A. Production of chondroitin sulphate from head, skeleton and fins of *Scyliorhinus canicula* by-products by combination of enzymatic, chemical precipitation and ultrafiltration methodologies. *Mar. Drugs* **2015**, *13*, 3287–3308. [CrossRef] [PubMed]
21. Safari, R.; Motamedzadegan, A.; Ovissipour, M.; Regenstein, J.M.; Gildberg, A.; Rasco, B. Use of hydrolysates from yellowfin tuna (*Thunnus albacares*) heads as a complex nitrogen source for lactic acid bacteria. *Food Bioprocess Technol.* **2012**, *5*, 73–79. [CrossRef]
22. Ahn, C.-B.; Kim, J.-G.; Je, J.-Y. Purification and antioxidant properties of octapeptide from salmon byproduct protein hydrolysate by gastrointestinal digestion. *Food Chem.* **2014**, *147*, 78–83. [CrossRef] [PubMed]
23. Vázquez, J.A.; Blanco, M.; Massa, A.E.; Amado, I.R.; Pérez-Martín, R.I. Production of fish protein hydrolysates from *Scyliorhinus canicula* discards with antihypertensive and antioxidant activities by enzymatic hydrolysis and mathematical optimization using response surface methodology. *Mar. Drugs* **2017**, *15*, 306. [CrossRef] [PubMed]
24. Vázquez, J.A.; Noriega, D.; Ramos, P.; Valcarcel, J.; Novoa-Carballal, R.; Pastrana, L.; Reis, R.L.; Pérez-Martín, R.I. Optimization of high purity chitin and chitosan production from *Illex argentinus* pens by a combination of enzymatic and chemical processes. *Carbohydr. Polym.* **2017**, *174*, 262–272. [CrossRef] [PubMed]
25. Kim, S.B.; Ji, C.I.; Woo, J.W.; Do, J.R.; Cho, S.M.; Lee, Y.B.; Kang, S.N.; Park, J.H. Simplified purification of chondroitin sulphate from scapular cartilage of shortfin mako shark (*Isurus oxyrinchus*). *Int. J. Food Sci. Technol.* **2012**, *47*, 91–99. [CrossRef]
26. Vázquez, J.A.; Blanco, M.; Fraguas, J.; Pastrana, L.; Pérez-Martín, R. Optimisation of the extraction and purification of chondroitin sulphate from head by-products of *Prionace glauca* by environmental friendly processes. *Food Chem.* **2016**, *198*, 28–35. [CrossRef] [PubMed]
27. Pinela, J.; Prieto, M.; Barreiro, M.F.; Carvalho, A.M.; Oliveira, M.B.P.; Vázquez, J.A.; Ferreira, I.C. Optimization of microwave-assisted extraction of hydrophilic and lipophilic antioxidants from a surplus tomato crop by response surface methodology. *Food Bioprod. Process.* **2016**, *98*, 283–298. [CrossRef]

28. Yu, F.; Zong, C.; Jin, S.; Zheng, J.; Chen, N.; Huang, J.; Chen, Y.; Huang, F.; Yang, Z.; Tang, Y. Optimization of extraction conditions and characterization of pepsin-solubilised collagen from skin of giant croaker (*Nibea japonica*). *Mar. Drugs* **2018**, *16*, 29. [CrossRef] [PubMed]
29. Suganthi, S.H.; Ramani, K. Microbial assisted industrially important multiple enzymes from fish processing waste: Purification, characterization and application for the simultaneous hydrolysis of lipid and protein molecules. *RSC Adv.* **2016**, *6*, 93602–93620. [CrossRef]
30. Liu, L.; Wang, Y.; Peng, C.; Wang, J. Optimization of the preparation of fish protein anti-obesity hydrolysates using response surface methodology. *Int. J. Mol. Sci.* **2013**, *14*, 3124–3139. [CrossRef] [PubMed]
31. Murado, M.A.; Fraguas, J.; Montemayor, M.I.; Vázquez, J.A.; González, P. Preparation of highly purified chondroitin sulphate from skate (*Raja clavata*) cartilage by-products. Process optimization including a new procedure of alkaline hydroalcoholic hydrolysis. *Biochem. Eng. J.* **2010**, *49*, 126–132. [CrossRef]
32. Shi, Y.G.; Meng, Y.C.; Li, J.R.; Chen, J.; Liu, Y.H.; Bai, X. Chondroitin sulfate: Extraction, purification, microbial and chemical synthesis. *J. Chem. Technol. Biotechnol.* **2014**, *89*, 1445–1465. [CrossRef]
33. Garnjanagoonchorn, W.; Wongekalak, L.; Engkagul, A. Determination of chondroitin sulfate from different sources of cartilage. *Chem. Eng. Process.* **2007**, *46*, 465–471. [CrossRef]
34. Lignot, B.; Lahogue, V.; Bourseau, P. Enzymatic extraction of chondroitin sulfate from skate cartilage and concentration-desalting by ultrafiltration. *J. Biotechnol.* **2003**, *103*, 281–284. [CrossRef]
35. Murado, M.A.; Montemayor, M.I.; Cabo, M.; Vázquez, J.A.; González, M. Optimization of extraction and purification process of hyaluronic acid from fish eyeball. *Food Bioprod. Process.* **2012**, *90*, 491–498. [CrossRef]
36. Lamarque, G.; Lucas, J.-M.; Viton, C.; Domard, A. Physicochemical behavior of homogeneous series of acetylated chitosans in aqueous solution: Role of various structural parameters. *Biomacromolecules* **2005**, *6*, 131–142. [CrossRef] [PubMed]
37. Ottøy, M.H.; Vårum, K.M.; Christensen, B.E.; Anthonsen, M.W.; Smidsrød, O. Preparative and analytical size-exclusion chromatography of chitosans. *Carbohydr. Polym.* **1996**, *31*, 253–261. [CrossRef]
38. Bertini, S.; Bisio, A.; Torri, G.; Bensi, D.; Terbojevich, M. Molecular weight determination of heparin and dermatan sulfate by size exclusion chromatography with a triple detector array. *Biomacromolecules* **2005**, *6*, 168–173. [CrossRef] [PubMed]
39. Li, L.; Li, Y.; Feng, D.; Xu, L.; Yin, F.; Zang, H.; Liu, C.; Wang, F. Preparation of low molecular weight chondroitin sulfates, screening of a high anti-complement capacity of low molecular weight chondroitin sulfate and its biological activity studies in attenuating osteoarthritis. *Int. J. Mol. Sci.* **2016**, *17*, 1685. [CrossRef] [PubMed]
40. Novoa-Carballal, R.; Pérez-Martín, R.; Blanco, M.; Sotelo, C.G.; Fassini, D.; Nunes, C.; Coimbra, M.A.; Silva, T.H.; Reis, R.L.; Vázquez, J.A. By-products of *Scyliorhinus canicula*, *Prionace glauca* and *Raja clavata*: A valuable source of predominantly 6S sulfated chondroitin sulfate. *Carbohydr. Polym.* **2017**, *157*, 31–37. [CrossRef] [PubMed]
41. Pomin, V.H. NMR chemical shifts in structural biology of glycosaminoglycans. *Anal. Chem.* **2013**, *86*, 65–94. [CrossRef] [PubMed]
42. Galeotti, F.; Maccari, F.; Volpi, N. Selective removal of keratan sulfate in chondroitin sulfate samples by sequential precipitation with ethanol. *Anal. Biochem.* **2014**, *448*, 113–115. [CrossRef] [PubMed]
43. Volpi, N. Purification of heparin, dermatan sulfate and chondroitin sulfate from mixtures by sequential precipitation with various organic solvents. *J. Chromatogr. B Biomed. Sci. Appl.* **1996**, *685*, 27–34. [CrossRef]
44. Mucci, A.; Schenetti, L.; Volpi, N. ^{1}H and ^{13}C nuclear magnetic resonance identification and characterization of components of chondroitin sulfates of various origin. *Carbohydr. Polym.* **2000**, *41*, 37–45. [CrossRef]
45. Pomin, V.H.; Park, Y.; Huang, R.; Heiss, C.; Sharp, J.S.; Azadi, P.; Prestegard, J.H. Exploiting enzyme specificities in digestions of chondroitin sulfates A and C: Production of well-defined hexasaccharides. *Glycobiology* **2012**, *22*, 826–838. [CrossRef] [PubMed]
46. Higashi, K.; Takeuchi, Y.; Mukuno, A.; Tomitori, H.; Miya, M.; Linhardt, R.J.; Toida, T. Composition of glycosaminoglycans in elasmobranchs including several deep-sea sharks: Identification of chondroitin/dermatan sulfate from the dried fins of *Isurus oxyrinchus* and *Prionace glauca*. *PLOS ONE* **2015**, *10*, e0120860. [CrossRef] [PubMed]
47. Ko, C.-S.; Huang, J.-P.; Huang, C.-W.; Chu, I.M. Type II collagen-chondroitin sulfate-hyaluronan scaffold cross-linked by genipin for cartilage tissue engineering. *J. Biosci. Bioeng.* **2009**, *107*, 177–182. [CrossRef] [PubMed]

48. Chang, C.-H.; Liu, H.-C.; Lin, C.-C.; Chou, C.-H.; Lin, F.-H. Gelatin–chondroitin–hyaluronan tri-copolymer scaffold for cartilage tissue engineering. *Biomaterials* **2003**, *24*, 4853–4858. [CrossRef]
49. Balakrishnan, B.; Joshi, N.; Jayakrishnan, A.; Banerjee, R. Self-crosslinked oxidized alginate/gelatin hydrogel as injectable, adhesive biomimetic scaffolds for cartilage regeneration. *Acta Biomater.* **2014**, *10*, 3650–3663. [CrossRef] [PubMed]
50. Wei, Y.; Hu, Y.; Hao, W.; Han, Y.; Meng, G.; Zhang, D.; Wu, Z.; Wang, H. A novel injectable scaffold for cartilage tissue engineering using adipose—Derived adult stem cells. *J. Orthop. Res.* **2008**, *26*, 27–33. [CrossRef] [PubMed]
51. Nair, M.B.; Baranwal, G.; Vijayan, P.; Keyan, K.S.; Jayakumar, R. Composite hydrogel of chitosan–poly(hydroxybutyrate-*co*-valerate) with chondroitin sulfate nanoparticles for nucleus pulposus tissue engineering. *Colloids Surf. B. Biointerfaces* **2015**, *136*, 84–92. [CrossRef] [PubMed]
52. Hui, J.H.; Chan, S.-W.; Li, J.; Goh, J.C.H.; Li, L.; Ren, X.F.; Lee, E.H. Intra-articular delivery of chondroitin sulfate for the treatment of joint defects in rabbit model. *J. Mol. Histol.* **2007**, *38*, 483–489. [CrossRef] [PubMed]
53. Tan, G.-K.; Tabata, Y. Chondroitin-6-sulfate attenuates inflammatory responses in murine macrophages via suppression of NF-κB nuclear translocation. *Acta Biomater.* **2014**, *10*, 2684–2692. [CrossRef] [PubMed]
54. AOAC. *Association of Official Analytical Chemistry. Methods of Analysis*, 15th ed.; AOAC: Washington DC, USA, 1997.
55. Lowry, O.H.; Rosebrough, N.J.; Farr, A.L.; Randall, R.J. Protein measurement with the Folin phenol reagent. *J. Biol. Chem.* **1951**, *193*, 265–275. [PubMed]
56. van den Hoogen, B.M.; van Weeren, P.R.; Lopes-Cardozo, M.; van Golde, L.M.; Barneveld, A.; van de Lest, C.H. A microtiter plate assay for the determination of uronic acids. *Anal. Biochem.* **1998**, *257*, 107–111. [CrossRef] [PubMed]
57. Murado, M.A.; Vázquez, J.A.; Montemayor, M.I.; Cabo, M.L.; de Pilar González, M. Two mathematical models for the correction of carbohydrate and protein interference in the determination of uronic acids by the *m*-hydroxydiphenyl method. *Biotechnol. Appl. Biochem.* **2005**, *41*, 209–216. [PubMed]
58. Box, G.E.; Hunter, J.S.; Hunter, W.G. *Statistics for Experimenters: Design, Innovation, and Discovery*; Wiley-Interscience: New York, NY, USA, 2005; Volume 2.
59. Adler-Nissen, J. *Enzymic Hydrolysis of Food Proteins*; Elsevier Applied Science Publishers: London, UK, 1986.
60. Amado, I.R.; Vázquez, J.A.; González, M.P.; Murado, M.A. Production of antihypertensive and antioxidant activities by enzymatic hydrolysis of protein concentrates recovered by ultrafiltration from cuttlefish processing wastewaters. *Biochem. Eng. J.* **2013**, *76*, 43–54. [CrossRef]
61. Volpi, N. Hyaluronic acid and chondroitin sulfate unsaturated disaccharides analysis by high-performance liquid chromatography and fluorimetric detection with dansylhydrazine. *Anal. Biochem.* **2000**, *277*, 19–24. [CrossRef] [PubMed]

© 2018 by the authors. Licensee MDPI, Basel, Switzerland. This article is an open access article distributed under the terms and conditions of the Creative Commons Attribution (CC BY) license (http://creativecommons.org/licenses/by/4.0/).

marine drugs

MDPI

Article

Supercritical Carbon Dioxide Extraction of Astaxanthin, Lutein, and Fatty Acids from *Haematococcus pluvialis* Microalgae

Giuseppe Di Sanzo [1], Sanjeet Mehariya [2,3], Maria Martino [1], Vincenzo Larocca [1], Patrizia Casella [2], Simeone Chianese [3], Dino Musmarra [3], Roberto Balducchi [1] and Antonio Molino [2,*]

1 ENEA, Italian National Agency for New Technologies, Energy and Sustainable Economic Development, Department of Sustainability, CR Trisaia SS Jonica 106, km 419+500, 75026 Rotondella, Italy; giuseppe.disanzo@enea.it (G.D.S.); maria.martino@enea.it (M.M.); vincenzo.larocca@enea.it (V.L.); roberto.baldicchi@enea.it (R.B.)

2 ENEA, Italian National Agency for New Technologies, Energy and Sustainable Economic Development, Department of Sustainability, CR Portici. P. Enrico Fermi, 1, 80055 Portici, Italy; smehariya@gmail.com (S.M.); patrizia.casella@enea.it (P.C.)

3 Department of Engineering, Università degli Studi della Campania "L. Vanvitelli", Real Casa dell'Annunziata, Via Roma 29, 81031 Aversa, Italy; sim.chianese@gmail.com (S.C.); dinomusmarra@gmail.com (D.M.)

* Correspondence: antonio.molino@enea.it; Tel.: +39-081-772-3276

Received: 12 August 2018; Accepted: 11 September 2018; Published: 13 September 2018

Abstract: *Haematococcus pluvialis* microalgae in the red phase can produce significant amounts of astaxanthin, lutein, and fatty acids (FAs), which are valuable antioxidants in nutraceutics and cosmetics. Extraction of astaxanthin, lutein, and FAs from disrupted biomass of the *H. pluvialis* red phase using carbon dioxide (CO_2) in supercritical fluid extraction (SFE) conditions was investigated using a bench-scale reactor in a semi-batch configuration. In particular, the effect of extraction time (20, 40, 60, 80, and 120 min), CO_2 flow rate (3.62 and 14.48 g/min) temperature (50, 65, and 80 °C), and pressure (100, 400, and 550 bar.) was explored. The results show the maximum recovery of astaxanthin and lutein achieved were 98.6% and 52.3%, respectively, at 50 °C and 550 bars, while the maximum recovery of FAs attained was 93.2% at 65 °C and 550 bars.

Keywords: microalgae; *Haematococcus pluvialis*; astaxanthin; lutein; fatty acids; supercritical fluid extraction; natural medicines

1. Introduction

In the last few years, microalgae have attracted growing attention for producing a wide range of "high value-added compounds", that are useful in several aspects of our life. Literature data show that microalgae are composed of molecules that can be used in many industrial sectors such as pharmaceutics, nutraceutics, food additives, and natural medicines, along with natural cosmetics [1–5]. These markets are characterized by high-quality safe-products at competitive prices. In this context, microalgae represent the starting point for the production of natural compounds with a sustainable approach characterized by low environmental impact [6,7]. Microalgae grow in diverse environments as freshwater/sea water and use sun light and carbon dioxide for photosynthesis [7,8]. They can be grown in photobioreactors or open ponds that can be located in marginal or unproductive land, and without the use of herbicides or pesticides, thus allowing for the reduction of the environmental impact related to cultivation system [9]. Another advantage of microalgae is that they can be used for carbon dioxide sequestration in their growth phase; in fact, each kilogram of dry biomass of microalgae could capture about 1.8–2 kg of CO_2. As a consequence, microalgae can be used to reduce CO_2 emission [1,10–13].

Astaxanthin, lutein, and fatty acids (FAs) naturally accumulate in several marine species including the microalgae *H. pluvialis*, which contains the highest levels per cell. Due to the strong antioxidant and antiaging properties from *H. pluvialis*, it has been cultivated by several industries [4,13–16]. *H. pluvialis* are unicellular representatives of the phylum Chlorophyta, which can be found in freshwater, marine, or even terrestrial environments [17]. Chekanov et al. [18] isolated *H. pluvialis* strain BM1 from the White Sea Coastal Rocks (66°29′47″ N, 33°24′22″ E) (Russia), which can accumulate a significant amount of astaxanthin under unfavourable environmental conditions. Moreover, the effect of salinity was analyzed on astaxanthin production in *H. pluvialis* growth [19]. Therefore, microalgae *H. pluvialis* could be found marine environments. However, the accumulation of these "high value-added products" within *H. pluvialis* cells is related to the hard cell wall that is highly resistant to both chemical and physical disruptions [20–22]. Unfortunately, the extraction of these compounds from *H. pluvialis* red microalgae is a major obstacle to recover these compounds with high purity in a cost-effective and eco-friendly manner. Therefore, the choice of a suitable extraction method depends on several aspects such as biomass, as well as extract, its end use, and its thermolability [23–25].

Conventional extraction techniques used for vegetables include squeezing, maceration, infusion, percolation, steam distillation, and solvent extraction. These techniques often have several issues related to the thermal degradation, which is due to their high extraction temperature; the solvent residues in the extracts can also compromise their end uses [24,26–28]. Moreover, in the last decade the scientific community has proposed advanced extraction techniques such as ultrasonic extraction, microwave extraction, accelerated solvent extraction, and extraction with supercritical fluid (SFE) to reduce these issues and minimize energy costs and the environmental impact [29–32]. Supercritical fluid extraction using CO_2 as an extraction fluid in supercritical condition (SFE-CO_2) represents a valid alternative to conventional techniques when it is necessary to guarantee thermal stability, and high-quality products (terms of purity and yield without solvent traces) [33]. Also, SFE-CO_2 is an eco-friendly technique for the obtaining of "high value-added compounds" from different matrices [14,28]. Moreover, CO_2 is not reactive at low temperatures, and it is easily recovered after each extraction stage [34]. Therefore, SFE-CO_2 is a novel technology with great potential for the extraction of bioactive compounds, which are used as food additives in the nutraceutical field [27,35–37]. Literature shows that several experimental tests have been carried out on the extraction of astaxantin from *H. pluvialis* using SFE-CO_2 [14,38–40]. Lutein extractions using SFE-CO_2 from other microalgal species, such as *Chlorella* [11,24,41] and *Scenedesmus* [9,42–45], have been investigated.

In this paper, the extraction performance of astaxanthin, lutein, and FAs from *H. pluvialis* in the red phase was assessed, using bench-scale SFE-CO_2 installation. In order to promote the extraction of astaxanthin, lutein, and FA, the cell wall of *H. pluvialis* red biomass was disrupted by mechanical (ball milling) pre-treatment [14], as optimized in our previous study [3]. The effect of different operative conditions, i.e., CO_2 flow rate (3.62 g/min and 14.48 g/min), run time (20–120 min), extraction temperature (50–80 °C), and pressure (100–550 bars) on the recovery and purity of astaxanthin, lutein, and FAs, was investigated, in order to find the best conditions to obtain the highest recovery and purity of all the compounds considered. Moreover, the characterization of the FAs extracted was performed, in terms of saturated fatty acids (SFAs), monounsaturated fatty acids (MFAs), and polyunsaturated fatty acids (PUFAs), in order to evaluate the effectiveness of the SFE-CO_2 extraction technique for the recovery of FAs species.

2. Materials and Methods

2.1. *H. pluvialis* Red Biomass and Chemicals

H. pluvialis in red phase (HPR) in powder was obtained by Micoperi Blue Growth®, an Italian company. HPR presented a mesh particle sieve lower than 50 μm, which contains 20 mg astaxanthin/$g_{dry\ biomass}$, 7.7 mg lutein/$g_{dry\ biomass}$, and 22.96 mg FAs/$g_{dry\ biomass}$. The lipid content was 2.6% by wt/wt of biomass, while the FAs content was 88.3% of total lipids. The saturated fatty acids (SFAs), monounsaturated fatty acids (MFAs), and polyunsaturated fatty acids (PUFAs) were 28.1%, 23.7%, and 48.2% of total FAs. Also, the chemical characterization of biomass was carried out using standard methods and summarized in our earlier study [3]. The biomass was stored at −20 °C and brought to room temperature before use. Carbon dioxide (Industrial grade) was obtained from Rivoira, Italy; astaxanthin, lutein, and FAs (analytical grade) were purchased from Sigma Aldrich, St. Louis, MO, USA. All other reagents were uHPLC grade unless otherwise stated.

2.2. Experimental Apparatus

Experimental tests were carried out using mechanically pre-treated dry microalgae and using the bench scale extractor SPE-ED SFE 2 by Applied Separations (Figure 1), which is characterized by a reactor volume of 30 mL. The mechanical pre-treatment of HPR biomass was carried out using a ball mill at 400 rpm for 5 min as described by Molino et al. [3]. The bench scale SFE-CO_2 is equipped with a heater able to achieve temperature up to 250 °C and a pumping system for the compression of carbon dioxide up to 680 bar. Two vessels are located inside the module: The first is used as CO_2 pre-heater, and the second one is the vessel where the extraction was carried out. In the extraction vessel there are two pressure controllers (Inlet and Outlet valves) and a Wika Transmitter with a precision of 0.6 mbar, whereas the CO_2 flow rate is monitored by using flow meter LPN/S80 AL G 2.5 by Sacofgas. The inlet flow rate is adjustable to 25 mL/min, and the flow control is done on the expanded gas. All parameters are controlled with a Distributed Control System (DCS). The temperature is monitored by thermocouples, while inlet and outlet flow are controlled by using micrometric valves.

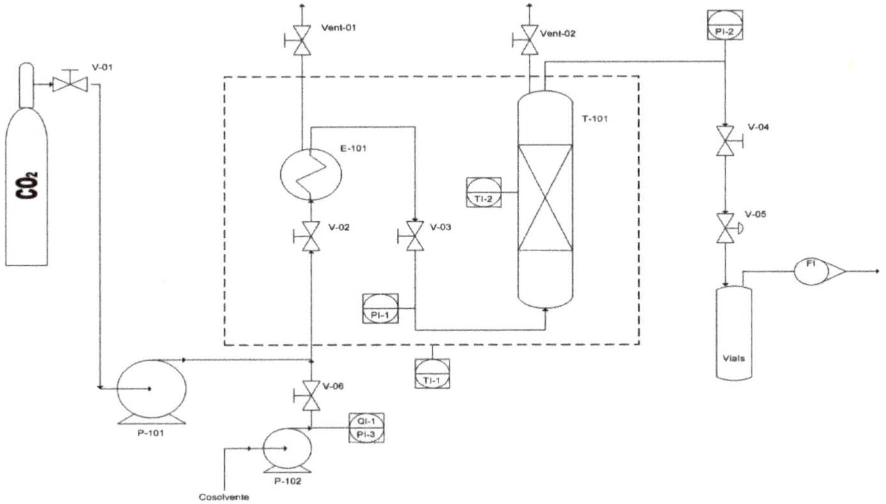

Figure 1. Schematization of the bench scale SFE-CO_2 experimental apparatus.

A picture of the extract is shown in Figure 2.

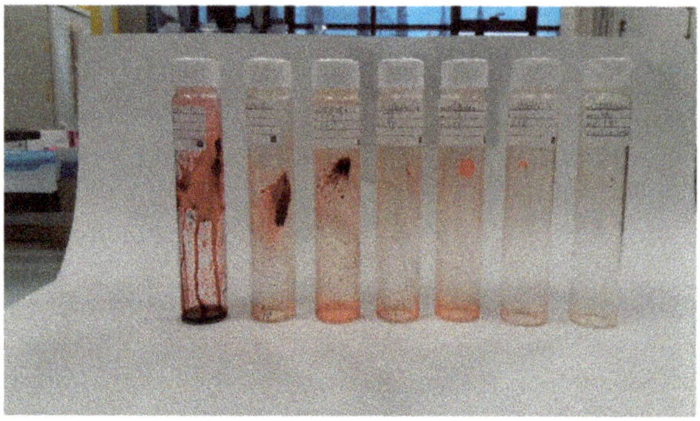

Figure 2. Extract from the bench scale SFE-CO_2 extractor.

2.3. Experimental Procedure

Before the extraction processes, to achieve uniform cell disruption and maximum product recovery [14] and to promote the extraction of astaxanthin, lutein, and FA, the cell wall of *H. pluvialis* red (HPR) biomass was disrupted by mechanical (ball milling) pre-treatment, as optimized in our pervious study [3]. In each run, around 1.4 g of biomass was mixed with 0.8 g of diatomaceous earth, which was disrupted and homogenized as described in earlier studies [3]. This quantity of mixture biomass/diatomaceous earth was loaded into the extraction cell, and free volume was filled by using diatomaceous earth till to complete the internal volume of the cell.

The disrupted cells were then extracted using SFE-CO_2 at different operative conditions. In particular, the effect of CO_2 flow rate (3.62 g/min and 14.48 g/min), time (20–120 min, extraction stage = 20 min), temperature (50–80 °C), and pressure (100–550 bar) were tested. These SFE-CO_2 parameters significantly influence the extraction efficiency, as well as selectivity of target compounds for extraction [14]. Therefore, these parameters have to be carefully considered and optimized for an efficient and selective recovery of target products. The experimental conditions are summarized in Table 1.

Table 1. The experimental plan.

Operative Conditions			
Temperature (°C)	**Pressure (bar)**	**CO_2 Flow Rate (g/min)**	**Biomass Load (g)**
50	100	3.62	1.38
50	100	14.48	1.36
50	400	3.62	1.37
50	400	14.48	1.38
50	550	3.62	1.38
50	550	14.48	1.36
65	100	3.62	1.34
65	100	14.48	1.34
65	400	3.62	1.33
65	400	14.48	1.32
65	550	3.62	1.35
65	550	14.48	1.34
80	100	3.62	1.35
80	100	14.48	1.34
80	400	3.62	1.31
80	400	14.48	1.38
80	550	3.62	1.34
80	550	14.48	1.34

Note: Biomass load is expressed on dry basis.

The effect of operative conditions on astaxanthin, lutein, and FAs extraction was expressed in terms of recovery and purity, which were calculated on the basis of initial weight of each compound in HPR [3] as reported in the following:

$$recovery\ (\%) = W_c/W_t \times 100 \quad (1)$$

$$purity\ (\%) = W_C/W_E \times 100 \quad (2)$$

in which W_C is the weight of the compound extracted (mg); W_T is the theoretical weight of the compound from conventional extraction (mg), which was calculated on the basis of the initial content of each compound in HPR, expressed as mg of extract per gram of dry weight of *H. pluvialis*, equal to = 20 mg/g for astaxanthin and equal to 7.7 mg/g for lutein; and W_E is the weight of the extract (mg).

Each experimental condition was replicated three to five times, and for each value standard deviation (SD) was calculated.

The extracted product was dissolved in acetone and stored at −30 °C with the exclusion of light prior to subsequent analysis.

2.4. Analytical Methods

The amount of astaxanthin and lutein in the extracts was measured by u-HPLC (Agilent 1290 Infinity II with Agilent Zorbax Eclipse plus C18 column 1.8 µm) [3]. The u-HPLC was equipped with a quaternary pump, thermostated oven column, and UV diode array detector (DAD) (measuring absorbance at 444–450–478 nm). A mixture of methanol/water (95:5%) was used as the mobile phase solvent in isocratic flow, while the sample was dissolved in a mixture of methanol/chloroform (90:10 containing 0.1% BHT as antioxidant agent). The flow rate and column temperature were kept constant at 0.4 mL/min and 28 °C, respectively. Gas chromatograph was used for the analysis of FAs, which was equipped with Flame Ionization detector (FID), a column HP-88 100 mt × 0.25 mm × 0.2 µm. This chromatographic column produced by Agilent is composed of a high polarity bis (Cyanopropyl) siloxane stationary phase and was chosen for its high resolution of positional and geometric isomers of fatty acid methyl esters. The column was maintained at 150 °C for 5 min and was followed by temperature ramping at 1.6 °C/min to 180 °C, then at 1.4 °C/min to 190 °C, and finally holding the temperature at 190 °C for 10 min. Nitrogen (purity $\geq$ 99.9999%) was used as carrier gas with a linear velocity of 30 cm/s and split ratio of 1:100. The injection port and detector were maintained at 250 °C. To quantify the concentration of the astaxanthin, lutein, and FAs compounds, the calibration curves were built by using chromatographic standards bought by Sigma Chemical Co., St Louis, MO, USA.

3. Result and Discussion

Total extraction yields for each operative condition are summarized in Table 1. The results are expressed as mg of extract per g dry weight of HPR, and values were obtained at the end of extraction (120 min, sum of each stage). At a pressure of 100 bars was measured the lowest exaction yields, which are among the values reported in Table 2; therefore, astaxanthin and lutein content at 100 bars for each stage were not analyzed.

3.1. Effect of Different CO_2 Flow Rate at Different Temperatures and Pressure on Astaxanthin Recovery and Purity over Extraction Time

The effects of CO_2 flow rate (3.62 g/min and 14.48 g/min), as a function of the extraction time, on SFE-CO_2 astaxanthin extraction were investigated by operating the temperature of the reaction chamber to 50 °C, 65 °C, and 80 °C and by keeping the pressure at 400 bar (Figure 3a–c) and at 550 bars (Figure 4a–c).

Table 2. Effect of temperature, pressure, and CO_2 flow rate on total extraction yield.

Operative Conditions			Total Extraction Yield (mg/g)
Temperature (°C)	Pressure (bar)	CO_2 Flow Rate (g/min)	
50	100	3.62	0.1
50	100	14.48	17.5
50	400	3.62	136.4
50	400	14.48	20.7
50	550	3.62	237.4
50	550	14.48	53.2
65	100	3.62	4.8
65	100	14.48	1.4
65	400	3.62	279.2
65	400	14.48	34.6
65	550	3.62	185.8
65	550	14.48	15.6
80	100	3.62	10.9
80	100	14.48	8.5
80	400	3.62	160.5
80	400	14.48	28.0
80	550	3.62	60.4
80	550	14.48	189.5

Note: Standard deviation was less than 5% in all operative conditions.

At 400 bars (Figure 3a–c), both the astaxanthin recovery and the astaxanthin purity were affected by the CO_2 flow rate. In particular, along with extraction time, for all the temperatures investigated, the lower the CO_2 flow rate, the higher the recovery, and for 50 °C and 65 °C, the higher CO_2 flow rate, the higher the purity. Around 70% astaxanthin recovery was achieved in first extraction cycle (20 min) with a CO_2 flow rate of 3.62 g/min and 35% at CO_2 flow rate of 14.48 g/min. A maximum purity of 68% astaxanthin was achieved at 50 °C with a CO_2 flow rate of 14.48 g/min and an extraction time of 80 min, while at the same temperature and pressure, the maximum amount of the total extract was achieved with a CO_2 flow rate of 3.62 g/min (136.4 mg/g).

At 550 bars (Figure 4a–c), for all the temperatures investigated, the astaxanthin recovery was affected by the CO_2 flow rate; for the first extraction cycle and the second extraction cycle (40 min), in particular, the lower the CO_2 flow rate, the higher the recovery. Around 90% astaxanthin recovery was achieved in first and second extraction cycles (40 min), with a CO_2 flow rate of 3.62 g/min and about 35% at CO_2 flow rate of 14.48 g/min. In terms of astaxanthin purity, the higher the CO_2 flow rate, the higher the purity. The maximum purity of astaxanthin of about 83% was achieved at 50 °C with a CO_2 flow rate of 14.48 g/min and an extraction time of 80 min, while at the same temperature and pressure, the maximum amount of the total extract was achieved with a CO_2 flow rate of 3.62 g/min (237.4 mg/g).

Machmudah et al. [46] suggested that the total extract slightly increased with increasing CO_2 flow rate, while the amount of astaxanthin recovery and the astaxanthin content in the extract almost did not change. Literature data also shows that the flow rate from 0.9 g/min to 1.8 g/min could not show clear influence on astaxanthin recovery and tended toward the same value at higher CO_2 consumption. In our study, investigations were carried out by using approximately 1.4 g of HPR. Furthermore, the clear effect of CO_2 flow rate were observed on astaxanthin recovery, as well as purity, due the range of tested flow rates (i.e., 3.62 and 14.48 g/min). A greater flow rate could be used to achieve the maximum purity, while a smaller flow rate could be used to achieve maximum recovery of astaxanthin from *H. pluvialis* red (HPR) biomass. Therefore, SFE-CO_2 with greater flow rate has the potential to be directly use in food products, avoiding the need for the solvent separation and purification [47].

By increasing temperature from 50 °C to 80 °C, both at 400 bars and at 550 bars, the recovery and purity decrease.

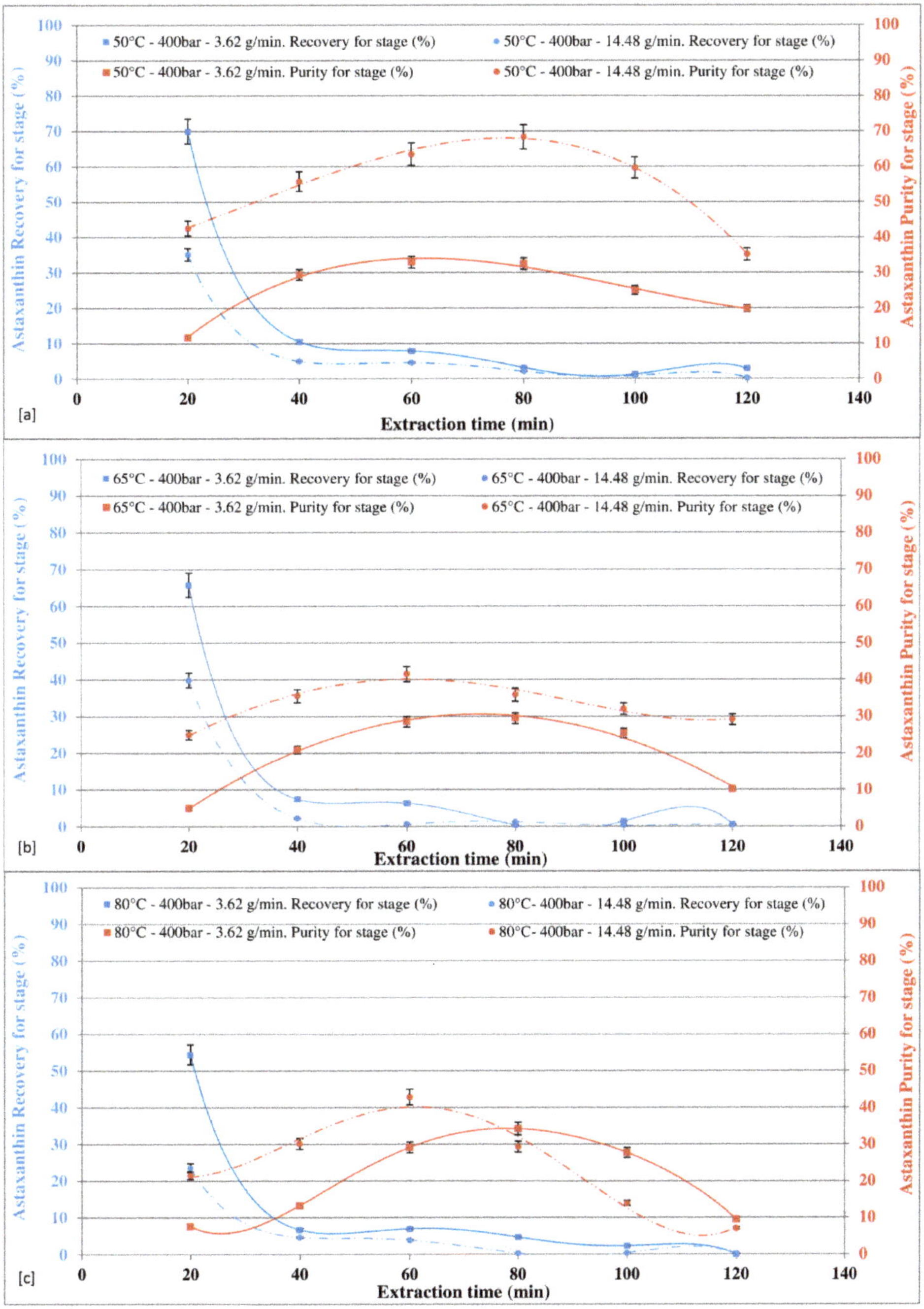

Figure 3. Effect of CO_2 flow rate at different temperatures on astaxanthin recovery and purity in extract at 400 bar.

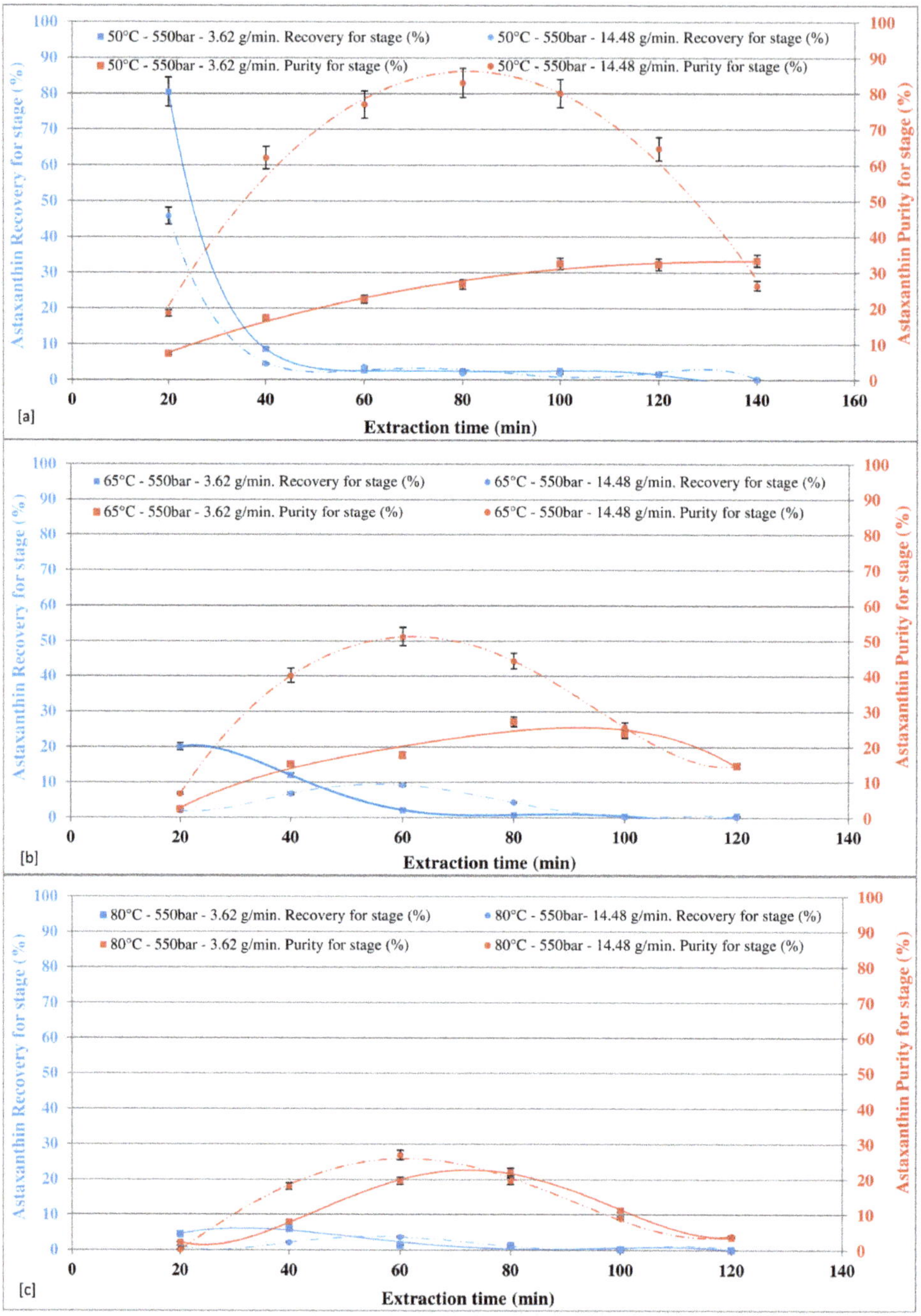

Figure 4. Effect of CO_2 flow rate at different temperature on astaxanthin recovery and purity in extract at 550 bar.

3.2. *Effect of Different CO_2 Flow Rate with Different Temperatures on Lutein Recovery and Purity over Extraction Time*

The effects of CO_2 flow rate (3.62 g/min and 14.48 g/min), as function of the extraction time, on SFE-CO_2 lutein extraction were investigated by operating the temperature of the reaction chamber to 50 °C, 65 °C, and 80 °C at 400 bar (Figure 5a–c) and at 550 bar (Figure 6a–c).

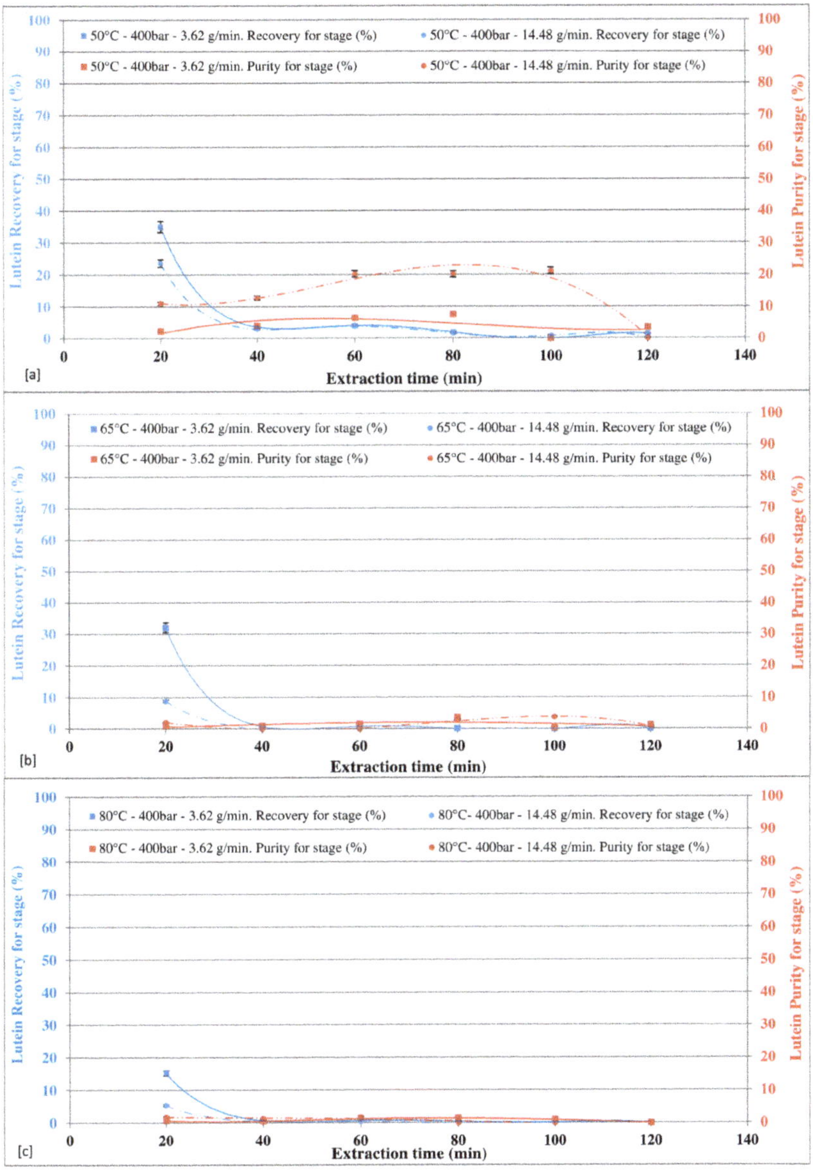

Figure 5. Effect of CO_2 flow rate at different temperatures on lutein recovery and purity in extract at 400 bar.

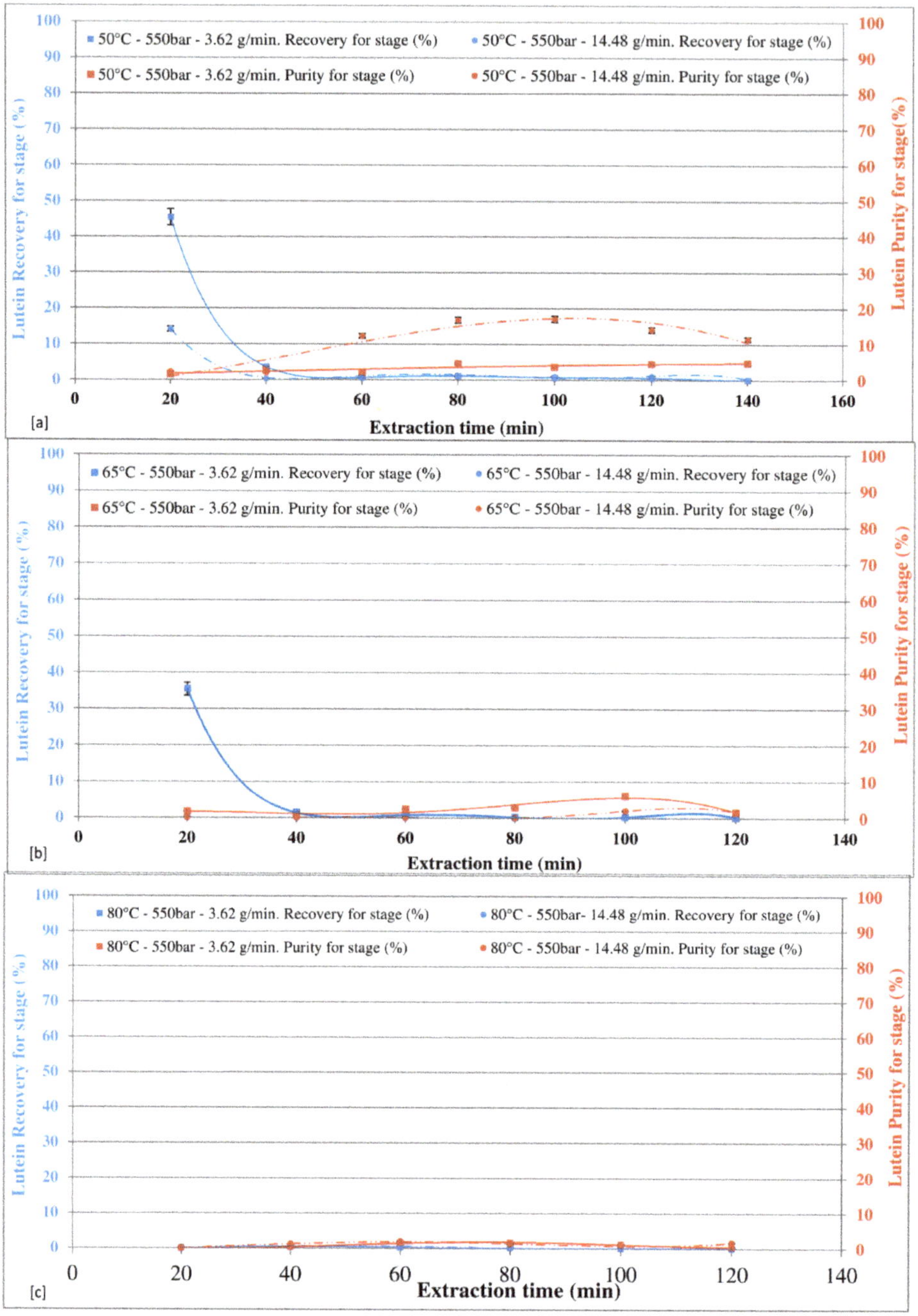

Figure 6. Effect of CO_2 flow rate at different temperatures on lutein recovery and purity in extract at 550 bar.

At 400 bar (Figure 5a–c), for all the temperatures investigated, the lutein recovery was affected by the CO_2 flow rate for the first extraction cycle (20 min), after which the effect of the CO_2 flow rate was negligible. In particular, around 40% lutein recovery was achieved in first extraction cycle (20 min), with a CO_2 flow rate of 3.62 g/min and about 25% at CO_2 flow rate of 14.48 g/min. The lutein purity was affected by the CO_2 flow rate at 50 °C, while at both 65 °C and 80 °C the effect of CO_2 flow rate was negligible. The maximum purity of about 20% lutein was achieved at 50 °C with a CO_2 flow rate of 14.48 g/min and an extraction time of 100 min.

At 550 bar (Figure 6a–c), the lutein recovery was affected by the CO_2 flow rate at 50 °C for the first extraction cycle (20 min), while at both 65 °C and 80 °C the effect of CO_2 flow rate was negligible for all the extraction stages. In particular, at 50 °C around 45% lutein recovery was achieved in first extraction cycle (20 min) with a CO_2 flow rate of 3.62 g/min and about 15% at CO_2 flow rate of 14.48 g/min. The lutein purity was affected by the CO_2 flow rate at 50 °C and 65 °C, while at 80 °C the effect of CO_2 flow rate was negligible. The maximum purity of about 20% lutein was achieved at 50 °C with a CO_2 flow rate of 14.48 g/min and an extraction time of 100 min.

The higher lutein recovery achieved in first extraction cycle with respect to the astaxanthin recovery in the similar experimental condition could be explained by considering the higher driving force of lutein mass transfer between the inside and outside the algal cell as reported by several research groups [24,30,46].

By increasing temperature from 50 °C to 80 °C, both at 400 bar and at 550 bar, the recovery and purity decrease.

3.3. *Effect of Temperature and Pressure on Global Recovery of Astaxanthin and Lutein*

The effect of temperature on astaxanthin total recovery, at the end of the extraction (120 min, sum of each stage), at different pressures with the CO_2 flow rate of 3.62 g/min is shown in Figure 7a, while Figure 7b shows the effect of the CO_2 flow rate of 14.48 g/min in the same conditions. By increasing temperature, a decrease in total astaxanthin recovery was observed. This finding may be explained by the possible increase of the thermal degradation rate of astaxanthin due to the increase of temperature. The opposite trend can be observed for the pressure, as the higher the pressure, the higher the astaxanthin extraction. It is evident that an increase in pressure increases the solubility of astaxanthin, and same trend was observed by Machmudah et al. [46]. In terms of CO_2 flow rate, the lower the CO_2 flow rate, the higher the astaxanthin recovery. The highest total recovery of astaxanthin, equal to 98.6%, was observed at 50 °C and 550 bar, with a CO_2 flow rate of 3.62 g/min. With a CO_2 flow rate of 3.62 g/min, increasing the extraction temperature to 65 °C and to 80 °C, the astaxanthin recovery drops to 36% and 14%, respectively. This effect may be explained considering the thermal degradation of subunits of astaxanthin as extensively reported in the literature [3,28,48,49]. These results show that relatively low temperature (50 °C) at 400 bars was optimum to effectively complete astaxanthin extraction.

The effect of temperature on lutein total recovery, at the end of extraction (120 min, sum of each stage), at different pressures with the CO_2 flow rate of 3.62 g/min is shown in Figure 7c, while Figure 7d shows the effect of the CO_2 flow rate of 14.48 g/min at the same conditions. The amount of lutein in the extract significantly decreased with increasing temperature, due to the thermal instability of carotenoids, as reported by several authors [50,51]. With a CO_2 flow rate of 3.62 g/min, at 50 °C and 65 °C, the higher recovery was found at 550 bar; at a temperature of 80 °C, the higher recovery was found at 400 bar. With a CO_2 flow rate of 14.48 g/min, for all the tested temperature, the higher recovery was found at 400 bar.

The highest total recovery of lutein, equal to 52%, was observed at 50 °C and 550 bar, with a CO_2 flow rate of 3.62 g/min. With a CO_2 flow rate of 3.62 g/min, increasing the extraction temperature to 65 °C and to 80 °C, the astaxanthin recovery drops to 35% and 14%, respectively. The lowest lutein recovery of 7% was achieved at 80 °C and 400 bar with a flow rate of 14.48 g/min.

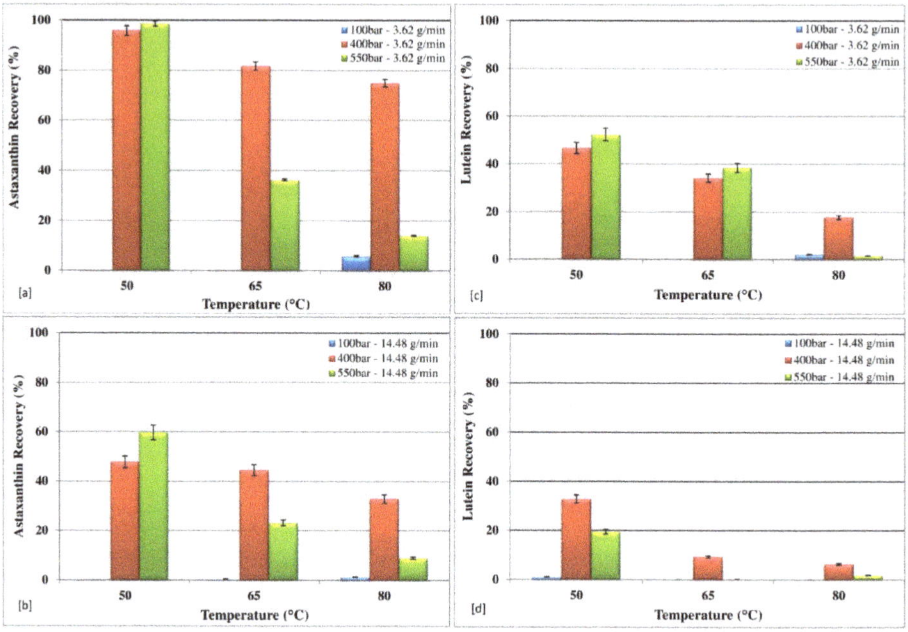

Figure 7. Effect of temperature and pressure on global recovery of astaxanthin and lutein.

3.4. *Effect of Temperature and Pressure on Recovery of FAs*

The recovery of FAs was investigated in two extracts, at 20 and 40 min, due to unavailability of FAs (lower than the detection limits) from the third extract (60 min), at different temperatures (50 °C, 65 °C and 80 °C) and pressures (100 bar, 400 bar and 550 bar) with both CO_2 flow rates (3.62 g/min, Figure 8a; 14.48 g/min Figure 8b). As shown in Figure 8, the higher the pressure, the higher the FAs recovery with both the CO_2 flow rates, for all the temperatures investigated, excluding the operative condition of a temperature of 65 °C and a CO_2 flow rate of 14.48 g/min, with which the FAs recoveries at 400 bar and at 550 bar were comparable. This trend is probably due to two opposite effects as the pressure rises at a constant temperature: an enhancement in the density of CO_2 in supercritical and a reduction CO_2 diffusion coefficient can be observed [28,44]. In particular, increase in the density leads to an increase in its solvating power and thus enhancement of the extraction yield. On the other hand, a decrease in the diffusion coefficient of CO_2 leads to a decrease in the ability of a fluid to penetrate the solid matrix, causing a reduction in the extraction yield. At the lowest temperature studied (50 °C), the dominant effect was the decrease in the diffusivity of CO_2 when the pressure increased, while at the optimum temperature (65 °C), an enhancement was observed in the solvating. The highest temperature (80 °C) reduced fatty acid recovery.

Experimental findings also highlight that the higher the CO_2 flow rate, the higher the FAs recovery; however, comparable FAs recoveries were achieved at 65 °C and 550 bar for both the CO_2 flow rates investigated.

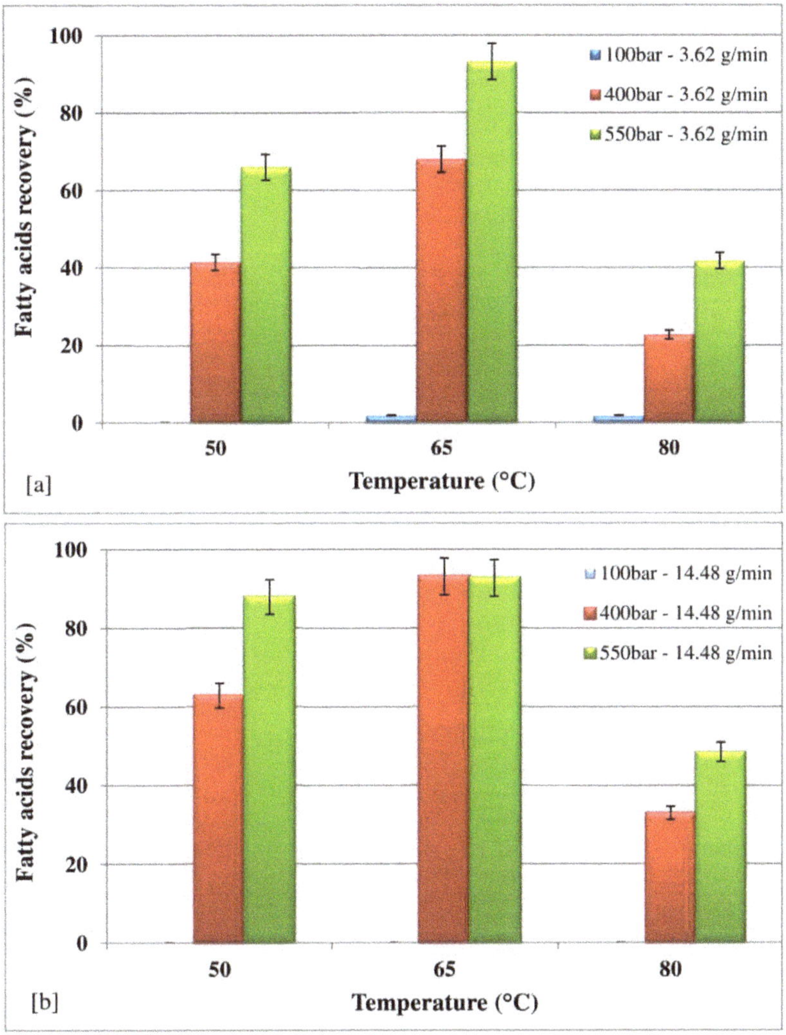

Figure 8. Effect of temperature and pressure on global recovery of fatty acids.

The characterization of the fatty acid (FA) extracted from *H. pluvialis* in red phase, including the effect of temperature and pressure on FAs classes at the CO_2 flow rates of 3.62 and 14.48 g/min, respectively, are reported in Table 3, in which the theoretical content for each FAs species is also enclosed. Comparing the extracted amounts with the theoretical contents, it is possible to observe that the highest recoveries of SFAs, MUFAs, and PUFAs with a CO_2 flow rate of 3.62 g/min were found at 65 °C and 550 bar, with values of about 86%, 90%, and 99%, respectively. With a CO_2 flow rate of 14.48 g/min, the highest recoveries of SFAs and PUFAs, equal to 86% and 98%, were found at 65 °C and 400 bar, while the highest recovery of MUFAs, equal to 91%, was found at 65 °C and 550 bar.

Table 3. Comparison of different operative conditions for fatty acid recovery at CO_2 flow rates of 3.62 g/min and 14.48 g/min.

Class of Fatty Acids (mg/g)	Operative Temperature (°C)									Theoretical Content
	50			65			80			
	Operative Pressure (bar) at CO_2 Flow Rate of 3.62 g/min									
	100	400	550	100	400	550	100	400	550	
SFAs	nd	0.64	5.5	0.42	4.8	5.57	0.41	0.38	0.47	6.45
MUFAs	nd	0.49	0.35	<Ldl	0.94	4.92	<Ldl	0.27	0.12	5.44
PUFAs	nd	8.38	9.3	<Ldl	9.87	10.92	<Ldl	4.57	8.98	11.06
	Operative Pressure (bar) at CO_2 Flow Rate of 14.48 g/min									
	100	400	550	100	400	550	100	400	550	
SFAs	nd	0.58	3.97	nd	5.57	5.46	nd	0.41	0.49	6.45
MUFAs	nd	4.56	5.25	nd	4.9	4.97	nd	0.84	2.57	5.44
PUFAs	nd	9.28	10.97	nd	10.9	10.85	nd	6.32	8.08	11.06

Note: nd = not detected; <Ldl = lower than the detection limit; standard deviation was less than 5% at all operative conditions.

3.5. Comparison of Astaxanthin, Lutein, and FAs Global Recovery at Different Operative Conditions

The comparison of the *H. pluvialis* extracts for total recovery of astaxanthin and lutein (120 min, sum of each extraction stage) and FAs (40 min, sum of first and second extraction stage) at different operative conditions shows that the FAs were a major component of the extract (Table 4). The maximum recoveries of astaxanthin (19.72 mg/g) and lutein (4.03 mg/g) were achieved with a CO_2 flow rate of 3.62 g/min at 50 °C and 550 bar. The maximum recovery of FAs (21.41 mg/g) was achieved with a CO_2 flow rate of 3.62 g/min at 65 °C and 550 bar.

The literature suggests that increasing temperature decreases the recovery of astaxanthin and lutein, while there is less thermal degradation of FAs with respect to astaxanthin and lutein [28,48,52–54].

Table 4. The recovery of astaxanthin, lutein, and FAs at different operative conditions.

Recovery ($mg/g_{dry\ biomass}$)	Temperature (°C)	CO_2 Flow Rate of 3.62 g/min			CO_2 Flow Rate of 14.48 g/min		
		Pressures (bar)					
		100	400	550	100	400	550
Astaxanthin	50	0.10	19.16	19.72	0.01	9.55	11.94
	65	0.06	16.34	7.24	0.07	8.91	4.62
	80	1.16	15.00	2.78	0.25	6.58	1.79
Lutein	50	0.08	3.60	4.03	0.08	2.53	1.50
	65	0.00	2.63	2.96	<Ldl	0.71	0.01
	80	0.16	1.36	0.12	<Ldl	0.49	0.15
FAs	50	nd	9.5	15.15	nd	14.43	20.19
	65	0.42	15.6	21.41	nd	21.37	21.29
	80	0.41	5.21	9.57	nd	7.57	11.14

Note: nd = not detected; <Ldl = lower than the detection limit; standard deviation was less than 5% at all operative conditions.

4. Conclusions

In this work, SFE-CO_2 extraction of astaxanthin, lutein, and FAs from *H. pluvialis* microalgae in red phase was investigated at different temperatures (50 °C, 65 °C, and 80 °C) and pressures (100 bar, 400 bar, and 550 bar) with CO_2 flow rates of 3.62 and 14.48 g/min. Experimental findings show that the SFE-CO_2 is more selective for the extraction of FAs with respect to astaxanthin and lutein. By using a single cell reactor, recoveries of astaxanthin, lutein, and FAs, which were equal to 98.62%, 52.32%, and 93.25%, were found at lower temperatures, and high pressure with the lower CO_2 flow rate. Results highlighting the influence of extraction operative conditions on the maximum recovery of these "high-value, added compounds". The maximum extractions of astaxanthin and lutein were achieved at 50 °C and 550 bar with a CO_2 flow rate of 3.62 g/min. The maximum extraction of FAs was found at 65 °C and 550 bar, with a CO_2 flow rate of 3.62 g/min. Among FAs species, PUFAs were extracted with the highest recovery.

Greater purities of astaxanthin and lutein were found when their recoveries were very low; therefore, this could represent a critical point for the development of this technology in the extraction of astaxanthin and lutein with respect to other carotenoids that have a similar polarity with CO_2.

Author Contributions: G.D.S. performed the supercritical extraction experiments with V.L. and M.M.; S.M. wrote and revised the manuscript; P.C. and S.C. performed the analysis of astaxanthin, lutein and fatty acid and. edited the manuscript; D.M., R.B. and A.M. supervised the project and conceived the experiments and supervised the work.

Funding: This research was funded by Bio Based Industries Joint Undertaking under the European Union's Horizon 2020 research and innovation program under grant agreement No 745695 (VALUEMAG).

Conflicts of Interest: The authors declare no conflict of interest.

References

1. Gordon, J.M.; Polle, J.E.W. Ultrahigh bioproductivity from algae. *Appl. Microbiol. Biotechnol.* **2007**, *76*, 969–975. [CrossRef] [PubMed]
2. Leu, S.; Boussiba, S. Advances in the Production of High-Value Products by Microalgae. *Ind. Biotechnol.* **2014**, *10*, 169–183. [CrossRef]
3. Molino, A.; Rimauro, J.; Casella, P.; Cerbone, A.; Larocca, V.; Chianese, S.; Karatza, D.; Mehariya, S.; Ferraro, A.; Hristoforou, E.; et al. Extraction of astaxanthin from microalga *Haematococcus pluvialis* in red phase by using Generally Recognized as Safe solvents and accelerated extraction. *J. Biotechnol.* **2018**, *283*, 51–61. [CrossRef] [PubMed]
4. Wang, H.-M.D.; Chen, C.-C.; Huynh, P.; Chang, J.-S. Exploring the potential of using algae in cosmetics. *Bioresour. Technol.* **2015**, *184*, 355–362. [CrossRef] [PubMed]
5. Wang, H.-M.D.; Li, X.-C.; Lee, D.-J.; Chang, J.-S. Potential biomedical applications of marine algae. *Bioresour. Technol.* **2017**, *244*, 1407–1415. [CrossRef] [PubMed]
6. Pulz, O.; Gross, W. Valuable products from biotechnology of microalgae. *Appl. Microbiol. Biotechnol.* **2004**, *65*, 635–648. [CrossRef] [PubMed]
7. Spolaore, P.; Joannis-Cassan, C.; Duran, E.; Isambert, A. Commercial applications of microalgae. *J. Biosci. Bioeng.* **2006**, *101*, 87–96. [CrossRef] [PubMed]
8. Mendes, R.L.; Coelho, J.P.; Fernandes, H.L.; Marrucho, I.J.; Cabral, J.M.S.; Novais, J.M.; Palavra, A.F. Applications of supercritical CO_2 extraction to microalgae and plants. *J. Chem. Technol. Biotechnol.* **1995**, *62*, 53–59. [CrossRef]
9. Yen, H.-W.; Chiang, W.-C.; Sun, C.-H. Supercritical fluid extraction of lutein from *Scenedesmus* cultured in an autotrophical photobioreactor. *J. Taiwan Inst. Chem. Eng.* **2012**, *43*, 53–57. [CrossRef]
10. Chauton, M.S.; Reitan, K.I.; Norsker, N.H.; Tveterås, R.; Kleivdal, H.T. A techno-economic analysis of industrial production of marine microalgae as a source of EPA and DHA-rich raw material for aquafeed: Research challenges and possibilities. *Aquaculture* **2015**, *436*, 95–103. [CrossRef]
11. Liu, J.; Chen, F. Biology and Industrial Applications of *Chlorella*: Advances and Prospects. In *Microalgae Biotechnology*; Posten, C., Feng Chen, S., Eds.; Springer International Publishing: Cham, Switzerland, 2016; pp. 1–35, ISBN 978-3-319-23808-1.
12. Rawat, I.; Ranjith Kumar, R.; Mutanda, T.; Bux, F. Biodiesel from microalgae: A critical evaluation from laboratory to large scale production. *Appl. Energy* **2013**, *103*, 444–467. [CrossRef]
13. Venkata Subhash, G.; Rajvanshi, M.; Navish Kumar, B.; Govindachary, S.; Prasad, V.; Dasgupta, S. Carbon streaming in microalgae: Extraction and analysis methods for high value compounds. *Bioresour. Technol.* **2017**, *244*, 1304–1316. [CrossRef] [PubMed]

14. Cheng, X.; Qi, Z.; Burdyny, T.; Kong, T.; Sinton, D. Low pressure supercritical CO_2 extraction of astaxanthin from *Haematococcus pluvialis* demonstrated on a microfluidic chip. *Bioresour. Technol.* **2018**, *250*, 481–485. [CrossRef] [PubMed]
15. Pan, J.-L.; Wang, H.-M.; Chen, C.-Y.; Chang, J.-S. Extraction of astaxanthin from *Haematococcus pluvialis* by supercritical carbon dioxide fluid with ethanol modifier. *Eng. Life Sci.* **2012**, *12*, 638–647. [CrossRef]
16. Brown, D.R.; Gough, L.A.; Deb, S.K.; Sparks, S.A.; McNaughton, L.R. Astaxanthin in Exercise Metabolism, Performance and Recovery: A Review. *Front. Nutr.* **2018**, *4*, 76. [CrossRef] [PubMed]
17. Heimann, K.; Huerlimann, R. Microalgal Classification: Major Classes and Genera of Commercial Microalgal Species. In *Handbook of Marine Microalgae*; Kim, S.-K., Ed.; Academic Press: Boston, MA, USA, 2015; pp. 25–41, ISBN 978-0-12-800776-1.
18. Chekanov, K.; Lobakova, E.; Selyakh, I.; Semenova, L.; Sidorov, R.; Solovchenko, A. Accumulation of Astaxanthin by a New *Haematococcus pluvialis* Strain BM1 from the White Sea Coastal Rocks (Russia). *Mar. Drugs* **2014**, *12*, 4504–4520. [CrossRef] [PubMed]
19. Sarada, R.; Tripathi, U.; Ravishankar, G.A. Influence of stress on astaxanthin production in *Haematococcus pluvialis* grown under different culture conditions. *Process Biochem.* **2002**, *37*, 623–627. [CrossRef]
20. Hagen, C.; Siegmund, S.; Braune, W. Ultrastructural and chemical changes in the cell wall of *Haematococcus pluvialis* (Volvocales, Chlorophyta) during aplanospore formation. *Eur. J. Phycol.* **2002**, *37*, 217–226. [CrossRef]
21. Lee, S.Y.; Cho, J.M.; Chang, Y.K.; Oh, Y.-K. Cell disruption and lipid extraction for microalgal biorefineries: A review. *Bioresour. Technol.* **2017**, *244*, 1317–1328. [CrossRef] [PubMed]
22. Show, K.-Y.; Lee, D.-J.; Tay, J.-H.; Lee, T.-M.; Chang, J.-S. Microalgal drying and cell disruption—Recent advances. *Bioresour. Technol.* **2015**, *184*, 258–266. [CrossRef] [PubMed]
23. De Melo, M.M.R.; Silvestre, A.J.D.; Silva, C.M. Supercritical fluid extraction of vegetable matrices: Applications, trends and future perspectives of a convincing green technology. *J. Supercrit. Fluids* **2014**, *92*, 115–176. [CrossRef]
24. Ruen-ngam, D.; Shotipruk, A.; Pavasant, P. Comparison of Extraction Methods for Recovery of Astaxanthin from *Haematococcus pluvialis*. *Sep. Sci. Technol.* **2010**, *46*, 64–70. [CrossRef]
25. Shah, M.M.R.; Liang, Y.; Cheng, J.J.; Daroch, M. Astaxanthin-Producing Green Microalga *Haematococcus pluvialis*: From Single Cell to High Value Commercial Products. *Front. Plant Sci.* **2016**, *7*, 531. [CrossRef] [PubMed]
26. Joana Gil-Chávez, G.; Villa, J.A.; Fernando Ayala-Zavala, J.; Basilio Heredia, J.; Sepulveda, D.; Yahia, E.M.; González-Aguilar, G.A. Technologies for Extraction and Production of Bioactive Compounds to be Used as Nutraceuticals and Food Ingredients: An Overview. *Compr. Rev. Food Sci. Food Saf.* **2013**, *12*, 5–23. [CrossRef]
27. Ameer, K.; Shahbaz, H.M.; Kwon, J.-H. Green Extraction Methods for Polyphenols from Plant Matrices and Their Byproducts: A Review. *Compr. Rev. Food Sci. Food Saf.* **2017**, *16*, 295–315. [CrossRef]
28. Poojary, M.M.; Barba, J.F.; Aliakbarian, B.; Donsì, F.; Pataro, G.; Dias, A.D.; Juliano, P. Innovative Alternative Technologies to Extract Carotenoids from Microalgae and Seaweeds. *Mar. Drugs* **2016**, *14*, 214. [CrossRef] [PubMed]
29. Crampon, C.; Boutin, O.; Badens, E. Supercritical Carbon Dioxide Extraction of Molecules of Interest from Microalgae and Seaweeds. *Ind. Eng. Chem. Res.* **2011**, *50*, 8941–8953. [CrossRef]
30. Mendes, R.L.; Fernandes, H.L.; Coelho, J.; Reis, E.C.; Cabral, J.M.S.; Novais, J.M.; Palavra, A.F. Supercritical CO_2 extraction of carotenoids and other lipids from *Chlorella vulgaris*. *Food Chem.* **1995**, *53*, 99–103. [CrossRef]
31. Mendes, R.L.; Nobre, B.P.; Cardoso, M.T.; Pereira, A.P.; Palavra, A.F. Supercritical carbon dioxide extraction of compounds with pharmaceutical importance from microalgae. *Inorg. Chim. Acta* **2003**, *356*, 328–334. [CrossRef]
32. Palavra, A.M.F.; Coelho, J.P.; Barroso, J.G.; Rauter, A.P.; Fareleira, J.M.N.A.; Mainar, A.; Urieta, J.S.; Nobre, B.P.; Gouveia, L.; Mendes, R.L.; et al. Supercritical carbon dioxide extraction of bioactive compounds from microalgae and volatile oils from aromatic plants. *J. Supercrit. Fluids* **2011**, *60*, 21–27. [CrossRef]

33. Sovová, H. Rate of the vegetable oil extraction with supercritical CO_2—I. Modelling of extraction curves. *Chem. Eng. Sci.* **1994**, *49*, 409–414. [CrossRef]
34. Kitzberger, C.S.G.; Lomonaco, R.H.; Michielin, E.M.Z.; Danielski, L.; Correia, J.; Ferreira, S.R.S. Supercritical fluid extraction of shiitake oil: Curve modeling and extract composition. *J. Food Eng.* **2009**, *90*, 35–43. [CrossRef]
35. Herrero, M.; Mendiola, J.A.; Cifuentes, A.; Ibáñez, E. Supercritical fluid extraction: Recent advances and applications. *J. Chromatogr. A* **2010**, *1217*, 2495–2511. [CrossRef] [PubMed]
36. Mattea, F.; Martín, Á.; Cocero, M.J. Carotenoid processing with supercritical fluids. *J. Food Eng.* **2009**, *93*, 255–265. [CrossRef]
37. Smith, R.M. Supercritical fluids in separation science—The dreams, the reality and the future. *J. Chromatogr. A* **1999**, *856*, 83–115. [CrossRef]
38. Nobre, B.; Marcelo, F.; Passos, R.; Beirão, L.; Palavra, A.; Gouveia, L.; Mendes, R. Supercritical carbon dioxide extraction of astaxanthin and other carotenoids from the microalga *Haematococcus pluvialis*. *Eur. Food Res. Technol.* **2006**, *223*, 787–790. [CrossRef]
39. Thana, P.; Machmudah, S.; Goto, M.; Sasaki, M.; Pavasant, P.; Shotipruk, A. Response surface methodology to supercritical carbon dioxide extraction of astaxanthin from *Haematococcus pluvialis*. *Bioresour. Technol.* **2008**, *99*, 3110–3115. [CrossRef] [PubMed]
40. Valderrama, J.O.; Perrut, M.; Majewski, W. Extraction of Astaxantine and Phycocyanine from Microalgae with Supercritical Carbon Dioxide. *J. Chem. Eng. Data* **2003**, *48*, 827–830. [CrossRef]
41. Kitada, K.; Machmudah, S.; Sasaki, M.; Goto, M.; Nakashima, Y.; Kumamoto, S.; Hasegawa, T. Supercritical CO_2 extraction of pigment components with pharmaceutical importance from *Chlorella vulgaris*. *J. Chem. Technol. Biotechnol.* **2008**, *84*, 657–661. [CrossRef]
42. Cerón-García, M.D.C.; Campos-Pérez, I.; Macías-Sánchez, M.D.; Bermejo-Román, R.; Fernández-Sevilla, J.M.; Molina-Grima, E. Stability of Carotenoids in *Scenedesmus almeriensis* Biomass and Extracts under Various Storage Conditions. *J. Agric. Food Chem.* **2010**, *58*, 6944–6950. [CrossRef]
43. Ishaq, A.G.; Matias-Peralta, H.M.; Basri, H. Bioactive Compounds from Green Microalga-*Scenedesmus* and Its Potential Applications: A Brief Review. *Pertanika J. Trop. Agric. Sci.* **2016**, *39*, 1–15.
44. Macías-Sánchez, M.D.; Fernandez-Sevilla, J.M.; Fernández, F.G.A.; García, M.C.C.; Grima, E.M. Supercritical fluid extraction of carotenoids from *Scenedesmus almeriensis*. *Food Chem.* **2010**, *123*, 928–935. [CrossRef]
45. Sánchez, J.F.; Fernández-Sevilla, J.M.; Acién, F.G.; Cerón, M.C.; Pérez-Parra, J.; Molina-Grima, E. Biomass and lutein productivity of *Scenedesmus almeriensis*: Influence of irradiance, dilution rate and temperature. *Appl. Microbiol. Biotechnol.* **2008**, *79*, 719–729. [CrossRef] [PubMed]
46. Machmudah, S.; Shotipruk, A.; Goto, M.; Sasaki, M.; Hirose, T. Extraction of Astaxanthin from *Haematococcus pluvialis* Using Supercritical CO_2 and Ethanol as Entrainer. *Ind. Eng. Chem. Res.* **2006**, *45*, 3652–3657. [CrossRef]
47. Krichnavaruk, S.; Shotipruk, A.; Goto, M.; Pavasant, P. Supercritical carbon dioxide extraction of astaxanthin from *Haematococcus pluvialis* with vegetable oils as co-solvent. *Bioresour. Technol.* **2008**, *99*, 5556–5560. [CrossRef] [PubMed]
48. Tachaprutinun, A.; Udomsup, T.; Luadthong, C.; Wanichwecharungruang, S. Preventing the thermal degradation of astaxanthin through nanoencapsulation. *Int. J. Pharm.* **2009**, *374*, 119–124. [CrossRef] [PubMed]
49. Ambati, R.R.; Phang, S.-M.; Ravi, S.; Aswathanarayana, R.G. Astaxanthin: Sources, Extraction, Stability, Biological Activities and Its Commercial Applications—A Review. *Mar. Drugs* **2014**, *12*, 128–152. [CrossRef] [PubMed]
50. Ruen-Ngam, D.; Shotipruk, A.; Pavasant, P.; Machmudah, S.; Goto, M. Selective extraction of lutein from alcohol treated *Chlorella vulgaris* by supercritical CO_2. *Chem. Eng. Technol.* **2012**, *35*, 255–260. [CrossRef]
51. Vasapollo, G.; Longo, L.; Rescio, L.; Ciurlia, L. Innovative supercritical CO_2 extraction of lycopene from tomato in the presence of vegetable oil as co-solvent. *J. Supercrit. Fluids* **2004**, *29*, 87–96. [CrossRef]
52. Shilpi, A.; Shivhare, U.S.; Basu, S. Supercritical CO_2 Extraction of Compounds with Antioxidant Activity from Fruits and Vegetables Waste—A Review. *Focus. Mod. Food Ind.* **2013**, *2*, 43–62.

53. Desbois, A.P.; Smith, V.J. Antibacterial free fatty acids: Activities, mechanisms of action and biotechnological potential. *Appl. Microbiol. Biotechnol.* **2010**, *85*, 1629–1642. [CrossRef] [PubMed]
54. Michalak, I.; Chojnacka, K. Algae as production systems of bioactive compounds. *Eng. Life Sci.* **2014**, *15*, 160–176. [CrossRef]

© 2018 by the authors. Licensee MDPI, Basel, Switzerland. This article is an open access article distributed under the terms and conditions of the Creative Commons Attribution (CC BY) license (http://creativecommons.org/licenses/by/4.0/).

marine drugs

MDPI

Article

Synthesis, Characterization, and Antifungal Property of Hydroxypropyltrimethyl Ammonium Chitosan Halogenated Acetates

Yingqi Mi [1,2], Wenqiang Tan [1,2], Jingjing Zhang [1,2], Lijie Wei [1,2], Yuan Chen [1,2], Qing Li [1], Fang Dong [1,*] and Zhanyong Guo [1,2,*]

1 Key Laboratory of Coastal Biology and Bioresource Utilization, Yantai Institute of Coastal Zone Research, Chinese Academy of Sciences, Yantai 264003, China; yqmi@yic.ac.cn (Y.M.); wqtan@yic.ac.cn (W.T.); jingjingzhang@yic.ac.cn (J.Z.); ljwei@yic.ac.cn (L.W.); yuanchen@yic.ac.cn (Y.C.); qli@yic.ac.cn (Q.L.)

2 University of Chinese Academy of Sciences, Beijing 100049, China

* Correspondence: fdong@yic.ac.cn (F.D.); zhanyongguo@hotmail.com (Z.G.); Tel.: +86-535-2109165 (F.D.); +86-535-2109171 (Z.G.); Fax: +86-535-2109000 (F.D.); +86-535-2109000 (Z.G.)

Received: 23 July 2018; Accepted: 31 August 2018; Published: 5 September 2018

Abstract: Hydroxypropyltrimethyl ammonium chitosan halogenated acetates were successfully synthesized from six different haloacetic acids and hydroxypropyltrimethyl ammonium chloride chitosan (HACC) with high substitution degree, which are hydroxypropyltrimethyl ammonium chitosan bromacetate (HACBA), hydroxypropyltrimethyl ammonium chitosan chloroacetate (HACCA), hydroxypropyltrimethyl ammonium chitosan dichloroacetate (HACDCA), hydroxypropyltrimethyl ammonium chitosan trichloroacetate (HACTCA), hydroxypropyltrimethyl ammonium chitosan difluoroacetate (HACDFA), and hydroxypropyltrimethyl ammonium chitosan trifluoroacetate (HACTFA). These chitosan derivatives were synthesized by two steps: first, the hydroxypropyltrimethyl ammonium chloride chitosan was synthesized by chitosan and 3-chloro-2-hydroxypropyltrimethyl ammonium chloride. Then, hydroxypropyltrimethyl ammonium chitosan halogenated acetates were synthesized via ion exchange. The structures of chitosan derivatives were characterized by Fourier transform infrared spectroscopy (FTIR), ^{1}H Nuclear magnetic resonance spectrometer (^{1}H NMR), ^{13}C Nuclear magnetic resonance spectrometer (^{13}C NMR), and elemental analysis. Their antifungal activities against *Colletotrichum lagenarium*, *Fusarium graminearum*, *Botrytis cinerea*, and *Phomopsis asparagi* were investigated by hypha measurement in vitro. The results revealed that hydroxypropyltrimethyl ammonium chitosan halogenated acetates had better antifungal activities than chitosan and HACC. In particular, the inhibitory activity decreased in the order: HACTFA > HACDFA > HACTCA > HACDCA > HACCA > HACBA > HACC > chitosan, which was consistent with the electron-withdrawing property of different halogenated acetates. This experiment provides a potential idea for the preparation of new antifungal drugs by chitosan.

Keywords: hydroxypropyltrimethyl ammonium chloride chitosan; halogenated acetate; antifungal activity; electronegativity

1. Introduction

Agricultural diseases resulted from plant pathogenic fungi may cause the large crop death, which limits crop production worldwide, and can lead to great financial losses to farmers [1,2]. There are various kinds of plant pathogenic fungi, with various modes of action. For instance, fusarium wilt in watermelon caused by *Fusarium oxysporum* (*F. oxysporum*) is a common disease in several countries including the China and United States, which can lead to massive loss to watermelon production [3].

Gibberella zeae (*G. zeae*) distributed all over the world is a devastating filamentous fungus. It can cause fusarium head blight disease in several economically important crops, such as maize, barley, and wheat [4,5]. How to prevent these diseases caused by plant pathogenic fungi is a thought-provoking question. Currently, the most common way to control the plant fungous diseases is to use massive chemical fungicides [6,7]. However, due to the excessive use of the chemical fungicides, the ecological environment has been seriously damaged [8]. So, it is urgent to research a kind of new drug with low toxicity and strong antifungal activity.

There are many bioactive compounds in the marine which can translate into fungicide alternatives [2]. Chitosan prepared by the *N*-deacetylation of chitin is one of the active substances in the ocean [9]. Chitosan, as a nontoxic and renewable natural polysaccharide, has good biocompatibility and biodegradability. In addition, it also has the characteristics of film-forming ability, low toxicity, antibacterial activity, and so on [10,11]. Therefore, chitosan has been drawing extensive attention in agriculture, medicine, food science, industry, and environmental protection due to its unique physical and chemical properties in recent years. However, compared with current fungicides, its relatively low antibacterial activity and poor solubility inhibit its feasibility as a kind of fungicide [12,13]. So, chemical modification of chitosan in order to obtain various chitosan derivatives which are active and water-soluble is the focus of research.

The structural modification sites of chitosan are mainly C_2-NH_2 and C_6-OH [14]. For instance, the C_2-NH_2 of chitosan can react with aldehydes or ketones to form the corresponding aldimines and ketimines, which is called Schiff base, and *O*-carboxymethyl chitosan can be formed by the introduction of carboxyl groups on the C_6-OH [15–17]. In general, chitosan derivatives with different activities can be synthesized through chemical modification such as acylation, alkylation, Schiff base reaction, quaternary ammonium reaction and so on. Among the above chemical modification, chitosan quaternary ammonium salt has attracted people's attention for its unique character. As one of the kind of chitosan quaternary ammonium salt, hydroxypropyltrimethyl ammonium chloride chitosan (HACC) is a polycationic compound, characterized by good water solubility, flocculation, moisture absorption, and antibacterial properties with low cytotoxicity to cells [11]. At the same time, HACC can be prepared by simple method with high synthesis efficiency and little harm to the environment. In recent years, many studies showed that HACC had potential applications in many fields. For instance, HACC has been reported as a chitosan derivative with enhanced antibacterial ability against *Escherichia coli*, *Candida albicans*, and *Staphylococcus aureus* [18]. And the antibacterial drugs made by HACC have been widely used. Meanwhile, it is reported that HACC can be used in other areas, such as nanofiltration, orthopedics, and drug delivery, due to its water solubility, low cytotoxicity to cells, and biocompatibility [19]. For example, HACC possesses the stronger electrostatic interaction with negatively charged tumor cells when it is used as a drug carrier for cancer treatment [20]. However, the antifungal activity of HACC is not optimistic according to the earlier studies [18]. Furthermore, it is reported that the halogens have good antifungal activity. It is assumed that the electron-withdrawing substitution—halogens can play a crucial part in the antifungal properties of compounds, which can destroy cell walls and membranes to lead to the death of fungus [21,22]. Chemical fungicides with halogens are widely used in recent years due to its effective antifungal activity. However, the chemical fungicides cause serious problems for the environment because of toxicities and residues. When the halogens are grafted to chitosan, they should be released slowly and may meet requirements of environmental safety.

On the basis of the above statement, we modified hydroxypropyltrimethyl ammonium chitosan via six different haloacetic acids to obtain high antifungal activity and water-soluble chitosan derivatives. Firstly, the hydroxypropyltrimethyl ammonium chloride chitosan was synthesized by chitosan and 3-chloro-2-hydroxypropyltrimethyl ammonium chloride. Then, hydroxypropyltrimethyl ammonium chitosan halogenated acetates were synthesized via ion exchange. The structures of chitosan derivatives were characterized by Fourier transform infrared spectroscopy (FTIR), ^{1}H Nuclear magnetic resonance spectrometer (^{1}H NMR), ^{13}C Nuclear magnetic resonance spectrometer (^{13}C NMR), and elemental analyses. Their antifungal activities against *Colletotrichum lagenarium* (*C. lagenarium*), *Fusarium oxysporum* (*F. oxysporum*), *Botrytis cinerea* (*B. cinerea*), and *Phomopsis asparagi* (*P. asparagi*) were investigated by hypha measurement in vitro. Based on the obtained data, the relationship between chitosan derivatives and antifungal activity was discussed briefly.

2. Results and Discussion

2.1. Chemical Synthesis and Characterization

The synthetic strategy of hydroxypropyltrimethyl ammonium chitosan halogenated acetates is shown in Scheme 1. Firstly, hydroxypropyltrimethyl ammonium chloride chitosan (HACC) was prepared by chitosan and 3-chloro-2-hydroxypropyltrimethyl ammonium chloride. Then, HACC was dissolved in 20% sodium halogenated acetate for purpose of replacing the chloride ions with haloacetic ions. Hydroxypropyltrimethyl ammonium chitosan halogenated acetates were obtained after drying in vacuo. The structures of chitosan derivatives were characterized by FTIR (Figure 1), ^{1}H NMR (Figure 2), ^{13}C NMR (Figure 3), and elemental analysis (Table 1), respectively.

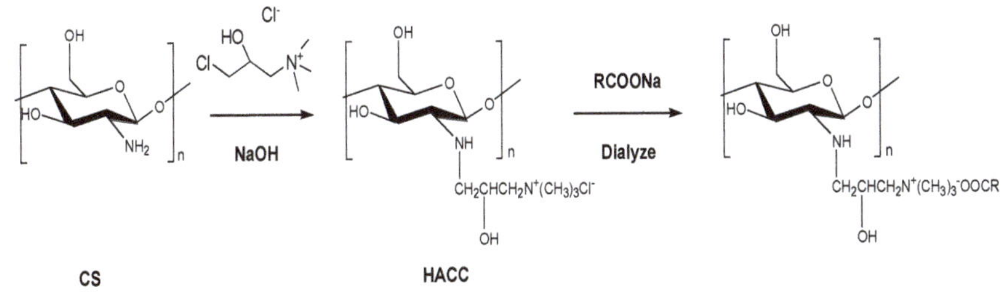

HACCA: R =CH_2Cl; HACDCA: R =$CHCl_2$; HACTCA: R =CCl_3; HACDFA: R =CHF_2; HACTFA: R =CF_3; HACBA: R =CH_2Br

Scheme 1. Synthesis routes for chitosan derivatives.

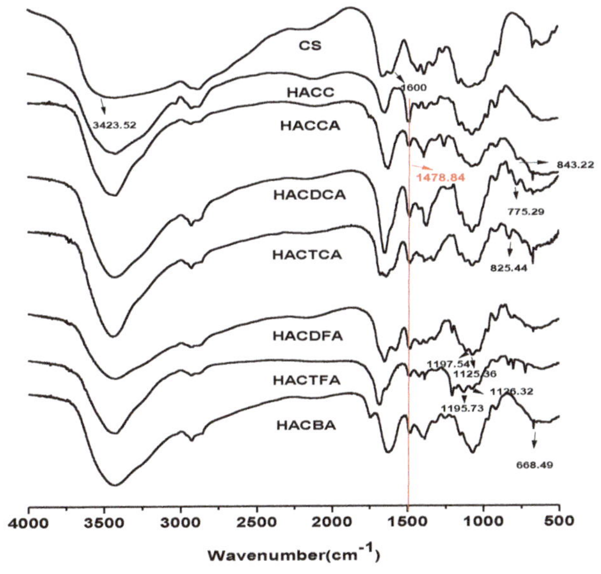

Figure 1. Fourier transform infrared spectroscopy (FTIR) spectra of chitosan and chitosan derivatives.

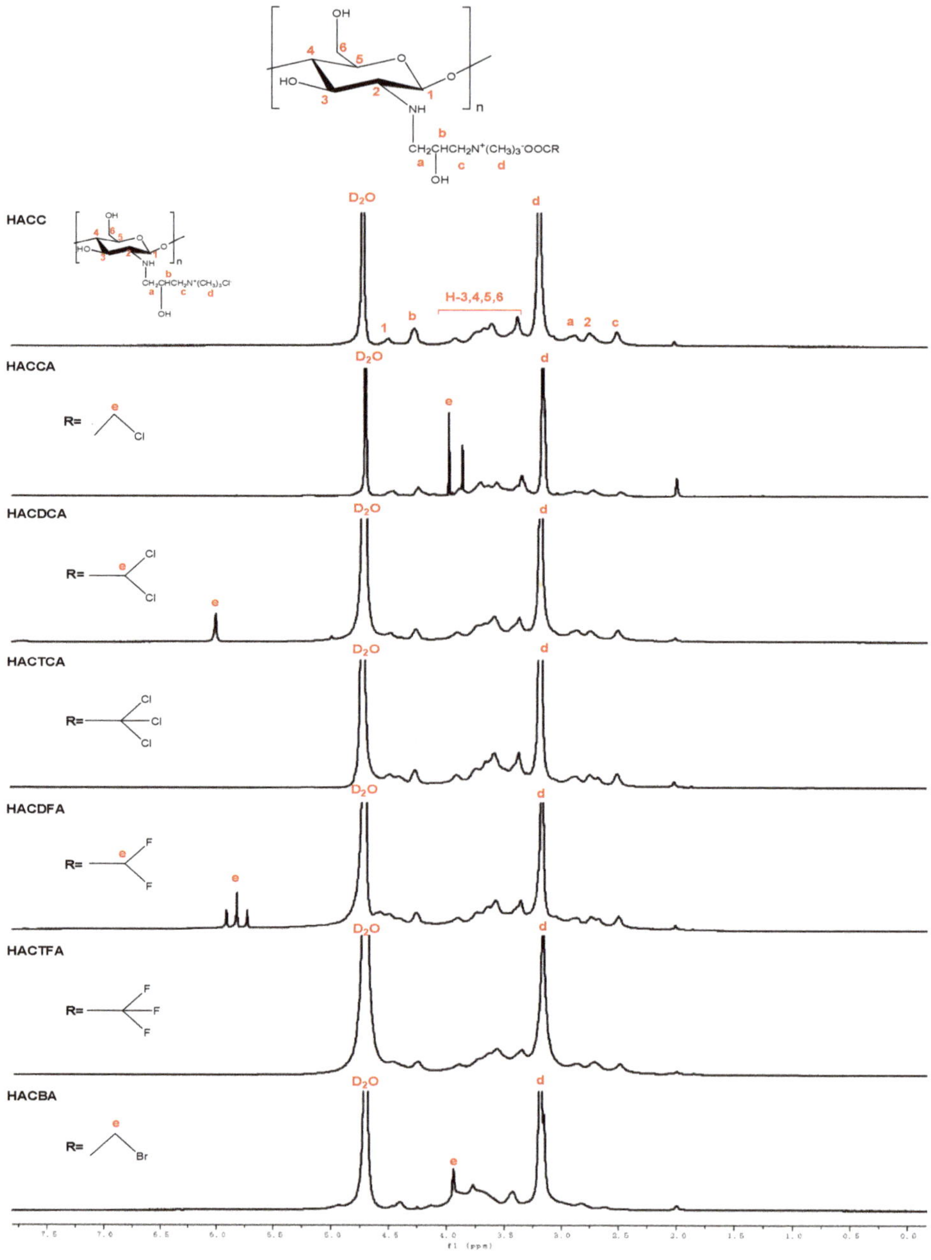

Figure 2. ^{1}H Nuclear magnetic resonance spectrometer (^{1}H NMR) spectra of chitosan derivatives.

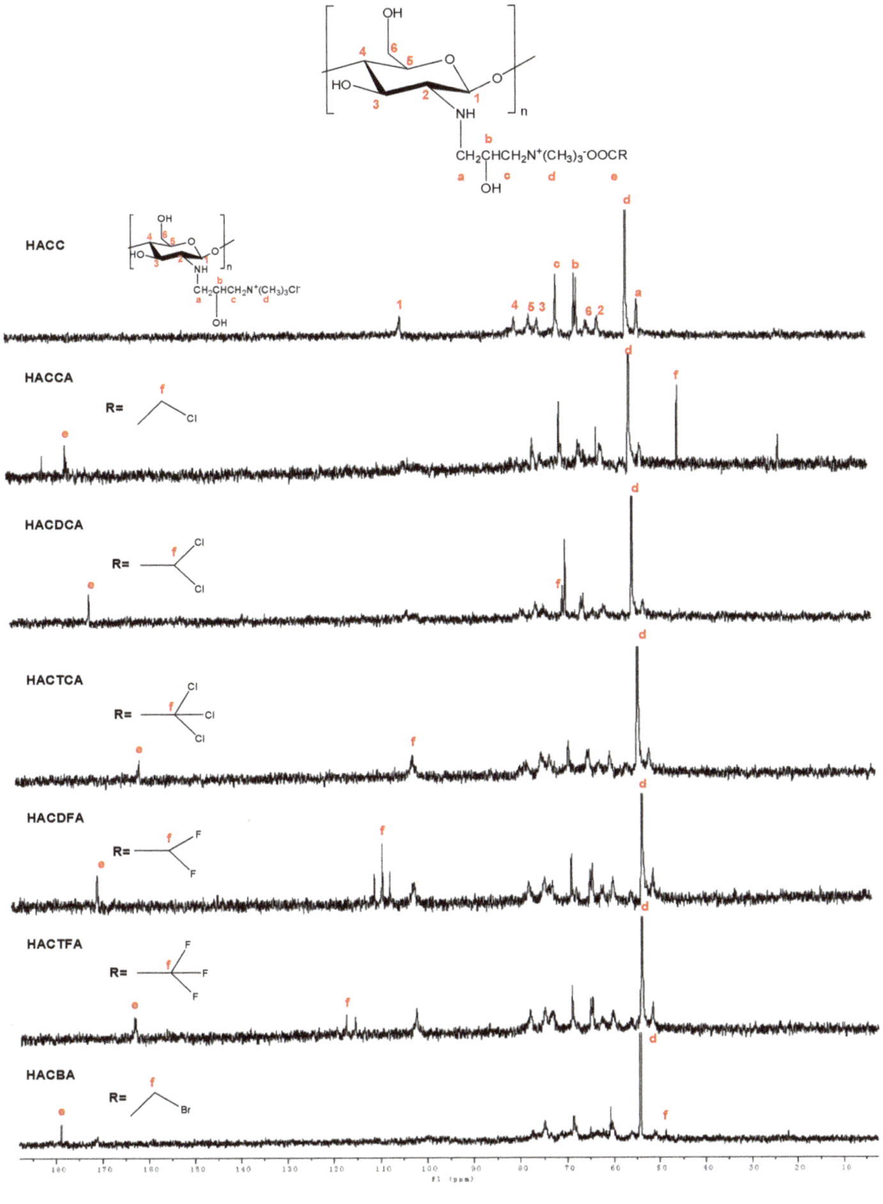

Figure 3. ^{13}C Nuclear magnetic resonance spectrometer (^{13}C NMR) spectra of chitosan derivatives.

Table 1. Yields and the degrees of substitution of chitosan derivatives.

Componds	Yields (%)	Elemental Analyses (%)			Degrees of Substitution (%)
		C	N	C/N	
CS	-	41.47	7.56	5.48	-
HACC	65.27	39.71	7.41	5.35	67.71
HACCA	69.43	38.10	6.27	6.05	67.31
HACDCA	50.86	38.86	6.63	5.86	56.23
HACTCA	64.85	37.22	6.07	6.13	71.97
HACDFA	58.97	40.86	7.13	5.73	48.64
HACTFA	67.56	38.27	6.25	6.12	71.39
HACBA	65.84	40.64	6.70	6.06	67.89

2.1.1. Fourier Transform Infrared Spectroscopy (FTIR) Spectra

Figure 1 shows the spectra of chitosan, intermediate product, and chitosan derivatives respectively. For chitosan, the peaks appear at 3423.62, 2922.51, 1650.24, 1600.21, and 1072.24 cm^{-1} [23]. The peak of 3423.62 cm^{-1} presents the characteristic absorbance of -OH and $–NH_2$. The weak peak at 2922.51 cm^{-1} shows the stretching vibration of –CH [24,25]. The band at 1650.24 cm^{-1} can be attributed to C=O (the amide I) stretching vibration. The band at 1600.21 cm^{-1} can be attributed to $-NH_2$. The peak at 1072.24 cm^{-1} shows the stretching vibrations of the C–O [26,27]. The IR spectrum of HACC (Figure 1) shows the introduction of the quaternary ammonium salt group to the chitosan backbone. Compared to chitosan, a peak at 1478.84 cm^{-1} is attributed to the C-H bending of the trimethylammonium group [18], and a peak at 1600.21 cm^{-1} weakens greatly for the partial change of the primary amine of chitosan to the secondary amine. For HACCA, HACDCA, and HACTCA, new peaks appeared at 843.22, 776.28, 826.44 cm^{-1} respectively can be attributed to the C-Cl bending [28,29]. For HACDFA, new peaks appear at 1187.64 and 1126.38 cm^{-1} for the C-F bending. Meanwhile, new peaks appear at 1186.73 and 1128.32 cm^{-1} are assigned to the characteristic absorbance of C-F for HACTFA [10]. For HACBA, a new peak appears at 668.49 cm^{-1}, which can be attributed to the C-Br bending [25,30]. In addition, the peak at 1478.84 cm^{-1} attributed to the C–H bending of the trimethylammonium group still exists in the molecules of HACCA, HACDCA, HACTCA, HACDFA, HACTFA, and HACBA.

2.1.2. Nuclear Magnetic Resonance Spectrometer (NMR) Spectra

^{1}H NMR spectra of intermediate products HACC and chitosan derivatives are shown in Figure 2. As shown in the figure, chemical shifts at 4.47 ppm, 3.24–4.02 ppm, and 2.72 ppm are assigned to [H1], [H3]–[H6], and [H2] of chitosan [31]. In ^{1}H NMR spectrum of HACC, an obvious characteristic peak of hydrogen (3.16 ppm) of trimethyl ammonium groups is appeared [18]. At the same time, for HACC, the other signals can be well observed: δ = 2.41 ppm attributed to $–CH_2$, δ = 2.69 ppm (a), δ = 4.50 ppm (b) [21,24,32]. For HACCA, compared to HACC, a new peak appears at 4.21 ppm, which can be assigned to protons of halogenated acetic anions (e). Furthermore, for HACDCA, HACDFA, HACBA, new peaks appear at 6.12 ppm, 5.75–6.01 ppm, and 3.78 ppm, which can be attributed to protons of halogenated acetic anions (e) [10,29]. However, the spectra of HACTCA and HACTFA are similar to HACC, and no new peaks appear because of the lack of protons of halogenated acetic anions. In addition, the chemical shifts of trimethyl ammonium groups at about 3.16 ppm still exist in the spectra of HACCA, HACDCA, HACTCA, HACDFA, HACTFA, and HACBA.

^{13}C NMR spectra of intermediate products HACC and chitosan derivatives are shown in Figure 3. As shown in the figures, all spectra show signals at 55.10–105.68 ppm (^{13}C NMR spectra) [26], which are assigned to the diagnostic chemical shifts of chitosan. In ^{13}C NMR spectrum of HACC, an obvious characteristic peak of carbon (57.25 ppm) of trimethyl ammonium groups is appeared [18]. Meanwhile, for HACC, the other signals can be well observed: δ = 51.85 ppm attributed to $–CH_2$, δ = 64.81 ppm (b), δ = 69.19 ppm (c) [29]. For hydroxypropyltrimethyl ammonium chitosan halogenated acetates, compared to HACC, new peaks appear at 174.83, 170.80, 161.41, 169.86, 162.93, and 178.90 ppm, which can be assigned to carbons of COO^- groups in HACCA, HACDCA, HACTCA, HACDFA, HACTFA, and HACBA (e) [10,28]. Furthermore, for hydroxypropyltrimethyl ammonium chitosan halogenated acetates, new peaks appear at 43.91 ppm (CH_2Cl in HACCA), 69.47 ppm ($CHCl_2$ in HACDCA), 102.47 ppm (CCl_3 in HACTCA), 109.14 ppm (CHF_2 in HACDFA), 117.35 ppm (CF_3 in HACTFA), and 48.78 ppm (CH_2Br in HACBA), which can confirm the presence of the halogenated methyl carbons [10,26,28]. In addition, the chemical shifts of trimethyl ammonium groups at about 57.25 ppm still exist in the spectra of HACCA, HACDCA, HACTCA, HACDFA, HACTFA, and HACBA.

These data indicate that hydroxypropyltrimethyl ammonium chitosan halogenated acetates are successfully synthesized. And according to the ^1H NMR spectra, the degrees of substitution of chitosan derivatives were calculated by using the integration of [H2] as an integral standard peak [20]. The degrees of substitution of HACC, HACCA, HACDCA, HACDFA, and HACTFA was determined as 71.30, 66.00%, 61.00%, 48.00%, and 68.00%, respectively (Table S1). However, the degrees of substitution of HACTCA and HACTFA can not calculate by the ^1H NMR spectra. Therefore, we did the elemental analysis in order to calculate the degrees of substitution.

2.1.3. Elemental Analysis

The yields and the degrees of substitution of chitosan derivatives are shown in Table 1. The changes in $W_{C/N}$ indicate the functional groups grafting on chitosan successfully. From the data in Table 1, the intermediate HACC presents the highest degree of substitution. The degrees of substitution of the other six chitosan derivatives are different. HACTCA, for example, has a far lower degree of substitution than HACDFA, which is 48.64%.

2.2. Antifungal Activity

Antifungal assays against *C. lagenarium*, *F. oxysporum*, *B. cinerea*, and *P. asparagi* are performed by following the plate growth rate method. The antifungal activity of chitosan and its derivatives is shown in Figures 4–7.

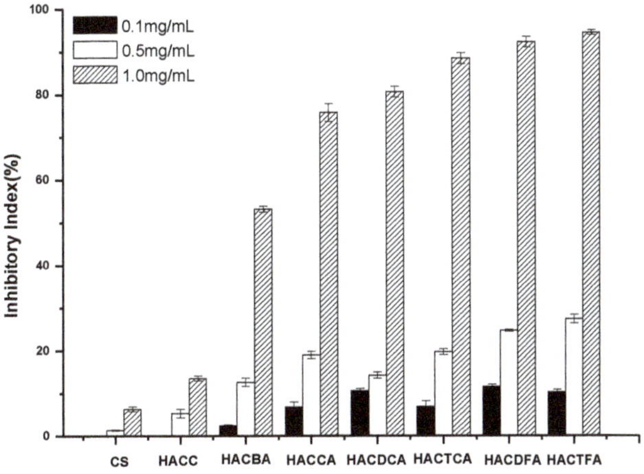

Figure 4. The antifungal activity of chitosan and chitosan derivatives against *Colletotrichum lagenarium*.

C. lagenarium, which is caused by the introduction of pathogenic bacteria in the seeds, has been increasingly harmful in recent years. It has a great impact on crop production, and is difficult to control. Figure 4 shows the antifungal activities of chitosan, intermediates, and target products against *C. lagenarium*. Chitosan and HACC have almost no inhibitory effect on *C. lagenarium*. However, the enhanced antifungal activities of the target products including HACCA, HACDCA, HACTCA,

HACDFA, HACTFA, and HACBA are very obvious. Specifically, the conclusions are as follows: firstly, all the target products including HACCA, HACDCA, HACTCA, HACDFA, HACTFA, and HACBA have much stronger antifungal activity. Secondly, with the augment of sample concentration, the antifungal activity of the target product increases gradually. For example, when the concentrations of HACTFA are 0.1 mg/mL, 0.5 mg/mL, and 1.0 mg/mL, the inhibition rates on *C. lagenarium* are 17.14%, 30.09%, and 96.57% respectively. Thirdly, the order of inhibition of *C. lagenarium* is: HACTFA > HACDFA > HACTCA > HACDCA > HACCA > HACBA. Meanwhile, it is clear that the inhibition rate of HACDFA with DS of 48.64% is 5.64 percent higher than that of HACDCA with degree of substitution of 56.23% at 1.0 mg/mL, which can reasonably suggest that higher inhibitory index of HACDFA should be possible if they have the same degree of substitution. Similarly, HACCA has better antifungal activity than HACBA, despite its low degree of substitution. Therefore, the expected order of inhibition should be as follows: HACTFA > HACDFA > HACTCA > HACDCA > HACCA > HACBA, which is identical to the experimental results. And this rule is consistent with the order of the electronegativity of halogen-containing substituents in the hydroxypropyltrimethyl ammonium chitosan halogenated acetates.

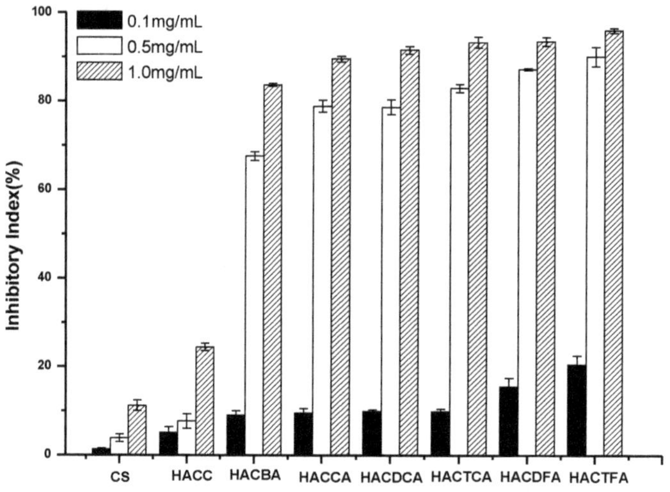

Figure 5. The antifungal activity of chitosan and chitosan derivatives against *Fusarium oxysporum*.

F. oxysporum is a common disease in several countries, which can lead to massive loss to watermelon production. Figure 5 shows the antifungal activities against *F. oxysporum* of chitosan and chitosan derivatives. Compared to chitosan and HACC, the antifungal activity against *F. oxysporum* of HACCA, HACDCA, HACTCA, HACDFA, HACTFA, and HACBA have been greatly improved. Specifically, antifungal activity increases with the augment of sample concentration. When the sample concentration is 1.0 mg/mL, and compared to chitosan with the inhibitory index 13.21%, the inhibitory indices of HACCA, HACDCA, HACTCA, HACDFA, HACTFA, and HACBA are 92.81%, 93.40%, 93.87%, 94.54%, 94.97%, and 97.50%, respectively. Meanwhile, after the introduction of active groups, chitosan derivatives have a particularly well antifungal effect on *F. oxysporum*, which inhibitory index reaches above 70.52% at the sample concentration of 0.5 mg/mL. Considering the relationships between degree of substitution and inhibitory index, the antifungal activities of chitosan derivatives are ranked as follows: HACTFA > HACDFA > HACTCA > HACDCA > HACCA > HACBA.

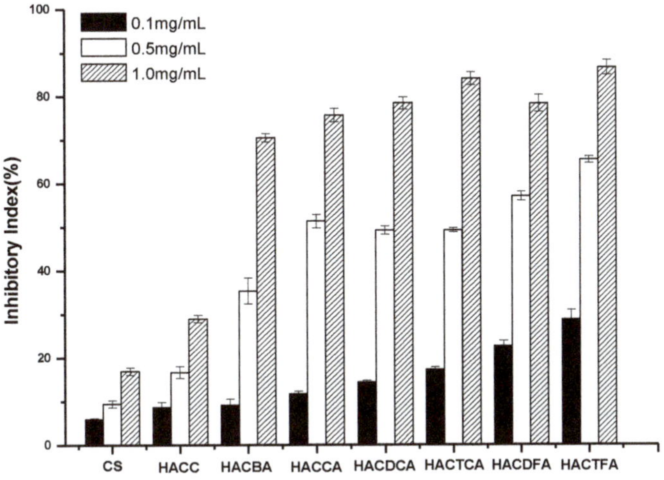

Figure 6. The antifungal activity of chitosan and chitosan derivatives against *Botrytis cinerea*.

As shown in Figure 6, chitosan and HACC possess little antifungal activity. However, hydroxypropyltrimethyl ammonium chitosan halogenated acetates have antifungal activity at all the tested concentration against *B. cinerea*. The inhibitory indices of all the samples mount up with the increasing concentration. After the introduction of active groups, the antifungal activity of all the target products is better than chitosan raw materials and intermediate product. Especially, this trend is apparently reinforced at 1.0 mg/mL, and compared to the inhibitory index of chitosan and HACC, the inhibitory indices of HACCA, HACDCA, HACTCA, HACDFA, HACTFA, and HACBA are 75.64%, 78.35%, 84.02%, 78.29%, 86.57%, and 70.46%, respectively. As previously described, the order of antifungal activity is HACTCA > HACDCA > HACCA. However, contrary to the previous description, the inhibitory property of HACDFA is slightly lower than HACTCA, which is possibly because of its lower substitution degree (Table 1) and less active ingredient.

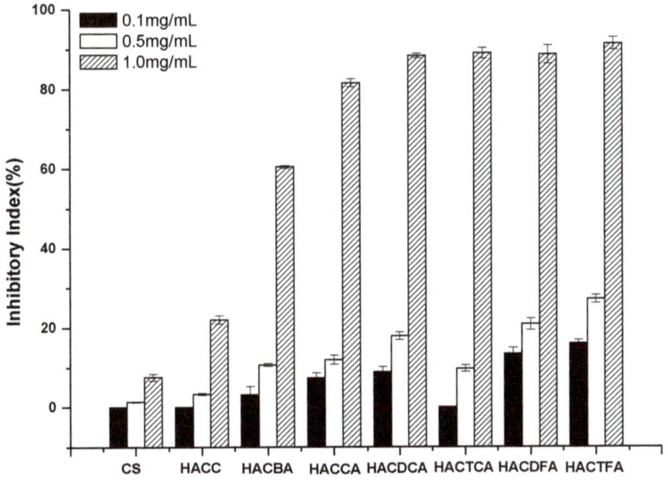

Figure 7. The antifungal activity of chitosan and chitosan derivatives against *Phomopsis asparagi*.

Asparagus stem blight is a highly destructive disease of asparagus in China and some Asian countries. Due to the filamentous fungus, *P. asparagi* is identified as the causing pathogen, it is particularly important to inhibit the activity of *P. asparagi*. As shown in Figure 7, apart from HACC, chitosan derivatives have outstanding antifungal activities at all the tested concentration against *P. asparagi*. The inhibitory indices of all the samples mount up with increasing concentration. All chitosan derivatives show stronger antifungal activity than chitosan and HACC. Especially, this trend reinforces apparently at 1.0 mg/mL, and compared to chitosan with the inhibitory index 7.59%, the inhibitory indices of HACBA, HACCA, HACDCA, HACTCA, HACDFA, and HACTFA are 60.47%, 81.58%, 88.42%, 89.05%, 88.69, and 90.45%, respectively. In summary, except for HACDFA and HACTCA, the antifungal activities are approximate, and the other antifungal activities are consistent with the previous description.

The results showed that the six different kinds of chitosan derivatives including HACCC, HACCDC, HACCTC, HACCDF, HACCTF, and HACCB, had much stronger inhibitory effect on *C. lagenarium*, *F. oxysporum*, *B. cinerea*, and *P. asparagi*. In a nutshell, the antifungal activity decreased in the order: HACTFA > HACDFA > HACTCA > HACDCA > HACCA > HACBA > HACC > chitosan. To be specific, the conclusions was as follows: firstly, all the target products including HACCA, HACDCA, HACTCA, HACDFA, HACTFA, and HACBA had much stronger antifungal activities on *C. lagenarium*, *F. oxysporum*, *B. cinerea*, and *P. asparagi*. The results confirmed that the introduction of halogen greatly enhanced the antifungal activity of chitosan derivatives. Because the halogen groups could inhibit synthesis of the cell membrane and cell wall to exhibit antifungal activity [24]. Specifically speaking, the halogen atoms, which had a high electron-withdrawing property, could increase the hydrophobicity of chitosan derivatives. The structures of the outer membranes as well as the internal membranes of microbial cells were impacted by the changes in hydrophobicity, and could prevent nutrient substances from entering cells [26]. The microorganisms would die for these reasons. Secondly, the antifungal activity of chitosan derivatives varies with the types and quantities of halogen atoms. On one hand, HACCA, HACDCA, HACTCA had the same types of halogen-Cl, and they exhibited different antifungal activities due to the different amounts of halogen groups. That was to say the capacity of electron-withdrawing would enhance with the amounts of halogen groups. So, the antifungal activities of the target products showed the order of HACTCA > HACDCA > HACCA. On the other hand, HACTFA and HACTCA, which had the same amount of halogens, demonstrated different antifungal activities. HACTFA showed stronger antifungal activity compared with HACTCA, which could be attributed to the higher electronegativity of fluorine atoms than chlorine atoms. Therefore, the antifungal potential of target products was related to the electronegativity of halogen substituents [11,30–32]. In short, the higher degree of electron-withdrawing property the halogen substituents possessed, the higher the positive charge density of cationic amino possessed. As a result, the chitosan derivatives showed stronger antifungal activity [33–35]; this was consistent with our experimental results.

3. Materials and Methods

3.1. Materials

Chitosan was purchased from Qingdao Baicheng Biochemical Corp. (Qingdao, China). Its degree of deacetylation was 85%, and the viscosity-average molecular weight was 2.0×10^5. 3-chloro-2-hydroxypropyltrimethyl ammonium chloride, isopropanol, chloroacetic acid, dichloroacetic acid, trichloroacetic acid, difluoroacetic acid, trifluoroacetic acid, and bromoacetic acid were purchased from Sigma-Aldrich Chemical Corp. (Shanghai, China). Ethanol and sodium hydroxide were all purchased from Sinopharm Chemical Reagent Co., Ltd. (Shanghai, China). The reagents were analytical grade and used without further purification. Fungi medium was purchased from Qingdao Hop Bio-Technogy Co., Ltd. (Qingdao, China). Agar powder was purchased from Beijing Chembase Technology Co., Ltd. (Beijing, China).

3.2. Analytical Methods

3.2.1. Fourier Transform Infrared (FTIR) Spectroscopy

FTIR spectra were performed ranging from 4000 cm^{-1} to 400 cm^{-1} using a Jasco-4100 (Tokyo, Japan), provided by JASCO China (Shanghai) Co. Ltd. (Shanghai, China). All samples were ground and mixed with KBr disks for testing.

3.2.2. Nuclear Magnetic Resonance (NMR) Spectroscopy

^{1}H NMR spectra and ^{13}C NMR spectra were recorded on samples dissolved in D_2O with a Bruker AVIII-500 Spectrometer (500 MHz, Fällanden, Switzerland, provided by Bruker Tech and Serv. Co., Ltd., Beijing, China) at 25 °C.

3.2.3. Elemental Analysis

The elemental analyses (C, H, and N) were performed on a Vario Micro Elemental Analyzer (Elementar, Hanau, Germany), and they can be used to evaluate the degree of substitution of chitosan derivatives. The degrees of substitution (DS) of chitosan derivatives were calculated according to the carbon nitrogen ratio, and the formula as follows [10,26]:

$$DS_1 = \frac{n_1 * M_C - M_N * W_{C/N}}{n_2 * M_C} \quad (1)$$

$$DS_2 = \frac{n_1 * M_C - n_2 * M_C * DS_1 - M_N * W_{C/N}}{M_N * W_{C/N} - n_3 * M_C} \quad (2)$$

$$DS_3 = \frac{M_N * W_{C/N} + M_N * DS_2 * W_{C/N} - n_1 * M_C * DS_2 - n_2 * M_C * DS_1}{n_4 * M_C} \quad (3)$$

where DS_1, DS_2, DS_3 represent the deacetylation degree of chitosan, the degrees of substitution of HACC, and degrees of substitution of hydroxypropyltrimethyl ammonium chitosan halogenated acetates; M_C and M_N are the molar masses of carbon and nitrogen, $M_C = 12$, $M_N = 14$, respectively; n_1, n_2, n_3 n_4 are the number of carbons of chitin, acetamido group, 2-chloromethyl ammonium chloride, and haloacetic acid group, $n_1 = 8$, $n_2 = 2$, $n_3 = 6$, $n_4 = 2$, respectively; $W_{C/N}$ represents the mass ratio between carbon and nitrogen in chitosan derivatives.

3.3. Synthesis of Chitosan Derivatives

3.3.1. Synthesis of Hydroxypropyltrimethyl Ammonium Chloride Chitosan (HACC)

The reaction scheme for the synthesis of HACC is shown in Scheme 1. HACC was prepared as follows: chitosan (5 g) was dissolved in 20 mL isopropanol prior to the addition of 9 mL 40% (w/v) NaOH aqueous solution, and stirred at 60 °C for 4 h. Then, 20 mL 60% (w/v) hydroxypropyl trimethyl ammonium chloride solution was dropped into the front mixture with stirring at 80 °C. After 10 h, the pH was adjusted to 7 at room temperature prior to filtering the mixture, and then the mixture was poured into substantial anhydrous ethanol. The leached compounds were rinsed thoroughly with 85% ethanol, dewatered with anhydrous ethanol, and dried in vacuo.

3.3.2. Synthesis of Hydroxypropyltrimethyl Ammonium Chitosan Halogenated Acetates

HACC was dissolved in 20% sodium halogenated acetate for purpose of replacing the chloride ions with haloacetic ions. The solution was dialyzed with distilled water for 48 h, and quaternary ammonium salts of chitosan bearing halogenated acetate including hydroxypropyltrimethyl ammonium chitosan bromacetate (HACBA), hydroxypropyltrimethyl ammonium chitosan chloroacetate (HACCA), hydroxypropyltrimethyl ammonium chitosan dichloroacetate (HACDCA), hydroxypropyltrimethyl ammonium chitosan trichloroacetate (HACTCA), hydroxypropyltrimethyl ammonium chitosan difluoroacetate (HACDFA), and hydroxypropyltrimethyl ammonium chitosan trifluoroacetate (HACTFA) were obtained after drying in vacuo (Scheme 1).

3.4. Antifungal Assays

Antifungal assay against *C. lagenarium*, *F. oxysporum*, *B. cinerea*, and *P. asparagi* was performed by following the plate growth rate method [34]. Firstly, the samples (chitosan and chitosan derivatives) were dissolved in distilled water at a concentration of 6.0 mg/mL. Then, in a sterile environment, 2.0 mL, 1.0 mL, and 0.2 mL sample solutions were shaken into the fungus culture medium and poured into a disposable culture dish respectively to solidify. Therefore, the final concentrations of the samples were 1.0 mg/mL, 0.5 mg/mL, and 0.1 mg/mL, respectively. Finally, the fungi mycelium of 5.0 mm diameter was inoculated into the solidified solid medium center with tweezers and cultured at 28 °C for three days. The unsampled deionized water was used as a blank control until the mycelia of the blank group grew to the edge of the dish. Next, the diameter of mycelium growth area was measured and the average value was taken. The inhibitory index was calculated as follows:

$$\text{Inhibitory index } (\%) = (1 - D_a/D_b) * 100 \tag{4}$$

where D_a is the diameter of the growth zone in the test plates, and D_b is the diameter of the growth zone in the control plate.

3.5. Statistical Analysis

The results of the antifungal activities were processed by Excel (2007, Microsoft Corporation, Redmond, WA, USA), Origin (8.0, OriginLab, Northampton, MA, USA), and the statistical software SPSS (19.0, SPSS, Chicago, IL, USA). Duncan's methods by SPSS were used to evaluate the differences in the inhibitory index in the antifungal tests. The data were analyzed by an analysis of variance. When $p < 0.05$, the results were considered statistically significant.

4. Conclusions

In this paper, hydroxypropyltrimethyl ammonium chitosan halogenated acetates were successfully synthesized from six different haloacetic acids and hydroxypropyltrimethyl ammonium chloride chitosan with high substitution degree. Through testing these antifungal activities against *C. lagenarium*, *F. oxysporum*, *B. cinerea*, and *P. asparagi*, we found that six different chitosan derivatives had better antifungal activities than chitosan and hydroxypropyltrimethyl ammonium chloride chitosan (HACC). In particular, the inhibitory activity decreased in the order: HACTFA > HACDFA > HACTCA > HACDCA > HACCA > HACBA > HACC > chitosan, which was consistent with the electron-withdrawing property of different halogenated acetate. In summary, halogen groups were introduced into the synthesized chitosan derivatives which contributed a lot to the antifungal action, and the magnitude of antifungal activity depended on the electronegativity of substituents. Meanwhile, considering the obvious toxicity of many halogenated fungicides, the sustained release action of chitosan could solve this problem to a certain extent, and it would largely remit the problem of environmental issue. In short, this paper provided a new way of preparing chitosan derivatives with excellent antifungal activity, which has the potential of becoming alternatives to some harmful pesticides for disease control.

Supplementary Materials: The following are available online at http://www.mdpi.com/1660-3397/16/9/315/s1, Table S1: The degrees of substitution (DS) of chitosan derivatives.

Author Contributions: Conceptualization, Y.M. and Z.G.; Formal analysis, F.D.; Methodology, J.Z. and Y.C.; Project administration, Y.M.; Software, W.T. and Q.L.; Supervision, L.W.; Writing—review & editing, Y.M.

Funding: This research was funded by the National Natural Science Foundation of China (41576156), Shandong Province Science and Technology Development Plan (2015GSF121045), Yantai Science and Technology Development Plan (2015ZH078), and Technology Research Funds Projects of Ocean (No. 2015418022-3).

Acknowledgments: We thank the National Natural Science Foundation of China (41576156), Shandong Province Science and Technology Development Plan (2015GSF121045), and Yantai Science and Technology Development Plan (2015ZH078), and Technology Research Funds Projects of Ocean (No. 2015418022-3) for financial support of this work.

Conflicts of Interest: The authors declare no conflict of interest.

References

1. Jones, D.A.; Bertazzoni, S.; Turo, C.J.; Syme, R.A.; Hane, J.K. Bioinformatic prediction of plant-pathogenicity effector proteins of fungi. *Curr. Opin. Microbiol.* **2018**, *46*, 43–49. [CrossRef] [PubMed]
2. Fan, Z.; Qin, Y.; Liu, S.; Xing, R.; Yu, H.; Chen, X.; Li, K.; Li, P. Synthesis, characterization, and antifungal evaluation of diethoxyphosphoryl polyaminoethyl chitosan derivatives. *Carbohydr. Polym.* **2018**, *190*, 1–11. [CrossRef] [PubMed]
3. Costa, A.E.S.; da Cunha, F.S.; Honorato, A.; Capucho, A.S.; Dias, R.; Borel, J.C.; Ishikawa, F.H. Resistance to *Fusarium Wilt* in watermelon accessions inoculated by chlamydospores. *Sci. Hortic.* **2018**, *228*, 181–186. [CrossRef]
4. Garmendia, G.; Umpierrez-Failache, M.; Ward, T.J.; Vero, S. Development of a PCR-RFLP method based on the transcription elongation factor 1-alpha gene to differentiate *Fusarium graminearum* from other species within the *Fusarium graminearum* species complex. *Int. J. Food. Microbiol.* **2018**, *70*, 28–32. [CrossRef] [PubMed]
5. Sevastos, A.; Kalampokis, I.F.; Panagiotopoulou, A.; Pelecanou, M.; Aliferis, K.A. Implication of *Fusarium graminearum* primary metabolism in its resistance to benzimidazole fungicides as revealed by ^{1}H NMR metabolomics. *Pestic. Biochem. Phys.* **2018**, *148*, 50–61. [CrossRef] [PubMed]
6. Kheiri, A.; Moosawi Jorf, S.A.; Malihipour, A.; Saremi, H.; Nikkhah, M. Application of chitosan and chitosan nanoparticles for the control of Fusarium head blight of wheat (*Fusarium graminearum*) in vitro and greenhouse. *Int. J. Biol. Macromol.* **2016**, *93 Pt A*, 1261–1272. [CrossRef]
7. Heneberg, P.; Svoboda, J.; Pech, P. Benzimidazole fungicides are detrimental to common farmland ants. *Biol. Conserv.* **2018**, *221*, 114–117. [CrossRef]
8. Yang, G.; Jin, Q.; Xu, C.; Fan, S.; Wang, C.; Xie, P. Synthesis, characterization and antifungal activity of coumarin-functionalized chitosan derivatives. *Int. J. Biol. Macromol.* **2018**, *106*, 179–184. [CrossRef] [PubMed]
9. Divya, K.; Smitha, V.; Jisha, M.S. Antifungal, antioxidant and cytotoxic activities of chitosan nanoparticles and its use as an edible coating on vegetables. *Int. J. Biol. Macromol.* **2018**, *114*, 572–577. [CrossRef] [PubMed]
10. Tan, W.; Li, Q.; Dong, F.; Wei, L.; Guo, Z. Synthesis, characterization, and antifungal property of chitosan ammonium salts with halogens. *Int. J. Biol. Macromol.* **2016**, *92*, 293–298. [CrossRef] [PubMed]
11. Huczynski, A.; Antoszczak, M.; Kleczewska, N.; Lewandowska, M.; Maj, E.; Stefanska, J.; Wietrzyk, J.; Janczak, J.; Celewicz, L. Synthesis and biological activity of salinomycin conjugates with floxuridine. *Eur. J. Med. Chem.* **2015**, *93*, 33–41. [CrossRef] [PubMed]
12. He, G.; Ke, W.; Chen, X.; Kong, Y.; Zheng, H.; Yin, Y.; Cai, W. Preparation and properties of quaternary ammonium chitosan-*g*-poly(acrylic acid-*co*-acrylamide) superabsorbent hydrogels. *React. Funct. Polym.* **2017**, *111*, 14–21. [CrossRef]
13. Demetgul, C.; Beyazit, N. Synthesis, characterization and antioxidant activity of chitosan-chromone derivatives. *Carbohydr. Polym.* **2018**, *181*, 812–817. [CrossRef] [PubMed]
14. Zhang, J.; Tan, W.; Zhang, Z.; Song, Y.; Li, Q.; Dong, F.; Guo, Z. Synthesis, characterization, and the antifungal activity of chitosan derivatives containing urea groups. *Int. J. Biol. Macromol.* **2018**, *109*, 1061–1067. [CrossRef] [PubMed]
15. Huber, D.; Grzelak, A.; Baumann, M.; Borth, N.; Schleining, G.; Nyanhongo, G.S.; Guebitz, G.M. Anti-inflammatory and anti-oxidant properties of laccase-synthesized phenolic-*O*-carboxymethyl chitosan hydrogels. *New. Biotechnol.* **2018**, *40*, 236–244. [CrossRef] [PubMed]
16. Yu, C.; Kecen, X.; Xiaosai, Q. Grafting Modification of Chitosan. In *Biopolymer Grafting*, 1st ed.; Thakur, V.K., Ed.; Elsevier: Amsterdam, The Netherlands, 2018; pp. 295–364. ISBN 9780128104613.
17. Bakshi, P.S.; Selvakumar, D.; Kadirvelu, K.; Kumar, N.S. Comparative study on antimicrobial activity and biocompatibility of *N*-selective chitosan derivatives. *React. Funct. Polym.* **2018**, *124*, 149–155. [CrossRef]

18. Peng, Z.-X.; Wang, L.; Du, L.; Guo, S.-R.; Wang, X.-Q.; Tang, T.-T. Adjustment of the antibacterial activity and biocompatibility of hydroxypropyltrimethyl ammonium chloride chitosan by varying the degree of substitution of quaternary ammonium. *Carbohydr. Polym.* **2010**, *81*, 275–283. [CrossRef]
19. Woraphatphadung, T.; Sajomsang, W.; Gonil, P.; Saesoo, S.; Opanasopit, P. Synthesis and characterization of pH-responsive *N*-naphthyl-*N*,*O*-succinyl chitosan micelles for oral meloxicam delivery. *Carbohydr. Polym.* **2015**, *121*, 99–106. [CrossRef] [PubMed]
20. Xu, X.; Li, Y.; Wang, F.; Lv, L.; Liu, J.; Li, M.; Guo, A.; Jiang, J.; Shen, Y.; Guo, S. Synthesis, in vitro and in vivo evaluation of new norcantharidin-conjugated hydroxypropyltrimethyl ammonium chloride chitosan derivatives as polymer therapeutics. *Int. J. Pharm.* **2013**, *453*, 610–619. [CrossRef] [PubMed]
21. Colombo, A.; Dragonetti, C.; Magni, M.; Roberto, D. Degradation of toxic halogenated organic compounds by iron-containing mono-, bi- and tri-metallic particles in water. *Inorg. Chim. Acta* **2015**, *431*, 48–60. [CrossRef]
22. Luo, J.; Hu, J.; Wei, X.; Fu, L.; Li, L. Dehalogenation of persistent halogenated organic compounds: A review of computational studies and quantitative structure-property relationships. *Chemosphere* **2015**, *131*, 17–33. [CrossRef] [PubMed]
23. Song, R.; Zhong, Z.; Lin, L. Evaluation of chitosan quaternary ammonium salt-modified resin denture base material. *Int. J. Biol. Macromol.* **2016**, *85*, 102–110. [CrossRef] [PubMed]
24. Li, Q.; Tan, W.; Zhang, C.; Gu, G.; Guo, Z. Synthesis of water soluble chitosan derivatives with halogeno-1,2,3-triazole and their antifungal activity. *Int. J. Biol. Macromol.* **2016**, *91*, 623–629. [CrossRef] [PubMed]
25. Zhang, S.; Liu, X.; Jin, X.; Li, H.; Sun, J.; Gu, X. The novel application of chitosan: Effects of cross-linked chitosan on the fire performance of thermoplastic polyurethane. *Carbohydr. Polym.* **2018**, *189*, 313–321. [CrossRef] [PubMed]
26. Liu, W.; Qin, Y.; Liu, S.; Xing, R.; Yu, H.; Chen, X.; Li, K.; Li, P. Synthesis, characterization and antifungal efficacy of chitosan derivatives with triple quaternary ammonium groups. *Int. J. Biol. Macromol.* **2018**, *114*, 942–949. [CrossRef] [PubMed]
27. Guo, Z.; Li, Q.; Wang, G.; Dong, F.; Zhou, H.; Zhang, J. Synthesis, characterization, and antifungal activity of novel inulin derivatives with chlorinated benzene. *Carbohydr. Polym.* **2014**, *99*, 469–473. [CrossRef] [PubMed]
28. Zhang, J.; Tan, W.; Luan, F.; Yin, X.; Dong, F.; Li, Q.; Guo, Z. Synthesis of quaternary ammonium salts of chitosan bearing halogenated acetate for antifungal and antibacterial activities. *Polymers* **2018**, *10*, 530. [CrossRef]
29. Kaushal, J.; Seema; Singh, G.; Arya, S.K. Immobilization of catalase onto chitosan and chitosan-bentonite complex: A comparative study. *Biotechnol. Rep.* **2018**, *18*, 251–258.
30. Rui, L.; Xie, M.; Hu, B.; Zhou, L.; Saeeduddin, M.; Zeng, X. Enhanced solubility and antioxidant activity of chlorogenic acid-chitosan conjugates due to the conjugation of chitosan with chlorogenic acid. *Carbohydr. Polym.* **2017**, *170*, 206–216. [CrossRef] [PubMed]
31. Tan, W.; Li, Q.; Li, W.; Dong, F.; Guo, Z. Synthesis and antioxidant property of novel 1,2,3-triazole-linked starch derivatives via 'click chemistry'. *Int. J. Biol. Macromol.* **2016**, *82*, 404–410. [CrossRef] [PubMed]
32. Sun, L.; Du, Y.; Fan, L.; Chen, X.; Yang, J. Preparation, characterization and antimicrobial activity of quaternized carboxymethyl chitosan and application as pulp-cap. *Polymer* **2006**, *47*, 1796–1804. [CrossRef]
33. Dananjaya, S.H.S.; Erandani, W.; Kim, C.H.; Nikapitiya, C.; Lee, J.; De Zoysa, M. Comparative study on antifungal activities of chitosan nanoparticles and chitosan silver nano composites against *Fusarium oxysporum* species complex. *Int. J. Biol. Macromol.* **2017**, *105*, 478–488. [CrossRef] [PubMed]
34. Sajomsang, W.; Gonil, P.; Tantayanon, S. Antibacterial activity of quaternary ammonium chitosan containing mono or disaccharide moieties: Preparation and characterization. *Int. J. Biol. Macromol.* **2009**, *44*, 419–427. [CrossRef] [PubMed]
35. Fan, L.; Yang, J.; Wu, H.; Hu, Z.; Yi, J.; Tong, J.; Zhu, X. Preparation and characterization of quaternary ammonium chitosan hydrogel with significant antibacterial activity. *Int. J. Biol. Macromol.* **2015**, *79*, 830–836. [CrossRef] [PubMed]

© 2018 by the authors. Licensee MDPI, Basel, Switzerland. This article is an open access article distributed under the terms and conditions of the Creative Commons Attribution (CC BY) license (http://creativecommons.org/licenses/by/4.0/).

marine drugs

Article

Elucidation of the Relationship between CD Cotton Effects and the Absolute Configuration of Sixteen Stereoisomers of Spiroheterocyclic-Lactams

Takeshi Yamada [1,*], Tetsuya Kajimoto [2], Takashi Kikuchi [1] and Reiko Tanaka [1]

1 Department of Medicinal Molecular Chemistry, Osaka University of Pharmaceutical Sciences, 4-20-1, Nasahara, Takatsuki, Osaka 569-1094, Japan; t.kikuchi@gly.oups.ac.jp (T.K.); tanakar@gly.oups.ac.jp (R.T)
2 Medicinal Organic Chemistry Laboratory, College of Pharmaceutical Sciences, Ritsumeikan University, 1-1-1, Nojihigshi, Kusatsu, Shiga 525-8577, Japan; kajimoto@fc.ritsumei.ac.jp
* Correspondence: yamada@gly.oups.ac.jp; Tel./Fax: +81-726-90-1085

Received: 12 June 2018; Accepted: 27 June 2018; Published: 29 June 2018

Abstract: As part of research to search for antitumor agents in fungi originating from marine organisms, cephalimysins E–L were isolated from a culture broth of *Aspergillus fumigatus* that was separated from the marine fish *Mugil cephalus*. One- and two-dimensional nuclear magnetic resonance spectra revealed their planar structures, which are diastereomers of each other. Their absolute stereostructures were established by epimerization at C-8 with acidic methanol, nuclear Overhauser effect spectroscopy (NOESY), and circular dichroism (CD) spectroscopy. These demonstrated the detailed relationships between absolute configuration and CD Cotton effects. Additionally, in the growth inhibition assay against P388, HL-60, L1210, and KB cell lines, some of the fungal metabolites or reaction products exhibited moderate activities.

Keywords: cephalimysins; *Aspergillus fumigatus*; marine microorganism; *Mugil cephalus*; spiro-heterocyclic γ-lactam; circular dichroism spectroscopy; cytotoxicity

1. Introduction

Our group searched for active antitumor compounds in microorganisms in marine environments [1–4]. We previously reported the isolation and structure determination of FD-838 and its three diastereomers, referred to as cephalimysins B–D, from a culture broth of the fungal strain *A. fumigatus* OUPS-T106B-5, which lives on the stomach wall of a marine fish, *M. cephalus* [5]. Since FD-838 has three chiral centers, it should have eight stereoisomers. However, naturally occurring spiroheterocyclic-lactams, including FD-838 and cephalimysins B–D isolated from this fungal strain, had the *S* absolute configuration at the methoxy acetal carbon in common. The treatment of FD-838 and its diastereomers with acidic methanol could provide each epimer at the methoxy acetal carbon, and we succeeded in obtaining a set of all the stereoisomers of FD-838. Thus, we unambiguously established the relationship between the absolute configuration and the CD Cotton effects for the spirofuranone-lactam skeleton [5]. Based on the above method, we succeeded in correcting the absolute configuration of pseurotin A_2 reported by F. Z. Wang and co-workers in 2011 [6,7].

During a further search for novel active antitumor compounds from this fungal strain, we isolated eight new spiroheterocyclic-lactams designated as cephalimysins E–L (**1**–**8**), and their treatment with acidic methanol gave a set of eight unnatural forms (**1′**–**8′**) to afford sixteen stereoisomers. The isolation of many structural or stereoisomers from one source often indicates that their biosynthesis, stereochemistry, and bioactivity are worth investigating. As a part of this research, we hypothesized that **1**–**8** were produced from a plausible precursor with an olefin side chain such as pseurotin A [7], and examined the biosynthetic pathway for an intramolecular annulation reaction using molecular orbital calculations. This examination showed that compounds **1–8** were more stably produced from the plausible precursor with an *E*-olefin side chain than one with a *Z*-olefin side chain, and provided a rational explanation why C-2, C-3, and C-13, three chiral centers newly generated by an intramolecular annulation reaction, have all *S* or all *R* absolute configurations [8].

Herein, we report the details of the relationship between the absolute configuration of the above compounds and the CD Cotton effect as well as the elucidation of the relative configurations by nuclear Overhauser effect spectroscopy (NOESY) experiments. Additionally, their cytotoxic activity against murine P388 leukemia, human HL-60 leukemia, murine L1210 leukemia, and human KB epidermoid carcinoma cell lines is described.

2. Results and Discussion

An ethyl acetate extract of the culture broth of *A. fumigatus* OUPS-T106B-5 was fractionated, employing a stepwise combination of Sephadex LH-20 and silica gel column chromatography, and purification by reverse-phase HPLC afforded cephalimysins E–L (**1–8**) (Figure 1) as reported previously [8].

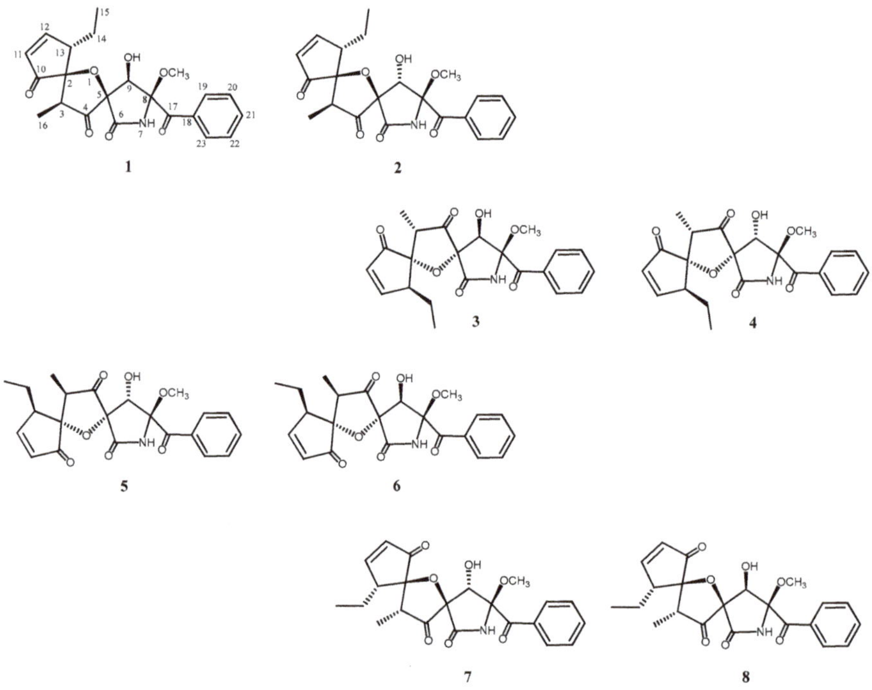

Figure 1. Structures of natural products from *A. fumigatus*.

Cephalimysins E–L (**1–8**) were assigned the same molecular formula, $C_{22}H_{23}NO_7$, based on deductions made from high-resolution fast atom bombardment mass spectral (HRFABMS) data. These ^{1}H and ^{13}C NMR spectra showed similar features except for differences in the chemical shifts at C-4, C-5, C-8, C-9, and C-10 (Tables 1 and 2), and HMBC analysis showed that they have the same planar structure. We previously isolated a series of diastereomers, cephalimysins B–D and FD-838, and reported their absolute stereostructures. Compounds **1–8** are a new series of diastereomers from the fungal metabolites, which have six chiral centers in their molecules.

Table 1. NMR Data for **1–4** in $CDCl_3$.

Position	1			2			3			4		
	δ_H [a]		δ_C	δ_H [a]		δ_C	δ_H [a]		δ_C	δ_H [a]		δ_C
1												
2			88.7 (s)			87.2 (s)			89.2 (s)			89.8 (s)
3	2.68	q	45.3 (d)	2.87	q	45.8 (d)	2.91	q	46.2 (d)	3.03	q	46.1 (d)
4			207.9 (s)			206.7 (s)			203.4 (s)			204.8 (s)
5			84.1 (s)			87.2 (s)			89.1 (s)			86.1 (s)
6			167.6 (s)			168.7 (s)			168.6 (s)			169.8 (s)
7	7.25	br s		6.65	br s		7.14	br s		7.12	br s	
8			91.6 (s)			87.8 (s)			90.8 (s)			94.8 (s)
9	4.15	d	73.9 (d)	4.54	s	82.1 (d)	4.36	d	76.1 (d)	4.95	d	76.4 (d)
10			204.0 (s)			204.5 (s)			211.0 (s)			209.0 (s)
11	6.28	dd	131.7 (d)	6.25	dd	131.5 (d)	6.23	dd	131.0 (d)	6.20	dd	130.9 (d)
12	7.78	dd	164.1 (d)	7.76	dd	164.7 (d)	7.84	dd	168.0 (d)	7.81	dd	167.1 (d)
13	3.10	ddq	52.2 (d)	3.09	ddt	51.9 (d)	3.12	ddt	51.1 (d)	3.16	ddt	50.2 (d)
14A	1.41	ddq	22.2 (t)	1.45	ddq	22.4 (t)	1.52	ddq	21.3 (t)	1.56	ddq	21.3 (t)
14B	1.91	dqd		1.90	dqd		1.97	dqd		2.00	d quint	
15	1.22	t	12.2 (q)	1.21	t	12.2 (q)	1.25	t	12.1 (q)	1.26	t	12.1 (q)
16	1.09	d	9.1 (q)	1.06	d	8.8 (q)	1.00	d	9.2 (q)	1.00	d	9.1 (q)
17			194.0 (s)			197.0 (s)			194.9 (s)			193.5 (s)
18			133.1 (s)			134.3 (s)			132.4 (s)			133.9 (s)
19	8.30	d	130.6 (d)	8.07	d	129.0 (d)	8.49	d	131.2 (d)	8.27	d	129.8 (d)
20	7.48	t	128.5 (d)	7.50	t	128.9 (d)	7.47	t	128.4 (d)	7.49	t	128.6 (d)
21	7.63	t	134.4 (d)	7.63	t	134.0 (d)	7.62	t	134.4 (d)	7.61	t	133.8 (d)
22	7.48	t	128.5 (d)	7.50	t	128.9 (d)	7.47	t	128.4 (d)	7.49	t	128.6 (d)
23	8.30	d	130.6 (d)	8.07	d	129.0 (d)	8.49	d	131.2 (d)	8.27	d	129.8 (d)
8-OCH_3	3.24	s	51.3 (q)	3.43	s	51.7 (q)	3.37	s	51.1 (q)	3.25	s	51.2 (q)
9-OH	3.53	d		5.05	br s		5.51	d		2.62	d	

a ^1H chemical shift values (δ ppm from $SiMe_4$) followed by multiplicity.

Table 2. NMR Data for **5**–**8** in $CDCl_3$.

Position	**5**			**6**			**7**			**8**		
	δ_H [a]		δ_C	δ_H [a]		δ_C	δ_H [a]		δ_C	δ_H [a]		δ_C
1												
2			87.0 (s)			86.3 (s)			88.5 (s)			89.4 (s)
3	2.88	q	44.0 (d)	2.90	q	45.6 (d)	3.09	q	47.2 (d)	3.19	q	46.2 (d)
4			202.7 (s)			205.0 (s)			209.4 (s)			205.8 (s)
5			85.1 (s)			88.9 (s)			83.0 (s)			85.0 (s)
6			168.7 (s)			167.7 (s)			170.5 (s)			169.4 (s)
7	7.32	br s		7.28	br s		7.14	br s		6.98	br s	
8			92.8 (s)			88.0 (s)			96.7 (s)			93.5 (s)
9	4.44	s	78.2 (d)	4.19	d	76.5 (d)	4.99	d	81.8 (d)	4.62	d	70.1 (d)
10			203.4 (s)			204.7 (s)			209.0 (s)			211.9 (s)
11	6.29	dd	131.6 (d)	6.27	dd	131.5 (d)	6.25	dd	131.1 (d)	6.27	dd	131.1 (d)
12	7.74	dd	164.4 (d)	7.74	dd	164.9 (d)	7.84	dd	167.4 (d)	7.84	dd	167.7 (d)
13	2.95	ddt	51.7 (d)	2.97	ddt	51.8 (d)	3.14	ddt	50.1 (d)	3.20	ddt	50.5 (d)
14A	1.54	ddq	22.3 (t)	1.43	ddq	22.4 (t)	1.54	ddq	21.2 (t)	1.56	ddq	21.0 (t)
14B	1.93	dqd		1.89	dqd		1.93	dqd		1.96	dqd	
15	1.14	t	12.3 (q)	1.15	t	12.2 (q)	1.22	t	12.2 (q)	1.25	t	12.1 (q)
16	1.10	d	8.7 (q)	1.06	d	8.6 (q)	0.97	d	8.6 (q)	0.96	d	8.8 (q)
17			192.2 (s)			194.1 (s)			192.7 (s)			194.1 (s)
18			133.9 (s)			132.9 (s)			133.9 (s)			132.7 (s)
19	8.20	d	129.5 (d)	8.18	d	130.2 (d)	8.25	d	129.7 (d)	8.48	d	131.2 (d)
20	7.49	t	128.7 (d)	7.48	t	128.7 (d)	7.48	t	128.6 (d)	7.49	t	128.4 (d)
21	7.62	t	134.0 (d)	7.63	t	134.3 (d)	7.61	t	133.8 (d)	7.63	t	134.4 (d)
22	7.49	t	128.7 (d)	7.48	t	128.7 (d)	7.48	t	128.6 (d)	7.49	t	128.4 (d)
23	8.20	d	129.5 (d)	8.18	d	130.2 (d)	8.25	d	129.7 (d)	8.48	d	131.2 (d)
8-OCH_3	3.25	s	50.9 (q)	3.38	s	51.2 (q)	3.20	s	51.2 (q)	3.33	s	51.8 (q)
9-OH	2.96	br s		3.55	d		4.44	d		4.52	d	

[a] As in Table 1.

As a first step toward examining their stereochemistry, we performed epimerization at C-8 with acidic methanol. We previously found that treatment of spiroheterocyclic-lactams with concentrated H_2SO_4 in MeOH reversed the absolute configuration at C-8, and the CD Cotton effect of the product showed an opposite sign to that of the reactant at a specific wavelength. Specifically, the CD spectra of cephalimysins B–D and FD-838 with an 8*S* configuration showed a negative Cotton effect at around 320 nm, whereas those of the reaction products, their 8*R* isomers, showed a positive Cotton effect at the same wavelength [5]. In this study, the same acid treatment of **1** gave the 8*R* isomer **5′** at a constant ratio (7.5%). The Cotton effects in the CD spectrum of **5′** reversed to positive at around 340 nm as shown by arrow in Figure 2. This result demonstrated that the Cotton effects at around 340 nm assigned the absolute configuration at C-8 in **1**; therefore, the negative Cotton effect ($\Delta\varepsilon_{340}$ −1.6) in the CD spectrum of **1** clearly indicated an *S* configuration at C-8 as for the cephalimysins isolated to date [5,7].

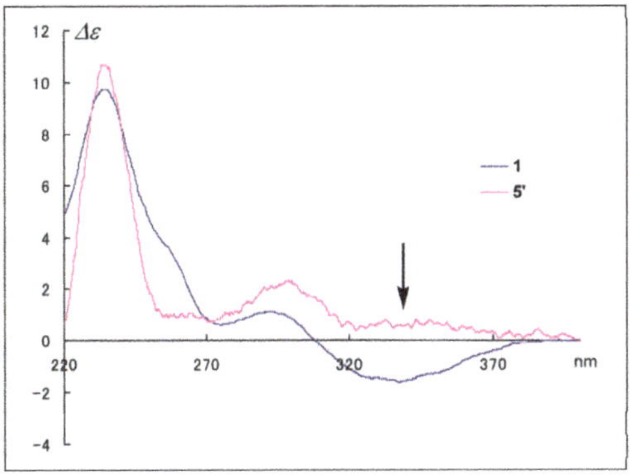

Figure 2. CD spectra of **1** and **5′**.

In the second step, the relative configuration between H-9 and 8-OCH_3 was deduced from the coupling constant between H-9 and 9-OH in the ^{1}H NMR spectrum. In the ^{1}H NMR spectrum of **1**, the coupling constant between H-9 and 9-OH was large (*J* = 12.6 Hz). This was due to a hydrogen bond between 9-OH and 8-OCH_3, which maintained the conformation of 9-OH; therefore, 9-OH was oriented *cis* to 8-OCH_3; i.e., **1** had the 9*R* configuration. Hayashi and co-workers reported that the hydrogen bond prevented racemization at C-9 in the last step of the synthesis of synerazol, which was the elimination of the protecting group [9].

In NOESY experiments of **1** as a final step, observed NOESY correlations (H-3/H-14 and H-16/H-14) revealed the relative configurations of C-2 and C-13. Additionally, when the H-9/H-3 and 9-OH/H-13 correlations were added, the relative configurations of C-2, C-3, C-5, C-9, and C-13 were deduced as shown in Figure 3. The above three steps demonstrated that **1** possessed the absolute configuration 2*S*,3*S*,5*R*,8*S*,9*R*,13*S*. In NOESY experiments with cephalimysins F–L (**2**–**8**), the observed NOESY correlations (H-3/H-14 and H-16/H-14) were the same as for **1**. Consequently, compounds **2**–**8** all have the same relative configuration of C-2, C-3, and C-13 as that of **1**. Additionally, the negative Cotton effects at around 340 nm in their CD spectra indicated that compounds **2**–**8** all possessed the 8*S* absolute configuration together with the natural spiroheterocyclic γ-lactams to date. If **1**–**8** are the stereoisomers at the two remaining stereogenic centers (C-5 and C-9), eight diastereomers cannot exist; therefore, we guessed that the absolute configurations at C-2, C-3, and C-13 formed two series (2*S*,3*S*,13*S* or 2*R*,3*R*,13*R*). For example, the acid treatment of **1** gave product **5′** as described above, for which the spectroscopic data were identical to that of **5** except that its $[\alpha]_D$ value ($[\alpha]_D$ −45.7) had the opposite sign to that of **5** ($[\alpha]_D$ +44.0). As expected, the same acid treatment transformed **2**, **3**, and **4** to 8-epimers **6′**, **7′**, and **8′** as enantiomers of **6**, **7**, and **8**, respectively. On the other hand, the same chemical transformation produced **1′** from **5**, **2′** from **6**, **3′** from **7**, and **4′** from **8**. CD spectra of the pairs of naturally occurring metabolites **1–8** and the reaction products **1′–8′** were observed with inverted signs (see a previous report [8] or Supplementary Materials, Figure S81), and demonstrated that compound **1–8** and **1′–8′** were the pairs of enantiomers, respectively. We then examined the absolute configuration at C-5 and C-9 in **2**, **3**, and **4** to match **1–8** to the eight assumed diastereomers shown in Figure 1. NOESY correlations for **2** (H-9/H-13, H-15, and 8-OCH_3) implied that **2** was an epimer of **1** at C-9, and the correlations for **3** (9-OH/H-16) implied that **3** was a epimer of **1** at C-5. Additionally, the NOESY correlations for **4** (H-9/H-16 and H-9/8-OCH_3) implied that **4** was a stereoisomer of **1** at C-5 and C-9.

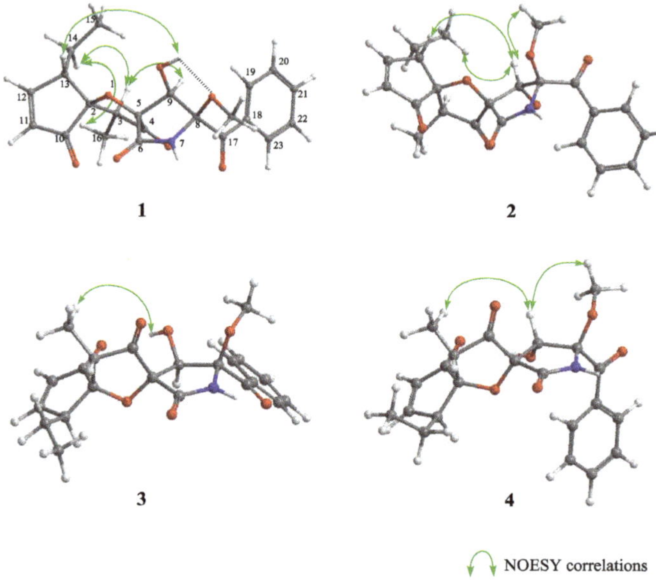

Figure 3. Key NOESY correlations of **1–4**.

The CD spectra of compounds **1–8** can be roughly divided into two groups according to the absolute configuration at C-2; i.e., 2*S*,3*S*,13*S* isomers as **1** showed positive Cotton effects (Figure 4A), while 2*R*,3*R*,13*R* isomers as **5** showed negative Cotton effects (Figure 4B) at around 240 ($\pi \rightarrow \pi^*$) and 290 ($n \rightarrow \pi^*$) nm, respectively. We deduced that the screw sense of chromophores between the carbonyl (C-4) and the enone moiety (C-10–C-12) determined the signs of the CD Cotton effects as shown in Figure 4; therefore, the absolute configurations at C-2, C-3, and C-13 for **2–4** and **6–8** were revealed; i.e., compounds **2–4** were2*S*,3*S*,13*S* isomers, and compounds **6–8** were 2*R*,3*R*,13*R* isomers. The above evidence, including the information provided from the transformation to 8-epimers **1′–8′**, revealed the absolute stereostructures of **1–8**. No additional stereoisomers of **1–8** were found despite the six chiral centers in the structure, although further purification was carried out. In a previous study, we studied the biosynthetic pathway for an intramolecular annelation reaction using molecular orbital calculations and concluded that the absolute configurations for C-2, C-3, and C-13 are either all *S* or all *R*.

We successfully isolated sixteen stereoisomers, including eight reaction products, and subsequently deduced the relationship between their stereochemistry and NMR chemical shifts as described below. The absolute configurations at C-2 and C-5 influenced the ^{13}C NMR chemical shift of the carbonyl group at C-10; i.e., in 2*S*,5*R* or 2*R*,5*S* isomers (**1**, **2**, **5**, and **6**), the carbonyl group (C-10) and the amido carbonyl group (C-6) are very close; therefore, the carbon signal at C-10 shifted to high field (δ_C around 204 ppm) by the anisotropic effect. The relationship between the chemical shift and the absolute configuration at C-5 and C-9 is similar to those in cephalimysins B–D and FD-838 [9]; i.e., the ^{13}C chemical shift at C-9 for the 5*R*,9*S* isomer (**2** and **7**) is observed in the maximum value (δ_C around 82 ppm) for the 5*R*,9*S* isomer (**2** and **7**), while that for the 5*R*,9*R* isomer (**1** and **8**) is observed in the minimum value (δ_C around 70 ppm). These findings, including the CD data, are useful for examining the stereochemistry of spirofuranone-lactams.

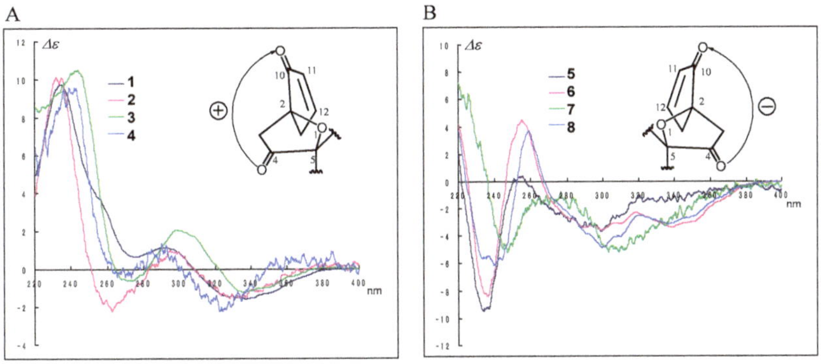

Figure 4. The difference of CD spectra of **1–4** twisting clockwise (**A**) and **5–8** twisting counterclockwise (**B**) between the carbonyl (C-4) and the enone moiety (C-10–C-12).

As a primary screening for antitumor activity, the inhibitory properties of natural products **1–8** and enantiomers **1′–8′** toward cancer cell growth were examined using murine P388 leukemia, human HL-60 leukemia, murine L1210 leukemia, and human KB epidermoid carcinoma cell lines. All compounds except **3′** and **6′** exhibited potent or moderate activity against the cell lines (Table 3). Compounds **3** and **6** exhibited the strongest activities (11.1 μM and 7.0 μM, respectively), equal to that of 5-fluorouracil against the KB cell line. Interestingly, **3′** and **6′**, the enantiomers of **3** and **6**, did not inhibit cell growth. To determine the bioactivity mechanism, molecular target screening for inhibitory effects on histone deacetylases, protein kinases, telomerases, and farnecyltransferases will be needed

Table 3. Cytotoxicity assay against P388, HL-60, L1210, and KB cells.

Compounds	Cell line P388 IC_{50} (μM) [a]	Cell line HL-60 IC_{50} (μM) [a]	Cell line L1210 IC_{50} (μM) [a]	Cell line KB IC_{50} (μM) [a]
1	58.5	57.9	60.5	33.9
2	56.9	55.7	62.2	60.5
3	26.6	15.7	58.1	11.1
4	55.2	52.5	12.8	35.1
5	69.0	55.2	14.3	31.5
6	51.2	50.8	57.6	7.0
7	56.9	53.9	22.5	53.3
8	57.5	58.1	60.5	52.1
1′	56.4	54.9	59.3	118.6
2′	53.5	67.8	55.9	198.5
3′	>200	>200	64.4	>200
4′	50.8	53.1	20.5	42.4
5′	54.5	55.7	20.3	53.0
6′	>200	>200	92.0	>200
7′	52.1	52.9	14.5	26.6
8′	53.3	54.5	12.3	52.3
5-fluorouracil [b]	2.8	3.2	2.0	8.5

[a] DMSO was used as vehicle; [b] Positive control.

3. Conclusions

In this study, we established the detailed relationships between absolute configuration and CD Cotton effects for new natural products, cephalimysins E–L (**1**–**8**), isolated a fungal strain separated from a marine fish together with unnatural products **1′**–**8′**. This result agreed well with the consideration derived from the orbital molecular calculation in the previous report [8]. In addition, the growth inhibition assay using P388, HL-60, L1210, and KB cell lines could not give the information of a structure-activity relationship well; however, **3** and **6** against KB cell, and **4**, **5**, **7′**, and **8′** against L1210 exhibited moderate activities.

4. Experimental Section

4.1. General Experimental Procedures

NMR spectra were recorded on an Agilent-NMR-vnmrs (Agilent Technologies, Santa Clara, CA, USA) 600 with tetramethylsilane (TMS) as an internal reference. FABMS was recorded using a JEOL JMS-7000 mass spectrometer (JEOL, Tokyo, Japan). IR spectra was recorded on a JASCO FT/IR-680 Plus (Tokyo, Japan). Optical rotations were measured using a JASCO DIP-1000 digital polarimeter (Tokyo, Japan). Silica gel 60 (230–400 mesh, Nacalai Tesque, Inc., Kyoto, Japan) was used for column chromatography with medium pressure. ODS HPLC was run on a JASCO PU-1586 (Tokyo, Japan) equipped with a differential refractometer RI-1531 (Tokyo, Japan) and Cosmosil Packed Column $5C_{18}$-MSII (25 cm × 20 mm i.d., Nacalai Tesque, Inc., Kyoto, Japan). Analytical TLC was performed on precoated Merck aluminum sheets (DC-Alufolien Kieselgel 60 F254, 0.2 mm, Merck, Darmstadt, Germany) with the solvent system CH_2Cl_2–MeOH (19:1) (Nacalai Tesque, Inc., Kyoto, Japan), and compounds were viewed under a UV lamp (AS ONE Co., Ltd., Osaka, Japan) and sprayed with 10% H_2SO_4 (Nacalai Tesque, Inc., Kyoto, Japan) followed by heating.

4.2. Fungal Material

A strain of *A. fumigatus* was initially isolated from a piece of the marine alga *Undaria pinnatifida* collected at collected in Osaka bay, Japan in May 2015. The fungal strain was identified by Techno Suruga Laboratory Co., Ltd., Shizuoka, Japan. The surface of the marine alga was wiped with EtOH (Nacalai Tesque, Inc., Kyoto, Japan) and its snip applied to the surface of nutrient agar layered in a Petri dish. Serial transfers of one of the resulting colonies provided a pure strain of *A. fumigatus*.

4.3. Culturing and Isolation of Metabolites

A strain of *A. fumigatus* was initially isolated from the marine fish *Mugil cephalus* captured in Katsuura Bay, Japan in October 2000. The fish was disinfected with EtOH and its gastrointestinal tract applied to the surface of nutrient agar layered in a Petri dish. Serial transfers of one of the resulting colonies provided a pure strain of *A. fumigatus*. The fungal strain was cultured at 27 °C for 6 weeks in a liquid medium (75 L) containing 1% soluble starch and 0.1% casein in 50% artificial seawater adjusted to pH 7.4. The culture was filtered under suction, and the culture filtrate was extracted three times with EtOAc (Nacalai Tesque, Inc., Kyoto, Japan). The combined extracts were evaporated in vacuo to afford a mixture of crude metabolites (18.8 g) that exhibited cytotoxicity against the P388 cell line (IC_{50} < 1 g/mL). The EtOAc extract was passed through a Sephadex LH-20 (GE Healthcare Japan, Tokyo, Japan) column using $CHCl_3$–MeOH (1:1) (Nacalai Tesque, Inc., Kyoto, Japan) as the eluent. The second fraction (14.6 g), exhibiting strong activity, was chromatographed on a silica gel column with a $CHCl_3$–MeOH gradient as the eluent to afford Fr. 1 (the 100% $CHCl_3$ eluate, 1.2 g) and Fr. 2 (the 1% MeOH in $CHCl_3$ eluate, 1.7 g). Fr. 1 was purified by HPLC using MeOH–H_2O (70:30) as the eluent to afford Fr. 3 (48.3 mg) and Fr. 4 (20.3 mg). Fr. 2 was purified by HPLC using MeOH–H_2O (70:30) as the eluent to afford Fr. 5 (359.0 mg) and Fr. 6 (263.7 mg). Fr. 3 was purified by ODS HPLC using MeCN–H_2O (45:55) as the eluent to afford Fr. 7 (2.8 mg) and Fr. 8 (2.1 mg). Fr. 7 and Fr. 8 were further purified by HPLC using MeCN–H_2O (43:57) as the eluent to afford **4** (1.1 mg, 0.006%) and **7**

(0.4 mg, 0.002%), respectively. Fr. 4 was purified by ODS HPLC using MeCN (Nacalai Tesque, Inc., Kyoto, Japan)–H_2O (45:55) as the eluent to afford Fr. 9 (4.5 mg) and Fr. 10 (3.5 mg). Fr. 9 and Fr. 10 were further purified by HPLC using MeCN–H_2O (40:60) as the eluent to afford **8** (2.0 mg, 0.011%) and **3** (1.8 mg, 0.009%), respectively. Fr. 5 was purified by ODS HPLC using MeCN–H_2O (45:55) as the eluent to afford Fr. 11 (17.1 mg) and Fr. 12 (4.5 mg). Fr. 11 was further purified by HPLC using MeCN–H_2O (30:70) as the eluent to afford **2** (0.8 mg, 0.004%). Fr. 12 was further purified by HPLC using MeCN–H_2O (40:60) as the eluent to afford **5** (0.3 mg, 0.002). Fr. 6 was purified by ODS HPLC using MeCN–H_2O (45:55) as the eluent to afford Fr. 13 (4.5 mg) and Fr. 14 (4.0 mg). Fr. 13 was further purified by HPLC using MeCN–H_2O (38:62) as the eluent to afford **6** (1.4 mg, 0.007%). Fr. 14 was further purified by HPLC using MeCN–H_2O (40:60) as the eluent to afford **1** (2.2 mg, 0.011%).

Cephalimysin E (1). Pale yellow oil; $[\alpha]_D^{24}$ +69.1 (*c* 0.16, EtOH); IR (liquid) ν_{max} 3342, 2923, 1770, 1729, 1680, 1596, 1490 cm^{-1}; UV (EtOH) λ_{max} (log ε) 249 (3.29), 288 (2.81), 343 (2.44) nm; NMR data, see Table 1 and Table S1 (Supplementary Materials); FABMS *m/z* (rel int) 414 ($[M + H]^+$, 100.0), 382 ($[M - OCH_3]^+$, 25.2); HRFABMS *m/z* 414.1554 $[M + H]^+$ (calcd for $C_{22}H_{24}NO_7$ 414.1552); CD (*c* 2.60 × 10^{-4} M, EtOH) λ_{max} ($\Delta\varepsilon$) 340 (−1.6), 292 (1.1), 234 (9.7) nm.

Cephalimysin F (2). Pale yellow oil; $[\alpha]_D^{24}$ +17.1 (*c* 0.10, EtOH); IR (liquid) ν_{max} 3274, 2923, 1771, 1731, 1700, 1615, 1597, 1580 cm^{-1}; UV (EtOH) λ_{max} (log ε) 242 (3.93), 284 (3.17), 334 (2.68) nm; NMR data, see Table 1 and Table S2 (Supplementary Materials); FABMS *m/z* (rel int) 436 ($[M + Na]^+$, 8.2); HRFABMS *m/z* 436.1369 $[M + Na]^+$ (calcd for $C_{22}H_{23}NO_7Na$ 436.1372); CD (*c* 1.94 × 10^{-4} M, EtOH) λ_{max} ($\Delta\varepsilon$) 331 (−1.6), 295 (1.0), 235 (10.0) nm.

Cephalimysin G (3). Pale yellow oil; $[\alpha]_D^{24}$ +77.7 (*c* 0.15, EtOH); IR (liquid) ν_{max} 3330, 2937, 1769, 1729, 1682, 1625, 1597, 1579 cm^{-1}; UV (EtOH) λ_{max} (log ε) 248 (3.86), 284 (3.43), 334 (3.28) nm; NMR data, see Table 1 and Table S3 (Supplementary Materials); FABMS *m/z* (rel int) 436 ($[M + Na]^+$, 76.4), 382 ($[M - OCH_3]^+$, 100.0); HRFABMS *m/z* 436.1375 $[M + Na]^+$ (calcd for $C_{22}H_{23}NO_7Na$ 436.1372); CD (*c* 1.97 × 10^{-4} M, EtOH) λ_{max} ($\Delta\varepsilon$) 336 (−1.2), 299 (1.8), 241 (10.3) nm.

Cephalimysin H (4). Pale yellow oil; $[\alpha]_D^{24}$ +110.1 (*c* 0.13, EtOH); IR (liquid) ν_{max} 3322, 2925, 1764, 1731, 1695, 1615, 1597, 1579 cm^{-1}; UV (EtOH) λ_{max} (log ε) 241 (4.05), 285 (3.17), 332 (2.71) nm; NMR data, see Table 1 and Table S4 (Supplementary Materials); FABMS *m/z* (rel int) 414 ($[M + H]^+$, 7.89), 382 ($[M - OCH_3]^+$, 39.85); HRFABMS *m/z* 414.1562 $[M + H]^+$ (calcd for $C_{22}H_{24}NO_7$ 414.1552); CD (*c* 1.09 × 10^{-4} M, EtOH) λ_{max} ($\Delta\varepsilon$) 323 (−2.2), 292 (1.2), 238 (9.5) nm.

Cephalimysin I (5). Pale yellow oil; $[\alpha]_D^{24}$ −45.7 (*c* 0.15, EtOH); IR (liquid) ν_{max} 3333, 2932, 1770, 1732, 1691, 1621, 1597, 1577 cm^{-1}; UV (EtOH) λ_{max} (log ε) 241 (4.08), 283 (3.67), 349 (3.23) nm; NMR data, see Table 2 and Table S5 (Supplementary Materials); FABMS *m/z* (rel int) 414 ($[M + H]^+$, 100.0), 382 ($[M-OCH_3]^+$, 7.87); HRFABMS *m/z* 414.1560 $[M + H]^+$ (calcd for $C_{22}H_{24}NO_7$ 414.1552); CD (*c* 1.99 × 10^{-4} M, EtOH) λ_{max} ($\Delta\varepsilon$) 335 (−1.6), 299 (−3.6), 234 (−9.5) nm.

Cephalimysin J (6). Pale yellow oil; $[\alpha]_D^{24}$ −36.9 (*c* 0.16, EtOH); IR (liquid) ν_{max} 3334, 2967, 1770, 1731, 1679, 1639, 1596, 1580 cm^{-1}; UV (EtOH) λ_{max} (log ε) 248 (3.76), 289 (3.10), 337 (3.06) nm; NMR data, see Table 2 and Table S6 (Supplementary Materials); FABMS *m/z* (rel int) 436 ($[M + Na]^+$, 100.0); HRFABMS *m/z* 436.1368 $[M + Na]^+$ (calcd for $C_{22}H_{23}NO_7Na$ 436.1372); CD (*c* 1.22 × 10^{-4} M, EtOH) λ_{max} ($\Delta\varepsilon$) 335 (−3.2), 299 (−3.6), 236 (−8.4) nm.

Cephalimysin K (7). Pale yellow oil; $[\alpha]_D^{24}$ −76.5 (*c* 0.06, EtOH); IR (liquid) ν_{max} 3325, 2924, 1767, 1717, 1695, 1616, 1595, 1576 cm^{-1}; UV (EtOH) λ_{max} (log ε) 240(4.07), 286 (3.41), 344 (3.02) nm; NMR data, see Table 2 and Table S7 (Supplementary Materials); FABMS *m/z* (rel int) 414 ($[M + H]^+$, 6.14), 382 ($[M - OCH_3]^+$, 57.67); HRFABMS *m/z* 414.1553 $[M + H]^+$ (calcd for $C_{22}H_{24}NO_7$ 414.1552) ; CD (*c* 1.06 × 10^{-4} M, EtOH) λ_{max} ($\Delta\varepsilon$) 335 (−3.2), 303 (−5.2), 247 (−5.2) nm.

Cephalimysin L (8). Pale yellow oil; $[\alpha]_D^{24}$ −18.6 (*c* 0.03, EtOH); IR (liquid) ν_{max} 3304, 2938, 1768, 1722, 1698, 1624, 1597, 1579 cm^{-1}; UV (EtOH) λ_{max} (log ε) 246 (3.96), 285 (3.54), 334 (3.53) nm; NMR data, see Table 2 and Table S8 (Supplementary Materials); FABMS m/z (rel int) 414 ([M + H]$^+$, 26.6), 382 ([M − OCH_3]$^+$, 100.0); HRFABMS m/z 414.1562 [M + H]$^+$ (calcd for $C_{22}H_{24}NO_7$ 414.1552); CD (*c* 8.33 × 10^{-5} M, EtOH) λ_{max} ($\Delta\varepsilon$) 336 (−3.2), 300 (−4.8), 240 (−6.1) nm.

4.4. Epimerization at C-8 in the Natural Occurred Compounds

Transformation of 1 to 5′: To a solution of cephalimysin E (**1**) (5.3 mg, 0.013 mmol) in MeOH (1.0 mL) was added concd H_2SO_4 (0.01 mL), and the reaction mixture was left at room temperature for 7 h. The mixture was diluted with water and extracted with diethyl ether, and the extract was evaporated under reduced pressure, and then the residue was purified by HPLC using MeCN–H_2O (38:62) as the eluent to afford **1** (2.7 mg, 50.9%) and **5′** (0.4 mg, 7.5%).
5′: pale yellow oil; $[\alpha]_D^{24}$ +44.0 (*c* 0.03, EtOH); CD (*c* 3.23 × 10^{-4} M, EtOH) λ_{max} nm ($\Delta\varepsilon$) 336 (0.6), 298 (2.3), 234 (10.7).

Transformation of 2 to 6′: Using the same procedure as above with **1**, a solution of cephalimysin F (**2**) (2.5 mg, 0.006 mmol) in MeOH (1.0 mL) was treated with concd H_2SO_4 (0.01 mL) and purified by HPLC using MeCN–H_2O (35:65) as the eluent to afford **2** (0.5 mg, 20.0%) and **6′** (0.6 mg, 24.0%).
6′: pale yellow oil; $[\alpha]_D^{24}$ +36.4 (*c* 0.02, EtOH); CD (*c* 3.15 × 10^{-5} M, EtOH) λ_{max} nm ($\Delta\varepsilon$) 336 (2.9), 300 (3.8), 236 (8.0).

Transformation of 3 to 7′: Using the same procedure as above with **1**, a solution of cephalimysin G (**3**) (6.1 mg, 0.015 mmol) in MeOH (1.0 mL) was treated with concd H_2SO_4 (0.01 mL) and purified by HPLC using MeCN–H_2O (43:57) as the eluent to afford **3** (3.1 mg, 50.8%) and **7′** (1.5 mg, 24.6%).
7′: pale yellow oil; $[\alpha]_D^{24}$ +76.3 (*c* 0.11, EtOH); CD (*c* 1.96 × 10^{-4} M, EtOH) λ_{max} nm ($\Delta\varepsilon$) 334 (2.1), 305 (3.1), 245 (6.1).

Transformation of 4 to 8′: Using the same procedure as above with **1**, a solution of cephalimysin H (**4**) (4.4 mg, 0.011 mmol) in MeOH (1.0 mL) was treated with concd H_2SO_4 (0.01 mL) and purified by HPLC using MeCN–H_2O (43:57) as the eluent to afford **4** (1.4 mg, 31.8%) and **8′** (0.4 mg, 9.1%).
8′: pale yellow oil; $[\alpha]_D^{24}$ +19.6 (*c* 0.05, EtOH); CD (*c* 6.47 × 10^{-5} M, EtOH) λ_{max} nm ($\Delta\varepsilon$) 337 (2.2), 300 (4.3), 240 (6.4).

Transformation of 5 to 1′: Using the same procedure as above with **1**, a solution of cephalimysin I (**5**) (4.5 mg, 0.011 mmol) in MeOH (1.0 mL) was treated with concd H_2SO_4 (0.01 mL) and purified by HPLC using MeCN–H_2O (40:60) as the eluent to afford **5** (1.1 mg, 24.4%) and **1′** (0.4 mg, 8.9%).
1′: pale yellow oil; $[\alpha]_D^{24}$ −64.0 (*c* 0.003, EtOH); CD (*c* 3.05 × 10^{-4} M, EtOH) λ_{max} nm ($\Delta\varepsilon$) 338 (1.2), 292 (−1.9), 233 (10.2).

Transformation of 6 to 2′: Using the same procedure as above with **1**, a solution of cephalimysin J (**6**) (3.7 mg, 0.009 mmol) in MeOH (1.0 mL) was treated with concd H_2SO_4 (0.01 mL) and purified by HPLC using MeCN–H_2O (36: 64) as the eluent to afford **6** (1.8 mg, 48.6%) and **2′** (0.2 mg, 5.4%).
2′: pale yellow oil; $[\alpha]_D^{24}$ −17.9 (*c* 0.07, EtOH); CD (*c* 1.15 × 10^{-4} M, EtOH) λ_{max} nm ($\Delta\varepsilon$) 332 (1.8), 286 (−2.9), 234 (10.6).

Transformation of 7 to 3′: Using the same procedure as above with **1**, a solution of cephalimysin K (**7**) (3.3 mg, 0.008 mmol) in MeOH (1.0 mL) was treated with concd H_2SO_4 (0.01 mL) and purified by HPLC using MeCN–H_2O (43:57) as the eluent to afford **7** (1.0 mg, 30.3%) and **3′** (0.4 mg, 12.1%).
3′: pale yellow oil; $[\alpha]_D^{24}$ −78.7 (*c* 0.01, EtOH); CD (*c* 2.57 × 10^{-4} M, EtOH) λ_{max} nm ($\Delta\varepsilon$) 335 (1.4), 298 (−2.3), 241 (−9.9).

Transformation of 8 to 4′: Using the same procedure as above with **1**, a solution of cephalimysin L (**8**) (7.2 mg, 0.017 mmol) in MeOH (1.0 mL) was treated with concd H_2SO_4 (0.01 mL) and purified by HPLC using MeCN–H_2O (45:55) as the eluent to afford **8** (1.2 mg, 16.7%) and **4′** (1.1 mg, 15.3%).
4′: pale yellow oil; $[\alpha]_D^{24}$ −112.0 (*c* 0.13, EtOH); CD (*c* 1.91 × 10^{-4} M, EtOH) λ_{max} nm ($\Delta\varepsilon$) 329 (2.0), 289 (−2.4), 238 (10.6).

4.5. Assay for Cytotoxicity

Cytotoxic activities of cephalimysins E–L (**1**–**8**), and epimers (**1′**–**8′**) were examined with the 3-(4,5-dimethyl-2-thiazolyl)-2,5-diphenyl-2H-tetrazolium bromide (MTT) method. P388, HL-60, L1210, and KB cells were cultured in RPMI 1640 Medium (10% fetal calf serum) at 37 °C in 5% CO_2. The test material was dissolved in DMSO to give a concentration of 10 mM, and the solution was diluted with the Essential Medium to yield concentrations of 200, 20, and 2 μM, respectively. Each sample solution (100 μL) was combined with each cell suspension (1×10^5 cells/mL, 100 μL) in the medium to make finally concentrations of 100, 10, and 1 μM, respectively. After incubating at 37 °C for 72 h in 5% CO_2, grown cells were labeled with 5 mg/mL MTT in phosphate buffered saline (PBS), and the absorbance of formazan dissolved in 20% sodium dodecyl sulfate (SDS) in 0.1 N HCl was measured at 540 nm with a microplate reader. Each absorbance value was expressed as percentage relative to that of the control cell suspension that was prepared without the test substance using the same procedure as that described above. All assays were performed three times, semilogarithmic plots were constructed from the averaged data, and the effective dose of the substance required to inhibit cell growth by 50% (IC_{50}) was determined.

Supplementary Materials: The following are available online at http://www.mdpi.com/1660-3397/16/7/223/s1, Table S1: Spectral data including 2D NMR data for **1**, Table S2: Spectral data including 2D NMR data for **2**, Table S3: Spectral data including 2D NMR data for **3**, Table S4: Spectral data including 2D NMR data for **4**, Table S5: Spectral data including 2D NMR data for **5**, Table S6: Spectral data including 2D NMR data for **6**, Table S7: Spectral data including 2D NMR data for **7**, Table S8: Spectral data including 2D NMR data for **8**, Figure S1: ^1H and ^{13}C NMR spectrum of **1** in $CDCl_3$, Figure S2: ^1H-^1H COSY of **1**, Figure S3: NOESY of **1**, Figure S4: HMQC of **1**, Figure S5: HMBC of **1**, Figure S6: IR Spectrum of **1**, Figure S7: FABMS of **1**, Figure S8: ^1H and ^{13}C NMR spectrum of **2** in $CDCl_3$, Figure S9: ^1H-^1H COSY of **2**, Figure S10: NOESY of **2**, Figure S11: HMQC of **2**, Figure S12: HMBC of **2**, Figure S13: IR Spectrum of **2**, Figure S14: FABMS of **2**, Figure S15: ^1H and ^{13}C NMR spectrum of **3** in $CDCl_3$, Figure S16: ^1H-^1H COSY of **3**, Figure S17: NOESY of **3**, Figure S18: HMQC of **3**, Figure S19: HMBC of **3**, Figure S20: IR Spectrum of **3**, Figure S21: FABMS of **3**, Figure S22: ^1H and ^{13}C NMR spectrum of **4** in $CDCl_3$, Figure S23: ^1H-^1H COSY of **4**, Figure S24: NOESY of **4**, Figure S25: HMQC of **4**, Figure S26: HMBC of **4**, Figure S27: IR Spectrum of **4**, Figure S28: FABMS of **4**, Figure S29: ^1H and ^{13}C NMR spectrum of **5** in $CDCl_3$, Figure S30: ^1H-^1H COSY of **5**, Figure S31: NOESY of **5**, Figure S32: HMQC of **5**, Figure S33: HMBC of **5**, Figure S34: IR Spectrum of **5**, Figure S35: FABMS of **5**, Figure S36: ^1H and ^{13}C NMR spectrum of **6** in $CDCl_3$, Figure S37: ^1H-^1H COSY of **6**, Figure S38: NOESY of **6**, Figure S39: HMQC of **6**, Figure S40: HMBC of **6**, Figure S41: IR Spectrum of **6**, Figure S42: FABMS of **6**, Figure S43: ^1H and ^{13}C NMR spectrum of **7** in $CDCl_3$, Figure S44: ^1H-^1H COSY of **7**, Figure S45: NOESY of **7**, Figure S46: HMQC of **7**, Figure S47: HMBC of **7**, Figure S48: IR Spectrum of **7**, Figure S49: FABMS of **7**, Figure S50: ^1H and ^{13}C NMR spectrum of **8** in $CDCl_3$, Figure S51: ^1H-^1H COSY of **8**, Figure S52: NOESY of **8**, Figure S53: HMQC of **8**, Figure S54: HMBC of **8**, Figure S55: IR Spectrum of **8**, Figure S56: FABMS of **8**, Figure S57: ^1H NMR spectrum of **1′** in $CDCl_3$, Figure S58: ^1H NMR spectrum of **2′** in $CDCl_3$, Figure S59: ^1H NMR spectrum of **3′** in $CDCl_3$, Figure S60: ^1H NMR spectrum of **4′** in $CDCl_3$, Figure S61: ^1H NMR spectrum of **5′** in $CDCl_3$, Figure S62: ^1H NMR spectrum of **6′** in $CDCl_3$, Figure S63: ^1H NMR spectrum of **7′** in $CDCl_3$, Figure S64: ^1H NMR spectrum of **8′** in $CDCl_3$, Figure S65: HPLC purification of Compound **1**, Figure S66: HPLC purification of Compound **2**, Figure S67: HPLC purification of Compound **3**, Figure S68: HPLC purification of Compound **4**, Figure S69: HPLC purification of Compound **5**, Figure S70: HPLC purification of Compound **6**, Figure S71: HPLC purification of Compound **7**, Figure S72: HPLC purification of Compound **8**, Figure S73: HPLC purification of Compound **5′**, Figure S74: HPLC purification of Compound **6′**, Figure S75: HPLC purification of Compound **7′**, Figure S76: HPLC purification of Compound **8′**, Figure S77: HPLC purification of Compound **1′**, Figure S78: HPLC purification of Compound **2′**, Figure S79: HPLC purification of Compound **3′**, Figure S80: HPLC purification of Compound **4′**, Figure S81: The CD spectra of the 16 stereoisomers **1**–**8** and **1′**–**8′**, symmetrical Cotton effects between enantiomers.

Author Contributions: Conceived and designed the experiments: T.Y., T.K. (Tetsuya Kajimoto), T.K. (Takashi Kikuchi), and R.T.; Performed the experiments: T.Y.; Analyzed the data: T.Y.; and Wrote the paper: T.Y.

Funding: This research received no external funding.

Acknowledgments: We thank Endo (Kanazawa University) for supply of the cancer cells. We are grateful to M. Fujitake and K. Minoura of this university for MS and NMR measurements, respectively.

Conflicts of Interest: The authors declare no conflict of interest.

References

1. Kitano, M.; Yamada, T.; Amagata, T.; Minoura, K.; Tanaka, R.; Numata, A. Novel pyridinopyrone sesquiterpene type pileotin produced by a sea urchin-derived *Aspergillus* sp. *Tetrahedron Lett.* **2012**, *53*, 4192–4194. [CrossRef]
2. Yamada, T.; Mizutani, Y.; Umebayashi, Y.; Inno, N.; Kawashima, M.; Kikuchi, T.; Tanaka, R. A novel ketoaldehyde decalin derivative, produced by a marine sponge-derived *Trichoderma harzianum*. *Tetrahedron Lett.* **2014**, *55*, 662–664. [CrossRef]
3. Suzue, M.; Kikuchi, T.; Tanaka, R.; Yamada, T. Tandyukisins E and F, novel cytotoxic decalin derivatives isolated from a marine sponge-derived fungus. *Tetrahedron Lett.* **2016**, *57*, 5070–5073. [CrossRef]
4. Yamada, T.; Suzue, M.; Arai, T.; Kikuchi, T.; Tanaka, R. Trichodermanins C–E, new diterpenes with a fused 6-5-6-6 ring system produced by a marine sponge-derived fungus. *Mar. Drugs* **2017**, *15*, 169. [CrossRef] [PubMed]
5. Yamada, T.; Kitada, H.; Kajimoto, T.; Numata, A.; Tanaka, R. The relationship between the CD Cotton effect and the absolute configuration of FD-838 and its seven stereoisomers. *J. Org. Chem.* **2010**, *75*, 4146–4153. [CrossRef] [PubMed]
6. Wang, F.Z.; Li, D.H.; Zhu, T.J.; Zhang, M.; Gu, Q.Q. Pseurotin A_1 and A_2, two new 1-oxa-7-azaspiro[4.4]non-2-ene-4,6-diones from the holothurian-derived fungus *Aspergillus fumigatus* WFZ-25. *Can. J. Chem.* **2011**, *89*, 72–76. [CrossRef]
7. Yamada, T.; Ohshima, M.; Yuasa, K.; Kikuchi, T.; Tanaka, R. Assignment of the CD cotton effect to the chiral center in pseurotins, and the stereochemical revision of pseurotin A2. *Mar. Drugs* **2016**, *14*, e74. [CrossRef] [PubMed]
8. Yamada, T.; Kimura, H.; Arimutsu, K.; Kajimoto, T.; Kikuchi, T.; Tanaka, R. Absolute configuration of eight cephalimysins isolated from the marine-derived *Aspergillus fumigatus*. *ChemistrySelect* **2017**, *2*, 10936–10940. [CrossRef]
9. Hayashi, Y.; Shoji, M.; Mukaiyama, T.; Gotoh, H.; Yamaguchi, S.; Nakata, M.; Kakeya, H.; Osada, H. First asymmetric total synthesis of synerazol, an antifungal antibiotic, and determination of its absolute stereochemistry. *J. Org. Chem.* **2005**, *70*, 5643–5654. [CrossRef] [PubMed]

© 2018 by the authors. Licensee MDPI, Basel, Switzerland. This article is an open access article distributed under the terms and conditions of the Creative Commons Attribution (CC BY) license (http://creativecommons.org/licenses/by/4.0/).

marine drugs

Article

Absolute Configuration Determination of Retroflexanone Using the Advanced Mosher Method and Application of HPLC-NMR

Caleb Singleton, Robert Brkljača and Sylvia Urban *

School of Science (Applied Chemistry and Environmental Science), RMIT University, GPO Box 2476, Melbourne, VIC 3001, Australia; caleb.taicho@gmail.com (C.S.); robert.brkljaca@rmit.edu.au (R.B.)
* Correspondence: sylvia.urban@rmit.edu.au

Received: 23 May 2018; Accepted: 7 June 2018; Published: 12 June 2018

Abstract: The absolute configuration of retroflexanone (**1**) and a closely related phlorogluinol (**2**) was established using the advanced Mosher method and by application of HPLC-NMR. HPLC-NMR permitted a small scale Mosher method analysis to be carried out on these unstable phloroglucinols.

Keywords: Mosher; retroflexanone; phloroglucinol; HPLC-NMR; secondary alcohol

1. Introduction

Retroflexanone (**1**) was recently reported from the dichloromethane extract of *Cystophora retroflexa* [1] using a combination of HPLC-NMR and HPLC-MS [2] while undertaking a phytochemical study of various southern Australian marine algae. Retroflexanone (**1**) contains a single stereogenic centre at the secondary alcohol, but to date, no efforts to confirm its absolute configuration have been undertaken. The Mosher ester analysis which was superseded by the advanced (or modified) Mosher ester analysis became a standard spectroscopic method for the determination of the absolute configuration of secondary alcohols [3–7]. The method relies upon comparing the changes and differences in chemical shifts observed in the ^{1}H NMR spectra of the prepared Mosher esters to those of the original natural product containing the secondary alcohol [3,5]. By observing the chemical shifts of each proton in the original secondary alcohol and each of the two prepared esters, the δ^{SR} value is able to be calculated for each individual proton. This value is simply the chemical shift of the protons in the natural product that is reacted with (*R*)-MTPA (which results in the *S*-MTPA derivative) subtracted from the chemical shift of the protons in the natural product that is reacted with (*S*)-MTPA (which results in the *R*-MTPA derivative). The changes in chemical shifts, together with consideration of the Cahn-Ingold-Prelog priority rules, allow for the absolute configuration to be elucidated.

Preliminary work carried out on this and related marine algae [1,8] indicated that retroflexanone (**1**) was significantly unstable and would most likely be unable to be purified directly from the crude extract in large quantities to perform the traditional advanced Mosher ester analysis.

In an attempt to address the supply and stability issues of retroflexanone (**1**), it was proposed to undertake the advanced Mosher method of retroflexanone, which was present in an enriched fraction, and then conduct HPLC-NMR to determine the absolute configuration by noting the changes in the ^{1}H NMR chemical shifts. The advanced or modified Mosher method has previously been carried out using HPLC-NMR in cases where only small amounts of compound were available [9–11]. In these instances, small amounts of compound were reacted with the Mosher reagents, and then subsequently purified, and ^{1}H NMR data acquired using HPLC-NMR.

This current work represents the fourth instance of the use of HPLC-NMR being used in conjunction with the advanced Mosher method to deduce the absolute configuration of a natural product [9–11]. The absolute configuration of the previously reported phloroglucinol (**2**) was determined by application of the advanced Mosher method on an enriched fraction followed by HPLC-NMR analysis of the mixture. The absolute configuration of retroflexanone (**1**) was determined after isolation of small quantities, application of the advanced Mosher method, followed by HPLC-NMR analysis. HPLC-NMR was essential for the determination of the absolute configuration of retroflexanone (**1**) as conventional NMR methods were found to result in the degradation of the retroflexanone Mosher esters before analysis could be carried out.

2. Results and Discussion

The dichloromethane crude extract of *C. retroflexa* was subjected to silica gel flash chromatography to yield retroflexanone (**1**), and a structurally related phloroglucinol analogue (**2**) in an enriched fraction (Scheme 1). The enriched fraction consisted of an approximate 3:1 ratio of the compounds (**2**) and (**1**) respectively. This enriched fraction was subjected to a complete 2D NMR analysis (via HPLC-NMR) whereby acquisition of the 2D NMR spectra for both compounds was achieved in the stop-flow mode. This permitted each compound to be structurally assigned. This approach would allow for rapid structure assignment of the Mosher esters based only on the ^{1}H NMR comparison of the Mosher esters to the natural compound.

The enriched fraction was subjected to the advanced Mosher method using α-methoxy-α-trifluoromethylphenylacetyl chloride (MPTA-Cl). As there was a greater amount of (**2**) present in the fraction, it was suspected that this would be derivatised preferentially over retroflexanone (**1**).

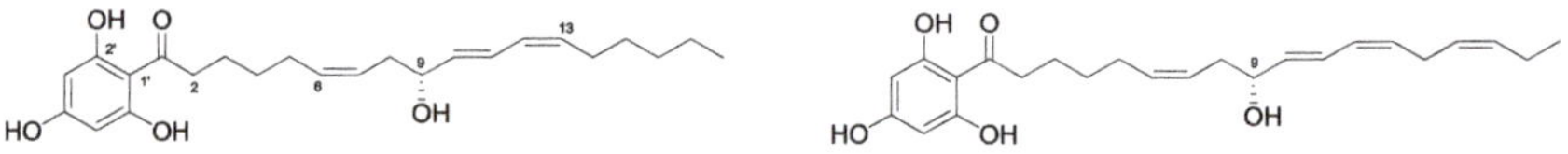

(**1**) - retroflexanone

(**2**)

Scheme 1. Phloroglucinols isolated from *Cystophora retroflexa.*

The enriched fraction was reacted with dry pyridine and (*R*)-(−)-MTPA-Cl and (*S*)-(+)-MTPA-Cl (α-methoxy-α-trifluoromethylphenylacetyl chloride) respectively to prepare the Mosher esters, paying particular attention to the fact that the (*R*)-(−)-MTPA-Cl gives the (*S*)-MTPA ester and vice versa [3]. Esterification yielded the diastereoisomeric (*S*)-MTPA and (*R*)-MTPA esters. The ^{1}H NMR chemical shift differences between the MTPA esters [$\Delta\delta_{SR} = \delta_s - \delta_R$] were established by comparing the ^{1}H NMR spectra of the esters to that of the original ^{1}H NMR spectrum of retraflexaonone, and are given in Table 1.

Each reaction was subsequently analysed individually via HPLC-NMR which revealed the presence of a new peak in the HPLC chromatogram, corresponding to the Mosher esters of the structurally related phloroglucinol analogue (**2a** and **2b**) respectively. The absolute configuration of (**2**) has previously been determined using the Horeau, and ozonolysis methods [12]. Analysis and interpretation of the ^{1}H NMR data for this compound provided a means to assess whether the formation of Mosher esters formed in a mixture could unequivocally provide the correct absolute configuration. By observing which of the proton chemical shifts and therefore which substituent is affected by the formation of each derivative, the absolute configuration of the secondary alcohol is able to be established. The ^{1}H NMR chemical shift differences between the MTPA esters [$\Delta\delta^{SR} = \delta_s - \delta_R$] were established for compound (**2**) (see Table 1). Despite some of the δ^{SR} values being unresolved or solvent suppressed in the HPLC-NMR analysis, the values that could be obtained were allocated within the same substituent based on their sign (positive or negative) and this permitted the absolute configuration of (**2**) to be deduced as being *R*, which was in agreement with the previous findings (refer to the retroflexanone example for complete details of the analysis and the supporting information file). With the methodology secured, the determination of retraflexonanone (**1**) was targeted.

Table 1. ^{1}H NMR data of compounds (**1**) and (**2**) and the characteristic chemical shift value differences $\Delta\delta^{SR}$ of the corresponding Mosher esters, recorded at 500 MHz (75% CH_3CN/D_2O).

Position	δ_H Retroflexanone (1) (ppm)	δ_H Retroflexanone Reacted with *R*-MTPA-Cl to Give *S*-MTPA Ester (1a) (ppm)	δ_H Retroflexanone Reacted with *S*-MTPA-Cl to Give *R*-MTPA Ester (1b) (ppm)	$\Delta\delta^{SR}$ (ppm)	$\Delta\delta^{SR}$ (Hz)
2	3.86, t (7.0)	3.85, t (7.5)	3.84, t (7.5)	+0.01	+6
3	2.44, p (7.0)	2.44, m	2.43, m	+0.01	+7
4	2.20, m	2.18, m	2.16, m	+0.02	+9
8a	3.09, m	3.33, m	3.26, m	+0.07	+42
8b	3.09, m	3.33, m	3.26, m	+0.07	+42
10	6.45, dd (6.5, 15.0)	6.14–6.45, m	6.52, dd (7.5, 15.5)	(negative value) [a]	(negative value) [a]
11	7.28, dd (11.0, 15.0)	7.36, dd (11.5, 13.0)	7.48, dd (11.0, 15.5)	−0.12	−62
12	6.78, dd (10.5, 10.5	6.76, dd (11.0, 11.5)	6.82, dd (10.5, 11.5)	−0.16	−26
14	3.09, m	ND	ND	n.a.	n.a.
18	1.70, t (7.0)	1.70, t (7.0)	1.70, m	0	0
Position	**δ_H Phloroglucinol (2) (ppm)**	**δ_H Phloroglucinol Reacted with *R*-MTPA-Cl to Give *S*-MTPA Ester (2a) (ppm)**	**δ_H Phloroglucinol Reacted with *S*-MTPA-Cl to Give *R*-MTPA ester (2b) (ppm)**	**$\Delta\delta^{SR}$ (ppm)**	**$\Delta\delta^{SR}$ (Hz)**
2	3.86, t (7.0)	3.84, t (7.5)	3.84, t (7.0)	0	0
3	2.45, p (7.0)	2.42, p (7.5)	2.41, p (7.0)	+0.01	+9
4	2.22, p (7.0)	2.19, p (7.5)	2.15, p (7.0)	+0.04	+20
8a	3.10, m	3.35, m	3.31, m	+0.04	+30
8b	3.10, m	3.29, m	3.24, m	+0.05	+31
10	6.47, dd (6.5, 15.0)	6.07–6.46, m	6.55, dd (7.5, 15.5)	(negative value) [a]	(negative value) [a]
11	7.32, dd (11.0, 15.0)	7.38, dd (11.5, 14.5)	7.52, dd (11.0, 15.5)	−0.14	−70
12	6.79, dd (11.0, 11.0)	6.76, dd (10.5, 11.5)	6.82, dd (10.5, 11.0)	−0.06	−30
14	3.74, dd (7.0, 14.5)	3.65, m	3.73, m	−0.08	−38
18	1.77, t (7.0)	1.75, t (7.5)	1.76, t (7.0)	−0.01	−3

ND—indicates signal was not detected due to signal suppression; n.a. $\Delta\delta^{SR}$ not available due to signal overlap or signal suppression; [a] exact $\Delta\delta^{SR}$ could not be determined due to signal overlap, but it was evident that the $\Delta\delta^{SR}$ value was negative.

It was noted during the HPLC-NMR analysis of the advanced Mosher reactions, that both retroflexanone (**1**) and the structurally related phloroglucinol (**2**) were still present in the enriched fraction, and that neither had completely reacted with the Mosher reagents. Moreover the Mosher esters of retroflexanone (**1**) were not observed. The reaction was carried out on a number of occasions using slightly different reaction conditions, but each time the Mosher esters of retroflexanone (**1**) were not observed.

An alternative approach was taken where retroflexanone (**1**) was rapidly purified from the enriched fraction by semi-preparative reversed phase HPLC. It was eventually established that retroflexanone (**1**) would remain intact long enough if kept in dichloromethane or methanol at −80 °C, but that it would degrade rapidly in the presence of chloroform or if kept at room temperature. Retroflexanone (**1**) was reacted with dry pyridine and the Mosher reagents (*R*)-(−)-MTPA-Cl and (*S*)-(+)-MTPA-Cl respectively. Subsequent HPLC-NMR analysis was performed on each of the reactions and this revealed the presence of the new Mosher ester derivatives of retroflexanone (**1a** and **1b**), together with residual retroflexanone (**1**) that had not reacted with the Mosher reagents. Stop-flow HPLC-NMR was carried out on the two Mosher esters (**1a** and **1b**) to obtain their corresponding ^{1}H NMR spectra. The ^{1}H NMR spectrum (Figure 1) of retroflexanone (**1**) was compared to the spectra obtained for the Mosher esters (**1a** and **1b**). Characteristic upfield and downfield shifts of the ^{1}H NMR chemical shifts were noted depending on their occurrence on either side of the stereogenic secondary alcohol.

Differences in the proton chemical shifts of **1a** and **1b** are given in Table 1. The majority of the $\Delta\delta^{SR}$ values could be calculated despite some unassigned or solvent suppressed signals. The two diastereomeric MTPA esters for retroflexanone are given in Figure 2, with R^1 and R^2 representing that alkyl chains on either side of the secondary alcohol moiety. It is shown in Figure 2 that the phenyl group from the MTPA will either shield the R^1 or R^2 group, depending on which diastereomer is present.

Using the conformations shown in Figure 2 for the MTPA esters of generic alcohols, the R^1 and R^2 substituents could be assigned. Protons that have positive $\Delta\delta^{SR}$ values reside within R^1, whereas those with negative values of $\Delta\delta^{SR}$ belong to the R^2 substituent [13]. Figure 2 shows that all of the positive $\Delta\delta^{SR}$ are located on the left hand side, while the negative $\Delta\delta^{SR}$ are located on the right hand side of the molecule. Specifically protons with positive $\Delta\delta^{SR}$ values (those in R^1) are all on one side (front) of the plane of the MTPA moiety, whereas those with negative values are all on the opposite (back) side of that plane. This, in conjunction with the Cahn Ingold Prelog convention, permitted the assignment of the original secondary alcohol absolute configuration to be assigned as *R*.

Since the structure of retroflexanone (**1**) had previously been successfully and unequivocally characterised by HPLC-NMR [1], an attempt was made to dissolve pure retroflexanone (**1**) in $CDCl_3$ to obtain conventional NMR data. Despite retroflexanone (**1**) being unstable in $CDCl_3$, this solvent was chosen to make the comparison to other related compounds in the literature easier. 1D and 2D NMR data was successfully obtained, however the methylene protons at position C-2 displayed unexpected splitting patterns. It was expected that these methylene protons would display a typical triplet. However the methylene at position C-2 appeared as a set of non-equivalent protons displaying a multiplet-type splitting. Initially it was thought that retroflexanone (**1**) may have degraded, but subsequent interpretation of the NMR data still supported the initial structure. It was proposed that when retroflexanone (**1**) and other structurally related compounds are dissolved in $CDCl_3$, that non-equivalent protons displaying multiplet-type splitting is observed rather than a typical triplet due to a pro-chiral effect created by the carbonyl group at C-1. To test this theory, the structurally related analogue (**2**) was placed into $CDCl_3$ and CD_3OD. The NMR data revealed that in $CDCl_3$ the methylene protons at position C-2 displayed multiplet-type splitting, but in CD_3OD the methylene protons appear as a typical triplet (see supporting information section). This confirmed that the appearance of these methylene protons is dependent on the NMR solvent used for acquisition. Detailed NMR data can be found in supporting materials.

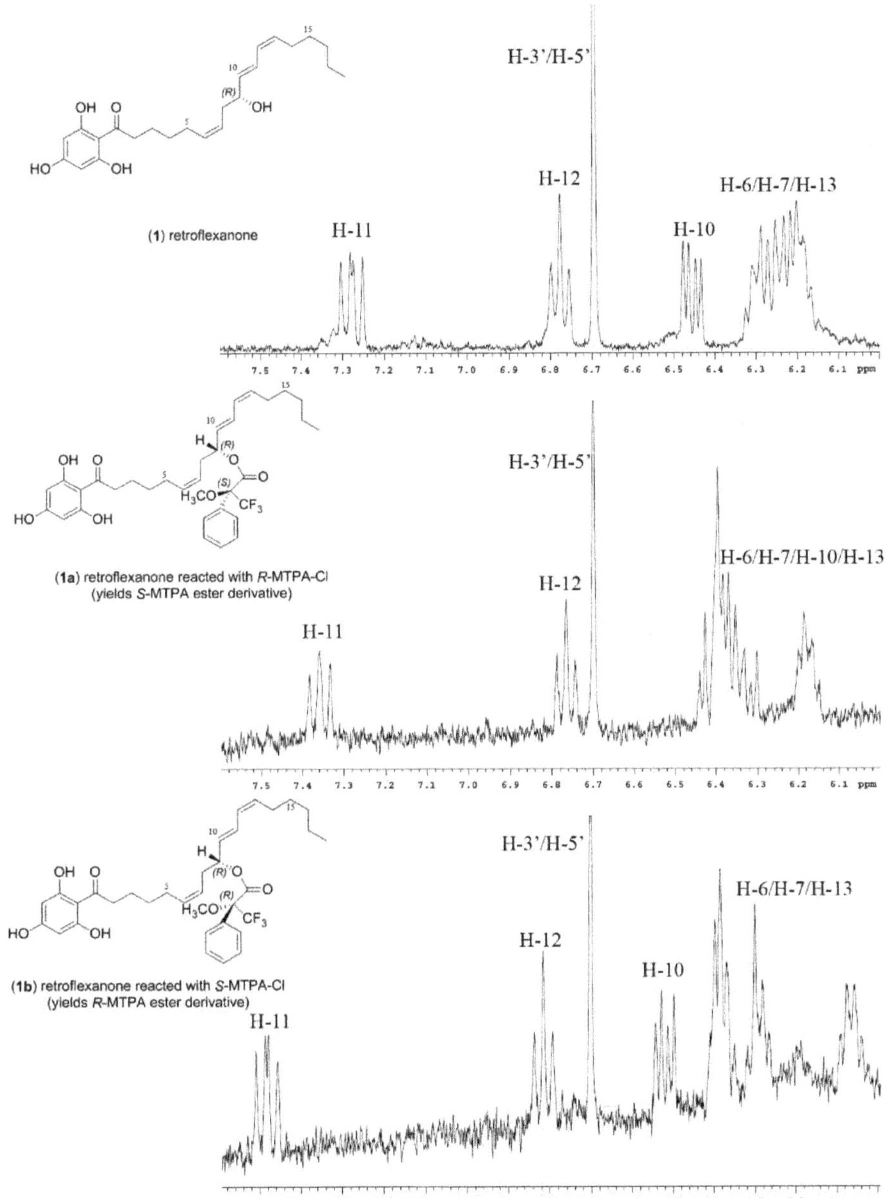

Figure 1. Stop-flow (HPLC-NMR) expansions of the ^{1}H NMR spectra of retroflexanone (**1**) and Mosher ester derivatives (**1a** and **1b**) showing characteristic chemical shift influences.

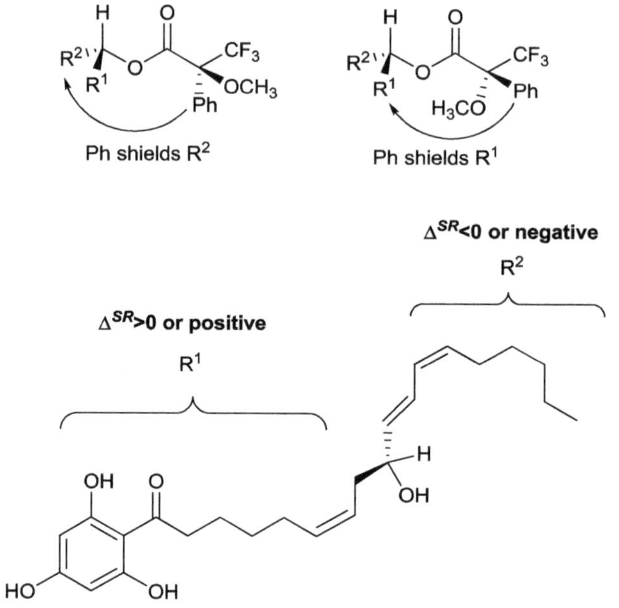

Figure 2. Diastereomeric MTPA esters of retroflexanone.

3. Materials and Methods

3.1. General Experimental Procedures

All organic solvents used were analytical reagent (AR or GR), UV spectroscopic, or HPLC grades with Milli-Q water also being used. ^{1}H (500 MHz) and ^{13}C (125 MHz) NMR spectra were acquired in $CDCl_3$ and CD_3OD on a 500 MHz Agilent DD2 NMR spectrometer, or a 300 MHz Bruker Avance III NMR spectrometer with referencing to solvent signals (δ_H 7.26; δ_C 77.0 and, δ_H 3.31; δ_C 49.0). Two-dimensional NMR experiments recorded included gradient correlation spectroscopy (gCOSY), heteronuclear single-quantum correlation spectroscopy with adiabatic pulses (HSQCAD), and gradient heteronuclear multiple-bond spectroscopy with adiabatic pulses (gHMBCAD).

3.2. Alga Material

C. retroflexa was collected via SCUBA on 21 April 2010 from Governor Reef (near Indented Head), Port Phillip Bay, Victoria, Australia. The alga was identified by Dr Gerry Kraft (The University of Melbourne) and a voucher specimen (designated the code number 2010-09) is deposited at the School of Science (Applied Chemistry and Environmental Science), RMIT University.

3.3. Fractionation of Dichloromethane Crude Extract

The alga (133 g, wet weight) was extracted with 3:1 $MeOH/CH_2Cl_2$ (1 L). The crude extract was decanted and concentrated under reduced pressure and sequentially solvent partitioned (triturated) into CH_2Cl_2 and MeOH soluble extracts, respectively. A portion of the CH_2Cl_2 crude extract (445 mg) of *C. retroflexa* was subjected to silica gel flash chromatography. Silica gel flash chromatography was carried out using Davisil LC35Å silica gel (40–60 mesh) using a 20% stepwise solvent elution from 100% petroleum spirits (60–80 °C) to 100% CH_2Cl_2 to 100% EtOAc and finally to 100% MeOH. The 60% $CH_2Cl_2/EtOAc$ fraction yielded a mixture which contained retroflexanone (**1**) and the structurally related phloroglucinol (**2**) (136.2 mg).

3.4. Advanced Mosher Derivatisation of Phloroglucinol (2) in an Enriched Fraction

The 60% CH_2Cl_2/EtOAc fraction (1 mg) was dissolved in CH_2Cl_2 (1 mL) to which (*R*)-(−)-MTPA-Cl (4.0 mg, 16 µmol) or alternatively (*S*)-(+)-MTPA-Cl (4.5 mg, 18 µmol) was added. Dry pyridine (200 µL, 760 µmol) was then added and the reaction stirred for 4 h. The reaction mixtures were then dried under a stream of nitrogen and reconstituted into HPLC-NMR grade CH_3CN.

3.5. HPLC Purification of Retroflexanone

Semi-preparative HPLC was carried out on a Dionex P680 (solvent delivery module) equipped with a Dionex UVD340U PDA detector and a Foxy Jr. automated fraction collector. An isocratic HPLC method (85% CH_3CN/H_2O) was employed using a Phenomenex Luna (2) 100 Å C18 250 × 10 mm (5 µm) HPLC column. The automatic fraction collector was programmed to collect the compounds based on their retention times at a flow rate of 4.0 mL/min. A portion of the 60% CH_2Cl_2/EtOAc fraction was subjected to reversed phase HPLC to yield retroflexanone (**1**) (2.8 mg) and the phloroglucinol (**2**) (6.0 mg).

3.6. Advanced Mosher Reaction of Retroflexanone

Retroflexanone (1.4 mg, 3.5 µmol) was dissolved in CH_2Cl_2 (1 mL) to which (*R*)-(−)-MTPA-Cl (50 mg, 198 µmol, 57 equiv.) or alternatively (*S*)-(+)-MTPA-Cl (50 mg, 198 µmol, 57 equiv.) was added. Dry pyridine (300 µL, 1140 µmol, 325 equiv.) was then added and the reaction stirred for 4 h. The reaction mixtures were then dried under a stream of nitrogen and reconstituted into HPLC-NMR grade CH_3CN.

3.7. HPLC-NMR Analysis

For HPLC-NMR details, please refer to Brkljaca and Urban [14]. For stop-flow HPLC-NMR modes, 50-µL injections of the reconstituted samples in CH_3CN were injected onto an Agilent Eclipse Plus C_{18} (150 × 4.6) 5-µ column using a solvent composition of 75% CH_3CN/D_2O at a flow rate of 1 mL/min. In the stop-flow HPLC-NMR mode WET1D NMR experiments were acquired.

3.8. On-Line NMR Data Obtained via HPLC-NMR

Retroflexanone or 9R-hydroxy-1-(2,4,6-trihydroxyphenyl)-6Z,10E,12Z-Octadecatrien-1-one reacted with (R)-(−)-MTPA-Cl yielding the S-MTPA ester (**1a**); ^{1}H NMR (500 MHz, 75% CH_3CN/D_2O) δ 8.28 (5H, m, MTPA-aromatic), 7.36 (1H, dd, *J* = 11.5, 13.0 Hz, H-11), 6.76 (1H, dd, *J* = 11.0, 11.5 Hz, H-12), 6.70 (2H, s, H-3′/H-5′), 6.14–6.45 (4H, m, H-6/H-7/H-10/H-13), 4.83 (1H, m, H-9), 4.35 (3H, s, MTPA-OCH_3), 3.85 (2H, t, *J* = 7.5 Hz, H-2), 3.33 (2H, m, H-8), 2.44 (2H, m, H-3), 2.18 (2H, m, H-4), 2.10 (2H, m, H-17), 1.70 (3H, t, *J* = 7.0 Hz, H-18), ND (11H, H-5/H-14/H-15/H-16,/2′-OH/4′-OH/6′-OH), ND indicates signal not detected.

Retroflexanone or 9R-hydroxy-1-(2,4,6-trihydroxyphenyl)-6Z,10E,12Z-Octadecatrien-1-one reacted with (S)-(+)-MTPA-Cl yielding the R-MTPA ester (**1b**); ^{1}H NMR (500 MHz, 75% CH_3CN/D_2O) δ 8.28 (5H, m, MTPA-aromatic), 7.48 (1H, dd, *J* = 11.0, 15.5 Hz, H-11), 6.82 (1H, dd, *J* = 10.5, 11.5 Hz, H-12), 6.70 (2H, s, H-3′/H-5′), 6.52 (1H, dd, *J* = 7.5, 15.5, H-10), 6.02–6.42 (3H, m, H-6/H-7/H-13), 4.83 (1H, m, H-9), 4.32 (3H, s, MTPA-OCH_3), 3.84 (2H, t, *J* = 7.5 Hz, H-2), 3.26 (2H, m, H-8), 2.43 (2H, m, H-3), 2.16 (2H, m, H-4), 2.10 (2H, m, H-17), 1.70 (3H, m, H-18), ND (11H, H-5/H-14/H-15/H-16/2′-OH/4′-OH/6′-OH), ND indicates signal not detected.

9R-hydroxy-1-(2,4,6-trihydroxy-phenyl)-6Z,10E,12Z,15Z-Octadecatetraen-1-one reacted with (R)-(−)-MTPA-Cl yielding the S-MTPA ester (**2a**); ^{1}H NMR (500 MHz, 75% CH_3CN/D_2O) δ 8.27 (5H, m, MTPA-aromatic), 7.38 (1H, dd, *J* = 11.5, 14.5 Hz, H-11), 6.76 (1H, dd, *J* = 10.5, 11.5 Hz, H-12), 6.69 (2H, s, H-3′/H-5′), 6.07–6.46 (6H, m, H-6/H-7/H-10/H-13/H-15/H-16), 4.34 (3H, s, MTPA-OCH_3), 3.84 (2H, t, *J* = 7.5 Hz, H-2), 3.65 (2H, m, H-14), 3.35 (1H, m, H-8a), 3.29 (1H, m, H-8b),

2.42 (2H, p, *J* = 7.5 Hz, H-3), 2.19 (2H, p, *J* = 7.5 Hz, H-4), 1.75 (3H, t, *J* = 7.5 Hz, H-18), ND (8H, H-5/H-9/H-17/2′-OH/4′-OH/6′-OH), ND indicates signal not detected.

9R-hydroxy-1-(2,4,6-trihydroxy-phenyl)-6Z,10E,12Z,15Z-Octadecatetraen-1-one reacted with (S)-(+)-MTPA-Cl to yield the R-MTPA ester (**2b**); ^{1}H NMR (500 MHz, 75% CH_3CN/D_2O) δ 8.30 (5H, m, MTPA-aromatic), 7.52 (1H, dd, *J* = 11.0, 15.5 Hz, H-11), 6.82 (1H, dd, *J* = 10.5, 11.0 Hz, H-12), 6.70 (2H, s, H-3′/H-5′), 6.55 (1H, dd, *J* = 7.5, 15.5 Hz, H-10), 6.04−6.42 (5H, m, H-6/H-7/H-13/H-15/H-16), 4.32 (3H, s, MTPA-OCH_3), 3.84 (2H, t, *J* = 7.0 Hz, H-2), 3.73 (2H, m, H-14), 3.31 (1H, m, H-8a), 3.24 (1H, m, H-8b), 2.41 (2H, p, *J* = 7.0 Hz, H-3), 2.15 (2H, p, *J* = 7.0 Hz, H-4), 1.76 (3H, t, *J* = 7.0 Hz, H-18), ND (8H, H-5/H-9/H-17/2′-OH/4′-OH/6′-OH), ND indicates signal not detected.

3.9. Off-Line NMR Data

Retroflexanone (**1**); unstable oil that darkened over time; ^{1}H NMR (500 MHz, $CDCl_3$) δ 6.52 (1H, dd, *J* = 11.5, 15.0 Hz, H-11), 5.97 (1H, dd, *J* = 11.0, 11.5 Hz, H-12), 5.88 (2H, s, H-3′/H-5′), 5.70 (1H, dd, *J* = 6.0, 15.0 Hz, H-10), 5.54 (1H, m, H-6), 5.45 (1H, dt, *J* = 7.0, 11.0 Hz, H-13), 5.39 (1H, m, H-7), 4.26 (1H, dt, *J* = 6.0, 6.5 Hz, H-9), 3.14 (1H, m, H-2a), 3.00 (1H, m, H-2b), 2.41 (1H, m, H-8a), 2.31 (1H, m, H-8b), 2.17 (2H, m, H-14), 2.12 (2H, m, H-5), 1.72 (2H, m, H-3), 1.48 (2H, m, H-4), 1.37 (2H, m, H-15), 1.29 (4H, m, H-16/H-17), 0.88 (3H, t, *J* = 7.0 Hz, H-18), ND (9-OH/2′-OH/4′-OH/6′-OH), ND indicates signal not detected; ^{13}C NMR (125 MHz, $CDC1_{3_3}$) δ 134.6 (CH, C-10), 133.5 (CH, C-6), 133.4 (CH, C-13), 127.5 (CH, C-12), 126.1 (CH, C-11), 124.7 (CH, C-7), 95.4 (CH, C-3′/C-5′), 72.5 (CH, C-9), 43.6 (CH_2, C-2), 35.2 (CH_2, C-8), 31.4 (CH_2, C-16), 29.3 (CH_2, C-4/C-15), 27.4 (CH_2, C-14), 26.8 (CH_2, C-5), 24.4 (CH_2, C-3), 22.6 (CH_2, C-17), 14.1 (CH_3, C-18), ND (C-1/C-1′/C-2′/C-4′/C-6′), ND indicates signal not detected.

9R-hydroxy-1-(2,4,6-trihydroxy-phenyl)-6Z,10E,12Z,15Z-Octadecatetraen-1-one (**2**); unstable oil that darkened over time; ^{1}H NMR (500 MHz, $CDCl_3$) δ 6.55 (1H, dd, *J* = 11.5, 15.0 Hz, H-11), 5.98 (1H, dd, *J* = 11.0, 11.0 Hz, H-12), 5.88 (2H, bs, H-3′/H-5′), 5.72 (1H, dd, *J* = 6.0, 14.5 Hz, H-10), 5.27−5.59 (5H, m, H-6/H-7/H-13/H-15/H-16), 4.27 (1H, dt, *J* = 6.0, 6.5 Hz, H-9), 3.11 (1H, m, H-2a), 3.00 (1H, m, H-2b), 2.93 (2H, dd, *J* = 7.0, 7.5 Hz, H-14), 2.39 (1H, m, H-8a), 2.32 (1H, m, H-8b), 2.12 (4H, m, H-5/H-17), 1.71 (2H, m, H-3), 1.48 (2H, p, *J* = 7.0 Hz, H-4), 0.97 (3H, t, *J* = 7.5 Hz, H-18), ND (9-OH/2′-OH′4′-OH/6′-OH), ND indicates signal not detected; ^{1}H NMR (300 MHz, CD_3OD) δ 6.55 (1H, dd, *J* = 11.1, 15.0 Hz, H-11), 5.97 (1H, dd, *J* = 10.8, 11.1 Hz, H-12), 5.83 (2H, s, H-3′/H-5′), 5.68 (1H, dd, *J* = 6.6, 15.0 Hz, H-10), 5.27−5.55 (5H, m, H-6/H-7/H-13/H-15/H-16), 4.15 (1H, dt, *J* = 6.3, 6.6 Hz, H-9), 3.06 (2H, t, *J* = 7.5 Hz, H-2), 2.94 (2H, dd, *J* = 7.0, 7.5 Hz, H-14), 2.32 (2H, m, H-8), 2.10 (4H, m, H-5/H-17), 1.69 (2H, p, *J* = 7.5 Hz, H-3), 1.45 (2H, p, *J* = 7.5 Hz, H-4), 0.98 (3H, t, *J* = 7.5 Hz, H-18), ND (9-OH/2′-OH′4′-OH/6′-OH), ND indicates signal not detected.

4. Conclusions

HPLC-NMR in conjunction with the advanced Mosher method was successful in confirming the absolute configuration of two related phloroglucinol compounds. The absolute configuration of retroflexanone (**1**) was achieved via off-line isolation followed by HPLC-NMR analysis, whilst compound (**2**) was secured via the advanced Mosher method HPLC-NMR analysis of an enriched fraction. Both compounds displayed an *R* absolute configuration at the secondary alcohol. This represents, to the best of our knowledge, the first instance of the modified Mosher method combined with HPLC-NMR being employed on an enriched fraction rather than individual purified compounds.

Supplementary Materials: The following are available online at http://www.mdpi.com/1660-3397/16/6/205/s1, supplementary materials S1–S12: NMR data of all compounds analyzed in this article.

Author Contributions: Conceptualization, S.U.; Methodology, C.S., R.B. and S.U.; Formal Analysis, C.S., R.B. and S.U.; Investigation, C.S.; Writing-Original Draft Preparation, C.S.; Writing-Review & Editing, R.B. and S.U.; Supervision, R.B. and S.U.

Conflicts of Interest: The authors declare no conflict of interest.

References

1. Brkljaca, R.; Goker, E.S.; Urban, S. Dereplication and chemotaxonomical studies of marine algae of the ochrophyta and rhodophyta phyla. *Mar. Drugs* **2015**, *13*, 2714–2731. [CrossRef] [PubMed]
2. Brkljaca, R.; Urban, S. Recent advancements in HPLC-NMR and applications for natural product profiling and identification. *J. Liquid Chromatogr. Relat. Technol.* **2011**, *34*, 1063–1076. [CrossRef]
3. Dale, J.A.; Mosher, H.S. Nuclear magnetic resonance enantiomer regents. Configurational correlations via nuclear magnetic resonance chemical shifts of diastereomeric mandelate, *O*-methylmandelate, and α-methoxy-α-trifluoromethylphenylacetate (MTPA) esters. *J. Am. Chem. Soc.* **1973**, *95*, 512–519. [CrossRef]
4. Ohtani, I.; Kusumi, T.; Kashman, Y.; Kakisawa, H. High-field FT NMR application of mosher's method. The absolute configurations of marine terpenoids. *J. Am. Chem. Soc.* **1990**, *113*, 4092–4096. [CrossRef]
5. Cimmino, A.; Masi, M.; Evidente, M.; Superchi, S. Application of Mosher's method for absolute configuration assignment to bioactive plants and fungi metabolites. *J. Pharm. Biomed. Anal.* **2017**, *144*, 59–89. [CrossRef] [PubMed]
6. Ohtani, I.; Kusumi, T.; Ishitsuka, M.O.; Kakisawa, H. Absolute configurations of marine diterpenes possessing a xenicane skeleton. An application of an advanced Mosher's method. *Tetrahedron Lett.* **1989**, *30*, 3147–3150. [CrossRef]
7. Ohtani, I.; Kusumi, T.; Kashman, Y.; Kakisawa, H. A new aspect of the high-field NMR application of Mosher's method. The absolute configuration of marine triterpene sipholenol A. *J. Org. Chem.* **1991**, *56*, 1296–1298. [CrossRef]
8. Brkljaca, R.; Urban, S. HPLC-NMR and HPLC-MS investigation of antimicrobial constituents in *Cystophora monilifera* and *Cystophora subfarcinata*. *Phytochemistry* **2015**, *117*, 200–208. [CrossRef] [PubMed]
9. Guilet, D.; Guntern, A.; Ioset, J.-R.; Queiroz, E.F.; Ndjoko, K.; Foggin, C.M.; Hostettmann, K. Absolute configuration of a tetrahydrophenanthrene fron *Heliotropium ovalifolium* by LC-NMR of its Mosher esters. *J. Nat. Prod.* **2003**, *66*, 17–20. [CrossRef] [PubMed]
10. Queiroz, E.F.; Wolfender, J.-L.; Raoelison, G.; Hostettmann, K. Determination of the absolute configuration of 6-alkylated a-pyrones from *Ravensara crassifolia* by LC-NMR. *Phytochem. Anal.* **2003**, *14*, 34–39. [CrossRef] [PubMed]
11. Seger, C.; Godejohann, M.; Spraul, M.; Stuppner, H.; Hadacek, F. Reaction product analysis by high-performance liquid chromatography-solid-phase extraction-nuclear magnetic resonance. Application to the absolute configuration determination of naturally occurring polyyne alcohols. *J. Chromatogr. A* **2006**, *1136*, 82–88. [CrossRef] [PubMed]
12. Kazlauskas, R.; King, L.; Murphy, P.T.; Warren, R.G.; Wells, R.J. New metabolites from the brown algal genus *Cystophora*. *Aust. J. Chem.* **1981**, *34*, 439–447. [CrossRef]
13. Hoye, T.R.; Jeffrey, C.S.; Shao, F. Mosher ester analysis for the determination of absolute configuration of stereogenic (chiral) carbinol carbons. *Nat. Protoc.* **2007**, *2*, 2451–2458. [CrossRef] [PubMed]
14. Brkljaca, R.; Urban, S. Chemical profiling (HPLC-NMR & HPLC-MS), isolation, and identification of bioactive meroditerpenoids from the southern Australian marine brown alga Sargassum paradoxum. *Mar. Drugs* **2015**, *13*, 102–127.

© 2018 by the authors. Licensee MDPI, Basel, Switzerland. This article is an open access article distributed under the terms and conditions of the Creative Commons Attribution (CC BY) license (http://creativecommons.org/licenses/by/4.0/).

marine drugs

MDPI

Article

Optimum Production Conditions, Purification, Identification, and Antioxidant Activity of Violaxanthin from Microalga *Eustigmatos* cf. *polyphem* (Eustigmatophyceae)

Feifei Wang †, Luodong Huang †, Baoyan Gao and Chengwu Zhang *

Institute of Hydrobiology, Department of Ecology, Jinan University, Guangzhou 510632, China; feifei2013360@126.com (F.W.); hld8124@sina.com (L.H.); gaobaoyan1211@126.com (B.G.)

* Correspondence: tzhangcw@jnu.edu.cn; Tel./Fax: +86-20-8522-4366

† These authors contributed equally to this work.

Received: 16 May 2018; Accepted: 30 May 2018; Published: 1 June 2018

Abstract: Violaxanthin is a major xanthophyll pigment in the microalga *Eustigmatos* cf. *polyphem*, but the amount produced after propagation can vary depending upon culture conditions. In this study, the effects of cultivation time, nitrogen concentration, light intensity, and culture mode on violaxanthin production were investigated. The results showed that this microalga vigorously grew and maintained a high level of violaxanthin in the fed-batch culture, and the highest violaxanthin productivity of 1.10 ± 0.03 mg L^{-1} d^{-1} was obtained under low light illumination with 18 mM of initial nitrogen supply for ten days. Additionally, violaxanthin was purified from *E.* cf. *polyphem* by silica gel chromatography and preparative high-performance liquid chromatography (PHPLC), and identified with high-resolution mass spectrometry (HRMS). The antioxidant activity of the purified violaxanthin was evaluated by three tests in vitro: reducing power assay, 2,2-diphenyl-1-picrylhydrazyl (DPPH), and 2,2-azobis-3-ethylbenzthiazoline-6-sulphonic acid (ABTS) radical assays. The strongest inhibition of purified violaxanthin occurred during the scavenging of $ABTS^{+}$ radicals, with EC_{50} of 15.25 μg mL^{-1}. In conclusion, this is the first report to investigate the effects of different culture conditions on violaxanthin accumulation in *E.* cf. *polyphem* and provide a novel source for the production of violaxanthin that can be used for food and pharmaceutical applications.

Keywords: *Eustigmatos* cf. *polyphem*; violaxanthin; culture conditions; purification; antioxidant activity

1. Introduction

Carotenoids belong to the isoprenoid group that is commonly characterized by a C_{40} tetraterpenoid structure built from eight C_5 isoprenoid units [1]. More than 750 carotenoids have been isolated from natural sources, and these carotenoids were divided into two different groups according to their chemical structures: (1) hydrocarbon carotenoids, generally named carotenes, which consist of only carbon and hydrogen, and (2) oxygenated carotenoids, which are called xanthophylls [2]. Carotenoids are rich in unsaturated groups, and many studies have confirmed that they exhibit strong activity in the scavenging of reactive oxygen species (ROS) [3,4]. Traditionally, carotenoids have been used as colorants in the food and feed industries. Carotenoids have also been formulated as dietary antioxidants, and extensive health-promoting characteristics, such as antioxidative, anti-arteriosclerosis, antiproliferative, and anticancer effects, as well as vision protection [5–7]. Since these protective functions were thought to be attributed to their strong antioxidant properties [8], various carotenoids were isolated and purified from natural sources for the evaluation of their potential antioxidant activity.

Microalgae contain abundant quantities of natural antioxidants, such as carotenoids [7,9]. In microalgae, the carotenoids usually function as accessory pigments and structural components of light-harvesting complexes in photosystems, and participate in photosynthetic reactions [10]. In addition, some carotenoids can serve as photoprotective agents to protect the photosynthetic apparatus from excess light damage by scavenging ROS, such as singlet oxygen and free radicals, and be responsible for phototaxis [11]. Various microalgae can accumulate large amounts of carotenoids, such as fucoxanthin, astaxanthin, lutein, canthaxanthin, and β-carotene, some of which have been commercialized, including β-carotene from the halophile green microalga *Dunaliella salina*, astaxanthin from the freshwater green microalga *Haematococcus lacustris* (formerly *Haematococcus pluvialis*), fucoxanthin from diatoms, and lutein from some Chlorophycean microalgae (class Chlorophyceae) [10,12]. At present, these main microalgal carotenoids have been used as colorants in food and nutraceuticals in human health care.

Apart from the above-mentioned primary carotenoids, microalgae may also accumulate other important carotenoids, such as violaxanthin and canthaxanthin. Violaxanthin is a natural xanthophyll pigment that is orange-colored. It is biosynthesized from zeaxanthin by epoxidation and has double 5,6-epoxy groups, which are found in orange-colored fruits, green vegetables, and microalgae [13,14]. Fu et al. [2] reported that violaxanthin purified from water spinach/water morning glory (*Ipomoea aquatica*, class Dicotyledonae) has a strong $ABTS^+$ radical scavenging activity, and it also demonstrated valid inhibition of lipid peroxidation and red blood cell hemolysis [2]. These actions indicated that violaxanthin has the potential to be widely applied in medical and health products. Among microalgal sources, there are only two studies reporting violaxanthin isolation; one described the isolation from the green microalga *Dunaliella tertiolecta* [15], and the other used *Chloroidium ellipsoideum* (formerly *Chlorella ellipsoidea*) [10] as the source. The violaxanthin purified from these two microalgae also exhibited anti-proliferative, anti-inflammatory, and proapoptotic activity against human cancer cell lines in vitro [16]. There are still additional microalgae resources that could be utilized, thus broadening the sources and new functional applications of violaxanthin.

Eustigmatos cf. *polyphem* (formerly determined as *Myrmecia bisecta*) is a yellow-green unicellular edaphic microalga belonging to the class Eustigmatophyceae [17]. Our previous work found that *E.* cf. *polyphem* can accumulate large quantities of lipids and β-carotene under stress conditions [18,19], and because of its high lipid productivity production, its photosynthetic apparatus is worthy of closer examination. The eustigmatophycean microalgae lack chlorophylls *b* and *c*, and they mainly contain chlorophyll *a*, violaxanthin, vaucheriaxanthin ester, and β-carotene as photosynthetic pigments [20]. Violaxanthin is the dominant carotenoid that usually combines with chlorophyll *a* and apoprotein to form violaxanthin-chorophyll-*a*-binding protein (VCP) complexes in the thylakoids of chloroplast, and takes part in light harvesting [21,22]. Violaxanthin is a structural component of the xanthophyll cycle that protects the photosynthetic apparatus against an excess of light via non-photochemical fluorescence quenching [23]. Demmig-Adams et al. [24] proved that the xanthophyll cycle is involved in light protection, and the amount of violaxanthin in microalgae varies with the light intensity. Pasquet et al. [15] reported that the low violaxanthin production in *Dunaliella tertiolecta* restricts its therapeutic applications, but the effects of culture conditions on violaxanthin accumulation in microalgae have not yet been investigated.

The content of violaxanthin in microalgae is variable, because it is affected by the external environment [25,26]. In the present study, the effects of different culture conditions on violaxanthin production in *E.* cf. *polyphem*, including culture time, initial nitrogen concentration in culture medium, light intensity, and culture mode, were investigated. Additionally, the violaxanthin was extracted, purified, and identified from the algal biomass, and its antioxidant activity was evaluated in vitro. This work is aimed at providing another new microalgal source of violaxanthin and maximizing the violaxanthin production in *E.* cf. *polyphem* for potential applications in food and pharmaceuticals.

2. Results and Discussion

2.1. Effect of Cultivation Time on Violaxanthin Production

The effect of cultivation time on violaxanthin production in *E.* cf. *polyphem* is shown in Figure 1A. The algal biomass concentration increased with the prolonging of culture time, and it reached 2.63 ± 0.04 g L^{-1} on the 11th day with low light illumination. However, the content of violaxanthin in *E.* cf. *polyphem* increased to the highest level of 0.39% (of DW) on the fifth day, and then gradually decreased to 0.30% on the 11th day. This result was in agreement with the reports of Sobrino et al. [27], who found that the violaxanthin content decreased with culture time in *Nannochloropsis* strains (class Eustigmatophyceae). Li et al. [18] reported that the violaxanthin content in *E.* cf. *polyphem* quickly decreased with prolonged culture time under high light illumination, while it decreased at a relatively slow rate in this study. Low light intensity was used in our study, which might slow the degradation of violaxanthin.

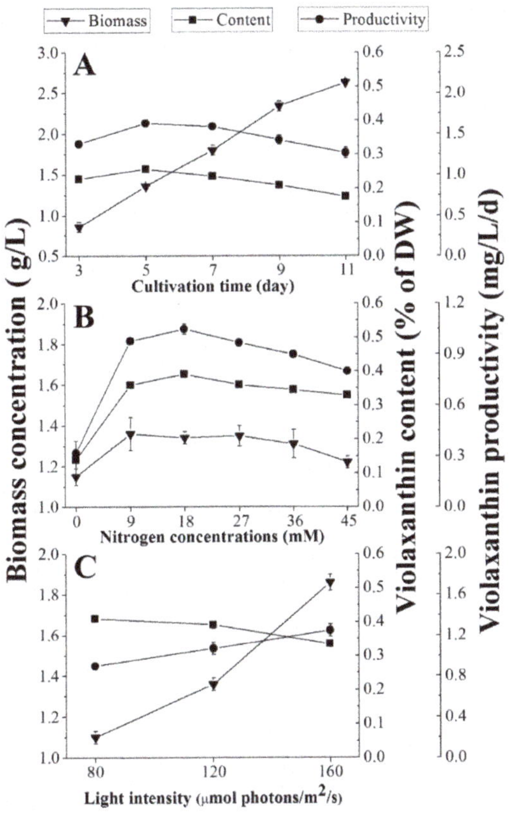

Figure 1. Effects of (**A**) cultivation time, (**B**) nitrogen concentration, and (**C**) light intensity on the violaxanthin production of *Eustigmatos* cf. *polyphem*. (**A** and **B**) The algae were cultured at a low light of 120 μmol photons m^{-2} s^{-1}. Values are expressed as the mean ± SD from three replicates; DW, dry weight.

Violaxanthin productivity is a suitable evaluation parameter for violaxanthin production due to the contradiction between algal biomass and violaxanthin content. The highest violaxanthin productivity of 1.07 ± 0.03 mg L^{-1} d^{-1} was obtained on the fifth day (Figure 1A) and, therefore, five days of culture time was selected and used for the next study.

2.2. Effect of Nitrogen Concentration on Violaxanthin Production

Nitrogen supply is essential for all microalgae growth, and its redundancy or limitation influences the biomass and biochemical composition of microalgae [28]. Therefore, the initial nitrogen concentration (0, 9, 18, 27, 36, and 45 mM) was designed to investigate its effect on violaxanthin production. As Figure 1B shows, the lowest nitrogen concentration group (LNCG, 0 mM) and the highest nitrogen concentration group (HNCG, 45 mM) adversely affected the microalgae growth and violaxanthin accumulation, especially the LNCG. The lowest biomass, violaxanthin content, and violaxanthin productivity, which were 1.15 ± 0.04 g L^{-1}, 0.14% ± 0.05 (of DW), and 0.32 ± 0.01 mg L^{-1} d^{-1}, respectively, were obtained at this nitrogen concentration (0 mM). The violaxanthin content increased with the higher nitrogen concentrations when the initial nitrogen concentration was between 0 mM and 18 mM. These results were consistent with the report of Gao et al. [26]. Then, the violaxanthin content gradually decreased when the initial nitrogen concentration ≥18 mM (Figure 1B). These results indicated that very high or insufficient nitrogen concentrations were disadvantageous to both algal growth and violaxanthin accumulation. In addition, the highest violaxanthin productivity (1.05 ± 0.03 mg L^{-1} d^{-1}) was achieved at 18 mM of the initial nitrogen despite a biomass concentration that was lower than 9 mM. Thus, 18 mM initial nitrogen concentration was shown to be more conducive to violaxanthin accumulation than the other investigated concentrations.

2.3. Effect of Light Intensity on Violaxanthin Production

Violaxanthin often exists in photosynthetic apparatus, and it is sensitive to light. In the xanthophyll cycle, violaxanthin transforms into zeaxanthin by de-epoxidation under high light, but zeaxanthin is epoxidated to violaxanthin under low light illumination [24]. Therefore, the amount of violaxanthin varies with the light intensity. In this study, three different light intensities of 80, 120, and 160 µmol photons m^{-2} s^{-1} were introduced to study the effect on violaxanthin production (Figure 1C).

As expected, the biomass accumulation was correlated with increasing light intensity, but the content of violaxanthin decreased with increasing light intensity, which was consistent with a previously published study [27]. Under the light intensity of 160 µmol photons m^{-2} s^{-1}, the highest biomass was 1.86 ± 0.05 mg L^{-1} with a high violaxanthin productivity of 1.25 ± 0.06 mg L^{-1} d^{-1}, but the violaxanthin content (0.33 ± 0.01% (of DW)) was significantly lower than that obtained at the light intensity of 80 and 120 µmol photons m^{-2} s^{-1} ($p < 0.05$). Moreover, we found that the violaxanthin content under high light illumination (160 µmol photons m^{-2} s^{-1}) quickly decreased beyond five days cultivation time in the preliminary experiment. Therefore, the lower light intensity was more suitable for the accumulation of violaxanthin, and 120 µmol photons m^{-2} s^{-1} was selected as the appropriate light intensity.

2.4. Effect of Culture Mode on Violaxanthin Production

As described earlier, the violaxanthin content in *E.* cf. *polyphem* was affected by the external environment and, therefore, fed-batch culture was used to overcome the effects of nutrient shortages and extracellular metabolite inhibition.

The effect of culture mode on violaxanthin production is presented in Table 1. In contrast with the control (the batch culture), the microalgae vigorously grew in the fed-batch culture, and the highest biomass (5.15 ± 0.03 g L^{-1}) was obtained on day 20. Moreover, as the culture time increased, the violaxanthin content was kept at a high level in the fed-batch culture and was significantly higher than that of the control. Although the violaxanthin productivity decreased with prolonged time in the fed-batch culture, it was still higher than that of the control, and the descent rate was much slower. Accordingly, the fed-batch culture was more suitable for violaxanthin production.

Table 1. Production of biomass and violaxanthin in *Eustigmatos* cf. *polyphem* grown in batch culture and fed-batch culture under low light illumination.

Culture Mode	Time (Day)	Biomass (g/L)	Violaxanthin Content (% of DW)	Violaxanthin Productivity (mg/L/d)
Batch culture (control)	5th	1.36 ± 0.03 [a]	0.39 ± 0.01 [a]	1.07 ± 0.03 [a]
	10th	2.53 ± 0.04 [b]	0.32 ± 0.01 [b]	0.82 ± 0.03 [b]
	15th	3.39 ± 0.06 [c]	0.27 ± 0.02 [c]	0.62 ± 0.04 [c]
	20th	4.37 ± 0.03 [d]	0.23 ± 0.01 [d]	0.51 ± 0.02 [d]
Fed-batch culture	5th	1.36 ± 0.03 [a]	0.39 ± 0.02 [a]	1.07 ± 0.03 [a]
	10th	2.92 ± 0.01 [e]	0.38 ± 0.01 [e]	1.10 ± 0.03 [a]
	15th	4.02 ± 0.05 [f]	0.36 ± 0.01 [f]	0.96 ± 0.02 [e]
	20th	5.15 ± 0.03 [g]	0.35 ± 0.02 [f]	0.90 ± 0.06 [be]

DW, dry weight. Values are expressed as the mean ± SD from three replicates. Values with different superscript letters (a, b, c, d, e, f, and g) in the same column are significantly different ($p < 0.05$).

2.5. Purification and Identification of Violaxanthin

Violaxanthin was extracted, isolated, and purified following the procedures illustrated in Figure 2. The pigment profile of the ethanol extract from *E.* cf. *polyphem* was obtained by high-performance liquid chromatography (HPLC). The result showed that violaxanthin, vaucheriaxanthin, chlorophyll *a*, and β-carotene were the major pigments (Figure 2A), which was consistent with the reports of Gao et al. [26]. Figure 2B showed that, after saponification, the peak of chlorophyll *a* was not detected, and this indicated that chlorophyll *a* was successfully removed. The concentrated ethyl acetate extract (2.77 g) was separated using silica gel column chromatography to obtain FB_2 (136 mg), and the purity of violaxanthin in FB_2 reached 62% (Figure 2C) based on the HPLC analysis. Further purification was performed using PHPLC, and $FB_{2\text{-}2}$ (10.0 mg) showed a single peak in the HPLC chromatogram at a purity ≥ 95% (Figure 2D).

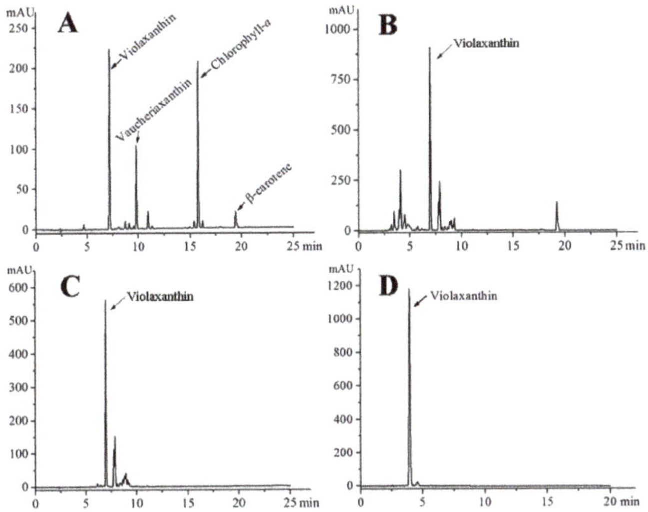

Figure 2. HPLC analysis of the pigment profile of the targeted fraction in each isolation and purification procedure. (**A**) ethanol extract; (**B**) saponification; (**C**) silica gel column chromatography; and (**D**) preparative HPLC.

Violaxanthin was then identified from $FB_{2\text{-}2}$ based on physicochemical properties, absorption spectra, and HRMS spectrum. The dried $FB_{2\text{-}2}$ powder was orange red, and it showed a characteristic UV–VIS spectrum. The maximum absorption peaks at 417.6 nm, 440.9 nm, and 470.1 nm in Figure 3A, were in agreement with those of previously published studies [10,15]. In addition, the HRMS spectrum showed two characteristic fragment ion peaks at m/z 601.4238 $[M + H]^+$ and m/z 602.4285 $[M + 2H]^+$, which corresponded to the molecular weight of the purified violaxanthin at 600.4 (Figure 3B). The results were consistent with previously published reports [2,15]. Therefore, this purified pigment was distinctly identified as 5,6,5′,6′-diepoxy-5,6,5′,6′-tetrahydro-β,β-carotene-3,3′-diol (Figure 3C).

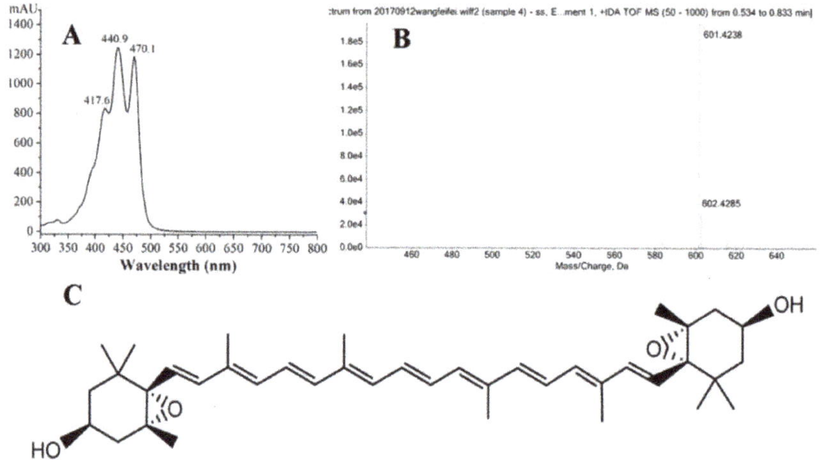

Figure 3. Identification of the purified violaxanthin from *Eustigmatos* cf. *polyphem*. (**A**) UV–VIS spectrum; (**B**) mass spectrum of violaxanthin; and (**C**) the chemical structure of violaxanthin.

2.6. Reducing Power of Purified Violaxanthin

The test sample with strong reducing power could serve as an electron donor to produce stable products and achieve the effect of scavenging radicals, and therefore the reducing power is an important indicator of the evaluation of antioxidant capacity [29]. In this study, the reducing power was determined by Fe^{3+}-Fe^{2+} transformation in the presence of different concentrations of violaxanthin. The Fe^{2+} was monitored by measuring the formation of Perl's Prussian blue at 700 nm, and the results are shown in Figure 4A. It was discernible that the reducing power of the purified violaxanthin and the positive control (ascorbic acid) increased in a concentration-dependent manner, but the purified violaxanthin showed weak reducing power in contrast with ascorbic acid. At 80 $\mu g\ mL^{-1}$, purified violaxanthin exhibited a reducing power of 0.32 ± 0.02 abs, while the reducing power of ascorbic acid reached 0.91 ± 0.02 abs. Additionally, we found that the reducing power of violaxanthin and ascorbic acid was low at 1.25 to 5 $\mu g\ mL^{-1}$ with no significant difference, but the reducing power of ascorbic acid notably increased when the concentration of ascorbic acid was greater than 10 $\mu g\ mL^{-1}$.

2.7. DPPH Radical-Scavenging Activity of Purified Violaxanthin

The DPPH radical assay is one of the most widely used methods for testing the antioxidant activity of various compounds [30]. DPPH is a stable nitrogen-centered radical, that is violet colored in ethanol and has a strong absorption peak at 517 nm. Therefore, this assay is based on the measurement of the absorbance change of the reaction solution at 517 nm after violaxanthin was mixed with DPPH, and the results are shown in Figure 4B. The DPPH-radical scavenging activity of purified violaxanthin was concentration-dependent. When the concentration was varied from 1.25–80 $\mu g\ mL^{-1}$, the inhibition percentage of purified violaxanthin ranged from 2.15% to 78.17%. Zhang et al. [31] reported that several natural pigments (lutein, lycopene, betalain, and capsanthin) showed an inhibition percentage of 25–60% in the scavenging of DPPH radicals, which were lower than the the inhibition activity of purified violaxanthin at the same concentration. Purified violaxanthin scavenged 50% of DPPH radicals with EC_{50} of 41.42 μg mL^{-1}, which was three times smaller compared to fucoxanthin isolated from *Odontella aurita* (phylum Bacillariophyta) (EC_{50} = 140 mg mL^{-1} [32]). Although the scavenging capacity of purified violaxanthin was inferior to the positive control (ascorbic acid), it always exhibited potent potential in the scavenging of DPPH radicals.

2.8. *ABTS Radical Scavenging Activity of the Purified Violaxanthin*

ABTS produces the stable glaucous cation radicals ($ABST^{+}$) by reacting with $K_2(SO_4)_2$, which has a characteristic peak absorbance at 734 nm. The absorbance of the reaction solution decreased from adding the antioxidants, which were used to assess its antioxidant activity.

As demonstrated in Figure 4C, purified violaxanthin and ascorbic acid both showed strong scavenging activities for $ABTS^{+}$ radicals. When the concentration $\geq$ 40 μg mL^{-1}, purified violaxanthin and ascorbic acid had the same $ABTS^{+}$ scavenging power, with the ability to almost completely scavenged $ABTS^{+}$ radicals. Between the concentrations of 1.25 and 40 μg mL^{-1}, the inhibition effect of the purified violaxanthin fortified with increasing concentration, and it showed an inhibition of 99.08 $\pm$ 0.32% at 40 μg mL^{-1}. The EC_{50} value of the purified violaxanthin was 15.25 μg mL^{-1}, and it clearly indicated that violaxanthin has a strong inhibitory effect on $ABTS^{+}$ radicals in comparison with that of fucoxanthin (EC_{50} = 30 μg/mL [32]). Fu et al. [2] reported that violaxanthin purified from water spinach scavenged $ABTS^{+}$ radicals more efficiently than the β-carotenoid and lutein, and that violaxanthin also inhibited a larger quantity of $ABTS^{+}$ radicals as compared to DPPH radicals. These findings were in accordance with our results.

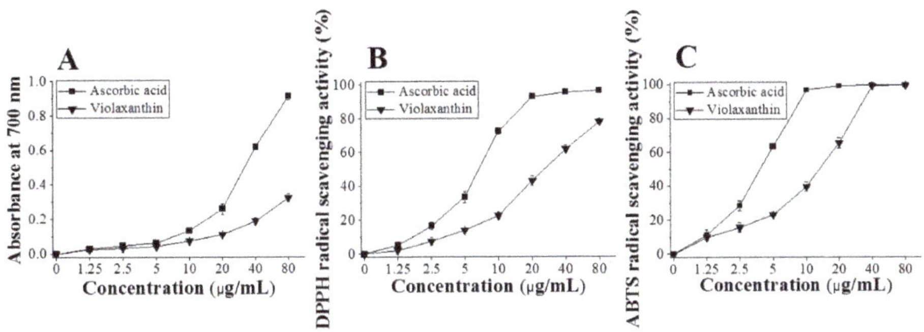

Figure 4. Antioxidant activity assays for purified violaxanthin from *Eustigmatos* cf. *polyphem*. (**A**) Reducing power; (**B**) scavenging of DPPH radicals; and (**C**) scavenging of ABTS radical. Ascorbic acid was used as a positive control. Values are shown as the mean ± standard deviation from three independent experiments.

3. Materials and Methods

3.1. *Chemicals and Reagents*

Pigment standards including chlorophyll *a*, violaxanthin, vaucheriaxanthin, and β-carotene were purchased from Sigma-Aldrich Chemical Co. (Shanghai, China; http://www.sigmaaldrich.com). Silica gel (200–300 mesh) was obtained from Qing Dao Marine Chemical Co. (Qingdao, China). HPLC-grade solvents used for HPLC analysis were purchased from Guangzhou Runhao Biotech Co. (Guangzhou, China), such as methanol, acetonitrile, acetic ether, and dichloromethane. Other analytical solvents (n-hexane, methanol, and acetone) used in extraction and isolation of violaxanthin were purchased from Guangzhou Runhao Biotech Co. (Guangzhou, China). Deionized water was prepared by a Milli-Q water purification system (Millipore Corp., Bedford, MA, USA).

Chemicals used for their antioxidant activity including 2,2-diphenyl-2-picrylhydrazyl hydrate (DPPH), 2,2′-azino-bis(3-ethylbenzothiazoline-6-sulfonic acid) (ABTS), potassium persulfate, ferrous chloride, potassium ferricyanide, trichloroacetic acid, hydrogen peroxide, ascorbic acid, sodium dihydrogen phosphate, and disodium hydrogen phosphate were obtained from Sangon Biotech Co. (Shanghai, China).

3.2. General Analytical Methods

For biomass measurement, 5.0 mL of algal cultures was filtered through a pre-weighed 0.45 μm GF/B filter paper. Then, the filter paper was dried in an oven at 105 °C overnight. The biomass (DW, g/L) was determined by the difference of the weight of the filter paper with microalgal cells (W_2) and the weight of filter paper (W_1) and was calculated as ($W_2 - W_1$) × 200.

For pigment profile analysis, 10.0 mg of freeze-dried microalgal powder mixed with 5 mL of methanol was extracted with a magnetic stirrer at 4 °C overnight until the algal residue was colorless. A certain volume of the pigment extracts was obtained by centrifugation (1940× *g*, 10 min) and filtration (Millipore, 0.45 μm), and analyzed by HPLC. The HPLC was conducted on a Dionex model U-3000 instrument equipped with a TC-C18 column (5 μm, 4.6 mm × 250 mm, Agilent, Santa Clara, CA, USA) and a UV–VIS detector (Waters 2998) at 445 nm. The mobile phase used for HPLC was a binary gradient solvent system (solvent A, acetonitrile/water = 9:1; solvent B, ethyl acetate) with a flow rate of 1 mL min^{-1}, and the elution program was as follows: 0 min, 100% A, 0% B; 20 min, 100% B, 0% A; 25 min, 100% B, 0% A; 27 min, 100% A, 0% B; 30 min, 100% A, 0% B.

A stock solution of the violaxanthin standard was prepared in methanol (HPLC grade), and then serially diluted to a final concentration of 60, 30, 15, 7.5, 3.75, and 1.875 μg mL^{-1}. A standard curve (y (μg mL^{-1}) = 3110.60x − 5.98, R^2 = 0.999) of violaxanthin was drawn on the basis of these concentrations by HPLC. Thus, the violaxanthin production in the *E.* cf. *polyphem* biomass was quantified by the following equations:

$$\text{Violaxanthin content (VC, \% of DW)} = \frac{C \times V \times 10^{-3}}{m} \times 100 \quad (1)$$

$$\text{Violaxanthin productivity}\left(\text{mg L}^{-1}\text{d}^{-1}\right) = \frac{DW \times VC\% \times 10^{3}}{t} \quad (2)$$

where m (mg) denotes the weight of microalgal powder, V (mL) denotes the volume of the extraction solvent; DW denotes the dry weight of biomass (g L^{-1}); t (day) denotes the cultivation time, and C (μg mL^{-1}) denotes the concentration of the extracted violaxanthin as determined by HPLC analysis.

3.3. Microalgae and Cultivation Conditions

The microalga *Eustigmatos* cf. *polyphem* (CAUP-H4302, formerly determined as *Myrmecia bisecta*) used in this study was obtained from the CAUP Culture Collection of Algae. *E.* cf. *polyphem* cells were maintained in a modified BG-11 (mBG-11) medium [26] and deposited in our laboratory. The inocula were prepared by culturing the microalgae in a bubble column glass photobioreactor (Ø6 × 60 cm) with 1.2 L of mBG-11 medium, and growing under continuous 60–70 μmol photons m^{-2} s^{-1} of white fluorescent light illumination at 25 ± 1 °C for 7–9 days. The seed cultures were then inoculated into the fresh mBG-11 medium for cultivation.

In order to investigate the effects of culture conditions on violaxanthin production in *E.* cf. *polyphem*, several important influencing factors were assessed, including culture time, nitrogen concentration, light intensity, and culture mode. The variation of biomass, violaxanthin content, and violaxanthin productivity were used to evaluate the effects of these factors on violaxanthin production in *E.* cf. *polyphem*. The detailed experimental design was as follows: (1) different cultivation times of 3, 5, 7, 9, and 11 days were set to culture the algal cells at a low light intensity of 120 μmol photons m^{-2} s^{-1}; (2) sodium nitrate was used as the nitrogen source, and different initial nitrogen supplementation levels (0, 9, 18, 27, 36, and 45 mM) were designed for the cultivation of *E.* cf. *polyphem* at a low light intensity of 120 μmol photons m^{-2} s^{-1}; (3) different light intensities of 80, 120, and 160 μmol photons m^{-2} s^{-1} were exploited to culture *E.* cf. *polyphem* with 18 mM of initial nitrogen supply; (4) *E.* cf. *polyphem* was grown in batch culture or fed-batch culture with low light irradiation of 120 μmol photons m^{-2} s^{-1}, and mBG-11medium was replaced at five-day intervals at the beginning of the fifth day in the fed-batch culture. All cultures were inoculated into Ø6 × 60 cm bubble column glass photobioreactors at the same initial cell density of 0.25–0.30 g/L and bubbled with 1% CO_2 (*v*/*v*) from the bottom of the column. The light intensity was measured with dual radiation meter (DRM-FQ, Apogee Instruments, Inc., Logan, UT, USA). Every experimental group was a set of three replicates.

At the end of the cultivation time, culture samples were harvested by centrifugation at 1940× *g* for 5 min, and then lyophilized in a vacuum freeze-dryer (Christ, Germany). The algal powder was stored at 4 °C prior to analysis.

3.4. Extraction, Isolation and Purification of Violaxanthin

The extraction, isolation and purification procedures for violaxanthin from *E.* cf. *polyphem* are shown in Figure 5. HPLC was used to analyze the pigment profile in each extraction and isolation procedure. All the processes were performed under weak light.

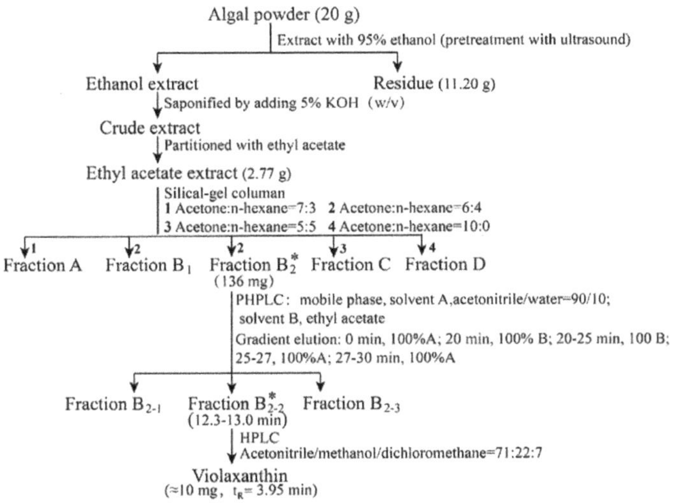

Figure 5. Flowchart of extraction, isolation, and identification of violaxanthin from *Eustigmatos* cf. *polyphem*. "*", denotes the fraction containing the highest violaxanthin content from the same row.

Freeze-dried microalgal powder (20 g, 0.38% of violaxanthin in dry weight) was mixed with 500 mL of 95% ethanol and subjected to ultrasound-assisted pretreatment in an ultrasonic cleaning bath for 2 h. After ultrasound treatment, the mixture was extracted with a magnetic stirrer in a 40 °C water bath for 4 h. This extraction procedure was repeated four times until the algal powder became colorless. The combined pigment extracts were collected by centrifugation at 1940× *g* for 10 min, and then saponified by adding 5% KOH (*w*/*v*, 100 g) at 50 °C for 30 min under continuous shaking. After the ethanol was removed using a rotary vacuum evaporator at 40 °C, the ethanol extract was re-dissolved in 300 mL of deionized water and partitioned with 400 mL of ethyl acetate in a separatory funnel (1 L) three times. The upper phases were combined and washed with deionized water several times until the KOH was completely removed. The concentrated ethyl acetate extract was obtained by evaporating, and then subjected to a silica-gel column (3 × 40 cm), which was continuously eluted with a stepwise gradient of n-hexane/acetone eluent (*v*/*v* = 7:3, 6:4, 5:5, 0:10) to obtain five fractions (FA, FB_1, FB_2, FC, and FD).

According to the HPLC analysis of pigment profiles from the five fractions, FB_2 was rich in violaxanthin, and was further separated by PHPLC to collect three fractions ($FB_{2\text{-}1}$, $FB_{2\text{-}2}$, and $FB_{2\text{-}3}$). PHPLC was conducted on an Agilent 1100 series instrument (Agilent, Santa Clara, CA, USA) equipped with a TC-C18 column (5 μm, 20 × 250 mm, Agilent, Santa Clara, CA, USA), and the mobile phase was the same as that used for HPLC analysis. The flow rate was 8 mL min^{-1}, and ultraviolet detection was a 445 nm. The target fraction ($FB_{2\text{-}2}$) was tracked and collected on the basis of the spectral characteristics of the standard.

3.5. HPLC Analysis and Identification of Purified Violaxanthin

Purity detection of the targeted fraction ($FB_{2\text{-}2}$, 15 μL) was performed using HPLC, and was applied with an isocratic mobile phase of acetonitrile/methanol/dichloromethane (71:22:7, *v*/*v*/*v*) at a flow rate of 1 mL min^{-1}; the other details have been previously described. The $FB_{2\text{-}2}$ powder was dissolved in methanol, and the accurate molecular weight was determined by high resolution mass spectrum (HRMS, SCIEX, X500R QTOF, Redwood city, CA, USA) using an instrument equipped with an electrospray ionization (ESI) source. Positive mode electrospray ionization ((+) ESI) was conducted to analyze the mass spectra over a mass range of 50–1000 *m*/*z* using a 0.1 unit step size.

3.6. Antioxidant Activity Assay

The antioxidant activity of purified violaxanthin was assessed in vitro by three tests, including the reducing power, DPPH radical scavenging activity, and $ABTS^+$ radical scavenging activity.

A stock solution (1.0 mg L^{-1}) of purified violaxantin was dissolved in ethanol, and then serially diluted with ethanol to a final concentration of 80, 40, 20, 10, 2.5, and 1.25 μg mL^{-1}, respectively. Ascorbic acid was used as the positive control, and it was dissolved in deionized water and prepared in a solution of the same concentration as violaxantin. The concentration (μg mL^{-1}) of a compound required to scavenge 50% of the radicals is expressed as EC_{50} for the evaluation of potency. All tests were run in triplicate, deionized water was used as a blank control, and the absorbance of the reaction solution was measured with an ultraviolet spectrophotometer (Thermo, Waltham, MA, USA).

Reducing power was determined using a method described by Xia et al. [32]. Briefly, 1.0 mL of different concentrations of purified violaxanthin (1.25–80 μg mL^{-1}) was mixed with 0.2 mL of phosphate buffered saline (PBS, 0.2 M, Ph = 6.6) and 1.5 mL of potassium ferricyanide (1%, *w*/*v*), respectively, and the mixture was incubated at 50 °C in a water bath for 20 min. Then, 1 mL of trichloroacetic acid (10%, *w*/*v*) was added to the mixture to quench the reaction. After centrifugation (1940× *g*, 10 min), 2 mL of the supernatant was diluted with 3 mL of deionized water and then reacted with 0.5 mL of ferric chloride (0.5%, *w*/*v*) for 6 min, and the absorbance was rapidly measured at 700 nm. A higher absorbance (A_{700}) of the reaction mixture indicated a stronger reducing power of violaxanthin.

DPPH radical scavenging activity of purified violaxanthin was evaluated according to the method of Bai et al. [33] with a slight modification. Two milliliters of DPPH methanolical solution (0.1 mM) was added to 1 mL of different concentrations of the purified violaxanthin (1.25–80 μg mL^{-1}). The mixture was vigorously shaken, and then maintained at room temperature in the dark for 30 min. The absorbance of the reaction solution was rapidly measured at 517 nm, and the scavenging ability was calculated using the following equation: DPPH radical scavenging activity (%) = $[(A_{control} - A_{test})/A_{control}] \times 100$, where $A_{control}$ was the absorbance of the blank control and A_{test} was the absorbance of a test reaction.

The scavenging ability of purified violaxanthin against the $ABTS^+$ radical was measured using a method by Chen et al. [34] with some modifications. The stock solutions of ABTS (7 mM) and potassium peroxydisulfate (2.45 mM) were firstly prepared with deionized water. One milliliter of ABTS solution and 1 mL of potassium peroxydisulfate solution were mixed and stored in the dark at room temperature for 12–16 h. Then, the mixed solution was diluted with ethanol to obtain an appropriate concentration of the $ABTS^+$ working solution (A_{734} = 0.70). Two milliliters of the $ABTS^+$ working solution was mixed with 1 mL of purified violaxanthin at concentrations ranging from 1.25–80 μg mL^{-1}, and the solution was incubated at room temperature for 6 min. The absorbance at 734 nm was rapidly measured, and the scavenging ability was calculated as: ABTS radical scavenging activity (%) = $[(A_{control} - A_{test})/A_{control}] \times 100$, where $A_{control}$ denotes the absorbance of the blank control, and A_{test} denotes the absorbance of the test reaction.

3.7. Statistical Analysis

All measurements were carried out at least in triplicate, and the experimental data are expressed as the mean ± SD (standard deviation). Student-Newman-Keul's test using one-way ANOVA was performed using a statistical analysis software package (SPSS 19.0, IBM Corporation, Armonk, NY, USA), and statistically significant difference were $p < 0.05$.

4. Conclusions

This work revealed that light intensity and nitrogen concentration were the main factors affecting the accumulation of violaxanthin in *Eustigmatos* cf. *polyphem*. The fed-batch culture was may be more suitable for maintaining the vigorous growth and a high level of violaxanthin under low-light irradiation. The violaxanthin purified from *Eustigmatos* cf. *polyphem* shows a potent efficacy in the scavenging of DPPH and $ABTS^+$ radicals, which indicates that violaxanthin could be used as a natural antioxidant agent for therapeutic or functional adjuvant purposes.

Author Contributions: C.Z. conceived and designed the experiments; F.W. and L.H. performed the experiments and analyzed the data; and F.W., B.G., and C.Z. wrote and revised the paper.

Acknowledgments: We would like to thank LetPub (www.letpub.com) for providing linguistic assistance during the preparation of this manuscript. This work was supported by the following funding: the National High Technology Research and Development Program of China (863 Program) (no. 2013AA065805); the Special Program for Low-Carbon, Reform and Development Commission of Guangdong Province (2011-051), and the Key Program of Zhouhai City (PC20081008).

Conflicts of Interest: The authors declare no conflict of interest.

References

1. Rodriguez-Amaya, D.B. *A Guide to Carotenoid Analysis in Foods;* ILSI Press: Washington, DC, USA, 2001.
2. Fu, H.; Xie, B.; Ma, S.; Zhu, X.; Fan, G.; Pan, S. Evaluation of antioxidant activities of principal carotenoids available in water spinach (*Ipomoea aquatica*). *J. Food. Compos. Anal.* **2011**, *24*, 288–297. [CrossRef]
3. Liu, D.; Shi, J.; Ibarra, A.C.; Kakuda, Y.; Xue, S.J. The scavenging capacity and synergistic effects of lycopene, vitamin E, vitamin C, and β-carotene mixtures on the DPPH free radical. *LWT-Food Sci. Technol.* **2008**, *41*, 1344–1349. [CrossRef]
4. Müller, L.; Fröhlich, K.; Böhm, V. Comparative antioxidant activities of carotenoids measured by ferric reducing antioxidant power (FRAP), ABTS bleaching assay (αTEAC), DPPH assay and peroxyl radical scavenging assay. *Food Chem.* **2011**, *129*, 139–148. [CrossRef]
5. Fraser, P.D.; Bramley, P.M. The biosynthesis and nutritional uses of carotenoids. *Prog. Lipid Res.* **2004**, *43*, 228–265. [CrossRef] [PubMed]
6. Milledge, J.J. Commercial application of microalgae other than as biofuels: A brief review. *Rev. Environ. Sci. Bio/Technol.* **2011**, *10*, 31–41. [CrossRef]
7. Rajauria, G.; Foley, B.; Abu-Ghannam, N. Characterization of dietary fucoxanthin from *Himanthalia elongata* brown seaweed. *Food Res. Int.* **2017**, *99*, 995–1001. [CrossRef] [PubMed]
8. Cano, M.; Gómez-Maqueo, A.; García-Cayuela, T.; Welti-Chanes, J. Characterization of carotenoid profile of Spanish *Sanguinos* and *Verdal* prickly pear (*Opuntia ficus-indica*, spp.) tissues. *Food Chem.* **2017**, *237*, 612–622. [CrossRef] [PubMed]

9. Hu, C.C.; Lin, J.T.; Lu, F.J.; Chou, F.P.; Yang, D.J. Determination of carotenoids in *Dunaliella salina* cultivated in Taiwan and antioxidant capacity of the algal carotenoid extract. *Food Chem.* **2008**, *109*, 439–446. [CrossRef] [PubMed]
10. Soontornchaiboon, W.; Joo, S.S.; Kim, S.M. Anti-inflammatory effects of violaxanthin isolated from microalga *Chlorella ellipsoidea* in RAW 264.7 macrophages. *Biol. Pharm. Bull.* **2012**, *35*, 1137–1144. [CrossRef] [PubMed]
11. Hagen, C.; Braune, W.; Vogel, K.; HÄDER, D.P. Functional aspects of secondary carotenoids in *Haematococcus lacustris* (Girod) Rostafinski (Volvocales). V. Influences on photomovement. *Plant Cell Environ.* **1993**, *16*, 991–995. [CrossRef]
12. Guedes, A.C.; Amaro, H.M.; Malcata, F.X. Microalgae as sources of carotenoids. *Mar. Drugs* **2011**, *9*, 625–644. [CrossRef] [PubMed]
13. Meléndez-Martínez, A.J.; Britton, G.; Vicario, I.M.; Heredia, F.J. The complex carotenoid pattern of orange juices from concentrate. *Food Chem.* **2008**, *109*, 546–553. [CrossRef]
14. Shukla, M.; Kumar, S. Algal biorefineries for biofuels and other value-added products. In *Biorefining of Biomass to Biofuels*; Springer: Cham, Switzerland, 2018; pp. 305–341.
15. Pasquet, V.; Morisset, P.; Ihammouine, S.; Chepied, A.; Aumailley, L.; Berard, J.-B.; Serive, B.; Kaas, R.; Lanneluc, I.; Thiery, V. Antiproliferative activity of violaxanthin isolated from bioguided fractionation of *Dunaliella tertiolecta* extracts. *Mar. Drugs* **2011**, *9*, 819–831. [CrossRef] [PubMed]
16. Talero, E.; García-Mauriño, S.; Ávila-Román, J.; Rodríguez-Luna, A.; Alcaide, A.; Motilva, V. Bioactive compounds isolated from microalgae in chronic inflammation and cancer. *Mar. Drugs* **2015**, *13*, 6152–6209. [CrossRef] [PubMed]
17. Zhang, J.; Wan, L.; Xia, S.; Li, A.; Zhang, C. Morphological and spectrometric analyses of lipids accumulation in a novel oleaginous microalga, *Eustigmatos* cf. *polyphem* (Eustigmatophyceae). *Bioprocess Biosyst. Eng.* **2013**, *36*, 1125–1130. [CrossRef] [PubMed]
18. Li, Z.; Ma, X.; Li, A.; Zhang, C. A novel potential source of β-carotene: *Eustigmatos* cf. *polyphem* (Eustigmatophyceae) and pilot β-carotene production in bubble column and flat panel photobioreactors. *Bioresour. Technol.* **2012**, *117*, 257–263. [CrossRef] [PubMed]
19. Gao, B.; Xia, S.; Lei, X.; Zhang, C. Combined effects of different nitrogen sources and levels and light intensities on growth and fatty acid and lipid production of oleaginous eustigmatophycean microalga *Eustigmatos* cf. *polyphem*. *J. Appl. Phycol.* **2018**, *30*, 215–229. [CrossRef]
20. Eliáš, M.; Amaral, R.; Fawley, K.P.; Fawley, M.W.; Němcová, Y.; Neustupa, J.; Přibyl, P.; Santos, L.M.; Ševčíková, T. *Handbook of the Protists*; Springer International Publishing: Basel, Switzerland, 2017; pp. 1–39.
21. Keşan, G.; Litvín, R.; Bína, D.; Durchan, M.; Šlouf, V.; Polívka, T. Efficient light-harvesting using non-carbonyl carotenoids: Energy transfer dynamics in the VCP complex from *Nannochloropsis oceanica*. *BBA-Bioenerg.* **2016**, *1857*, 370–379. [CrossRef] [PubMed]
22. Llansola-Portoles, M.J.; Litvin, R.; Ilioaia, C.; Pascal, A.A.; Bina, D.; Robert, B. Pigment structure in the violaxanthin–chlorophyll-a-binding protein VCP. *Photosynth. Res.* **2017**, *134*, 51–58. [CrossRef] [PubMed]
23. Bína, D.; Gardian, Z.; Herbstová, M.; Litvín, R. Modular antenna of photosystem I in secondary plastids of red algal origin: A *Nannochloropsis oceanica* case study. *Photosynth. Rese.* **2017**, *131*, 255–266. [CrossRef] [PubMed]
24. Demmig-Adams, B.; Adams, W.W. Xanthophyll cycle and light stress in nature: Uniform response to excess direct sunlight among higher plant species. *Planta* **1996**, *198*, 460–470. [CrossRef]
25. Uhrmacher, S.; Hanelt, D.; Nultsch, W. Zeaxanthin content and the degree of photoinhibition are linearly correlated in the brown alga *Dictyota dichotoma*. *Mar. Biol.* **1995**, *123*, 159–165. [CrossRef]
26. Gao, B.; Yang, J.; Lei, X.; Xia, S.; Li, A.; Zhang, C. Characterization of cell structural change, growth, lipid accumulation, and pigment profile of a novel oleaginous microalga, *Vischeria stellata* (Eustigmatophyceae), cultured with different initial nitrate supplies. *J. Appl. Phycol.* **2016**, *28*, 821–830. [CrossRef]
27. Lubián, L.M.; Montero, O.; Moreno-Garrido, I.; Huertas, I.E.; Sobrino, C.; González-del Valle, M.; Parés, G. *Nannochloropsis* (Eustigmatophyceae) as source of commercially valuable pigments. *J. Appl. Phycol.* **2000**, *12*, 249–255. [CrossRef]
28. Peccia, J.; Haznedaroglu, B.; Gutierrez, J.; Zimmerman, J.B. Nitrogen supply is an important driver of sustainable microalgae biofuel production. *Trends Biotechnol.* **2013**, *31*, 134–138. [CrossRef] [PubMed]

29. Dong, Y.R.; Cheng, S.J.; Qi, G.H.; Yang, Z.P.; Yin, S.Y.; Chen, G.T. Antimicrobial and antioxidant activities of *Flammulina velutipes* polysacchrides and polysacchride-iron (III) complex. *Carbohydr. Polym.* **2017**, *161*, 26–32. [CrossRef] [PubMed]
30. Sharma, O.P.; Bhat, T.K. DPPH antioxidant assay revisited. *Food Chem.* **2009**, *113*, 1202–1205. [CrossRef]
31. Zhang, J.; Hou, X.; Ahmad, H.; Zhang, H.; Zhang, L.; Wang, T. Assessment of free radicals scavenging activity of seven natural pigments and protective effects in AAPH-challenged chicken erythrocytes. *Food Chem.* **2014**, *145*, 57–65. [CrossRef] [PubMed]
32. Xia, S.; Wang, K.; Wan, L.; Li, A.; Hu, Q.; Zhang, C. Production, characterization, and antioxidant activity of fucoxanthin from the marine diatom *Odontella aurita*. *Mar. Drugs* **2013**, *11*, 2667–2681. [CrossRef] [PubMed]
33. Bai, K.; Xu, W.; Zhang, J.; Kou, T.; Niu, Y.; Wan, X.; Zhang, L.; Wang, C.; Wang, T. Assessment of free radical scavenging activity of dimethylglycine sodium salt and its role in providing protection against lipopolysaccharide-induced oxidative stress in mice. *PLoS ONE* **2016**, *11*, e0155393. [CrossRef] [PubMed]
34. Li, X.; Lin, J.; Gao, Y.; Han, W.; Chen, D. Antioxidant activity and mechanism of Rhizoma *Cimicifugae*. *Chem. Cent. J.* **2012**, *6*, 140–150. [CrossRef] [PubMed]

© 2018 by the authors. Licensee MDPI, Basel, Switzerland. This article is an open access article distributed under the terms and conditions of the Creative Commons Attribution (CC BY) license (http://creativecommons.org/licenses/by/4.0/).

marine drugs

MDPI

Article

Preparative Separation and Purification of Trichothecene Mycotoxins from the Marine Fungus *Fusarium* sp. LS68 by High-Speed Countercurrent Chromatography in Stepwise Elution Mode

Yong Liu [1], Xuezhen Zhou [1], C. Benjamin Naman [1,2,3], Yanbin Lu [4], Lijian Ding [1,2,*] and Shan He [1,2,*]

1 Li Dak Sum Yip Yio Chin Kenneth Li Marine Biopharmaceutical Research Center, Ningbo University, Ningbo 315211, China; 18892618896@163.com (Y.L.); zhouxuezhen@nbu.edu.cn (X.Z.); bnaman@gmail.com (C.B.N.)

2 Key Laboratory of Marine Biotechnology of Zhejiang Province, Ningbo University, Ningbo 315211, Zhejiang, China

3 Center for Marine Biotechnology and Biomedicine, Scripps Institution of Oceanography and Skaggs School of Pharmacy and Pharmaceutical Sciences, University of California, San Diego, La Jolla, CA 92093, USA

4 Institute of Seafood, Zhejiang Gongshang University, Hangzhou 310012, China; luyanbin@zjgsu.edu.cn

* Correspondences: dinglijian@nbu.edu.cn (L.D.); heshan@nbu.edu.cn (S.H.); Tel.: +86-574-8760-0458 (S.H.)

Received: 16 January 2018; Accepted: 16 February 2018; Published: 24 February 2018

Abstract: The contamination of foods and animal feeds with trichothecene mycotoxins is a growing concern for human and animal health. As such, large quantities of pure trichothecene mycotoxins are necessary for food safety monitoring and toxicological research. A new and effective method for the purification of trichothecene mycotoxins from a marine fungus, *Fusarium* sp. LS68, is described herein. Preparative high-speed countercurrent chromatography (HSCCC) was utilized for the scalable isolation and purification of four trichothecene mycotoxins for the first time in stepwise elution mode, with a biphasic solvent system composed of hexanes–EtOAc–CH_3OH–H_2O (6:4:5:5, *v*/*v*/*v*/*v*) and (8.5:1.5:5:5,*v*/*v*/*v*/*v*). This preparative HSCCC separation was performed on 200 mg of crude sample to yield four trichothecene mycotoxins, roridin E (**1**), roridin E acetate (**2**), verrucarin L acetate (**3**), and verrucarin J (**4**) in a single run, with each of >98% purity. These compounds were identified by MS, ^{1}H NMR, ^{13}C NMR, and polarimetry. The results demonstrate an efficient HSCCC method for the separation of trichothecene mycotoxins, which can be utilized to produce pure commercial and research standards.

Keywords: trichothecene mycotoxins; roridin; verrucarin; high-speed countercurrent chromatography; preparative separation; stepwise elution

1. Introduction

According to the Food and Agriculture Organization of the United Nations, about 25% of the food crops in the world are contaminated with mycotoxins, and these have adverse effects on humans, animals, and crops that result in serious illnesses and economic losses [1]. Among the major mycotoxins produced by *Fusarium* species, trichothecenes are pathogenic to important agricultural crops and foods [2], and these lead to serious economic losses by reducing yields and overall quality of North American agricultural products [3,4]. For example, *Fusarium* head blight disease, caused by trichothecene mycotoxins, has been shown to have contaminated cereals and grains [5,6].

Trichothecenes are a group of tetracyclic sesquiterpene mycotoxins that are produced by various fungi from the order *Hypocreales*, including those of the genera *Fusarium*, *Myrothecium*,

Verticimonosporium, *Stachybotrys*, *Trichoderma*, *Trichothecium*, *Cephalosporium*, and *Cylindrocarpon* [7–11]. These molecules are potent phytotoxins, and act as the virulence factors of pathogenic fungi on sensitive infected host plants, particularly wheat and barley [12–14]. The unfortunate contamination of botanical dietary supplements with mycotoxins has also been reported recently, representing a significant risk to public health [15]. One obstacle to the further investigation of these important topics has been the scarce quantity of pure compounds from the trichothecene class. Therefore, the preparative separation of high purity trichothecene mycotoxins is of great interest. At present, trichothecene mycotoxins are isolated from fungal extracts by conventional methods, such as macroporous resin separation followed by silica gel column chromatography. These methods can be considered costly, laborious, and time-consuming, and furthermore result in substantial sample loss due to irreversible adsorption to the silica [16,17]. It is therefore important to develop rapid and efficient methods for the separation and purification of trichothecene mycotoxins.

High-speed countercurrent chromatography (HSCCC) is a technique that uses liquid-liquid partition chromatography to improve recovery rates and efficiency, and which eliminates irreversible adsorption by solid support media [17–19]. HSCCC has been widely used for the preparative separation and purification of natural products, and this is a scalable technology [20,21]. Disclosed herein is the first preparative isolation and purification of trichothecene mycotoxins by HSCCC in stepwise elution mode, allowing for the purification of several compounds in one run. The trichothecene mycotoxins roridin E (**1**), roridin E acetate (**2**), verrucarin L acetate (**3**), and verrucarin J (**4**) were thus isolated from an epiphytic fungus, *Fusarium* sp. LS68, which was derived from the sponge *Haliclona* sp. The structures of **1–4** are presented in Figure 1.

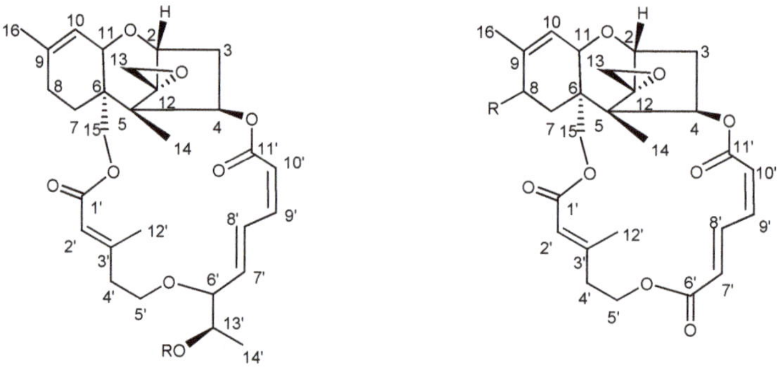

1 R = H   **3** R = OAc

2 R = Ac   **4** R = H

Figure 1. Structures of roridin E (**1**), roridin E acetate (**2**), verrucarin L acetate (**3**), verrucarin J (**4**).

2. Results and Discussion

2.1. HPLC Analysis of the Crude Extract

An HPLC method was developed to ensure the baseline separation of the target compounds and impurities. Different solvent systems, flow rates, detection wavelengths, and column temperatures were screened. The components of interest, **1–4**, were satisfactorily separated by a CH_3CN/H_2O gradient (flow rate 0.8 mL/min, 25–75% CH_3CN from 0–60 min) when the column temperature was set at 25 °C. The HPLC chromatogram of the crude extract is shown in Figure 2, Panel A. The same method was used to analyze HSCCC method development samples, and later HSCCC eluents (Figure 2, Panels B–E), for fraction pooling.

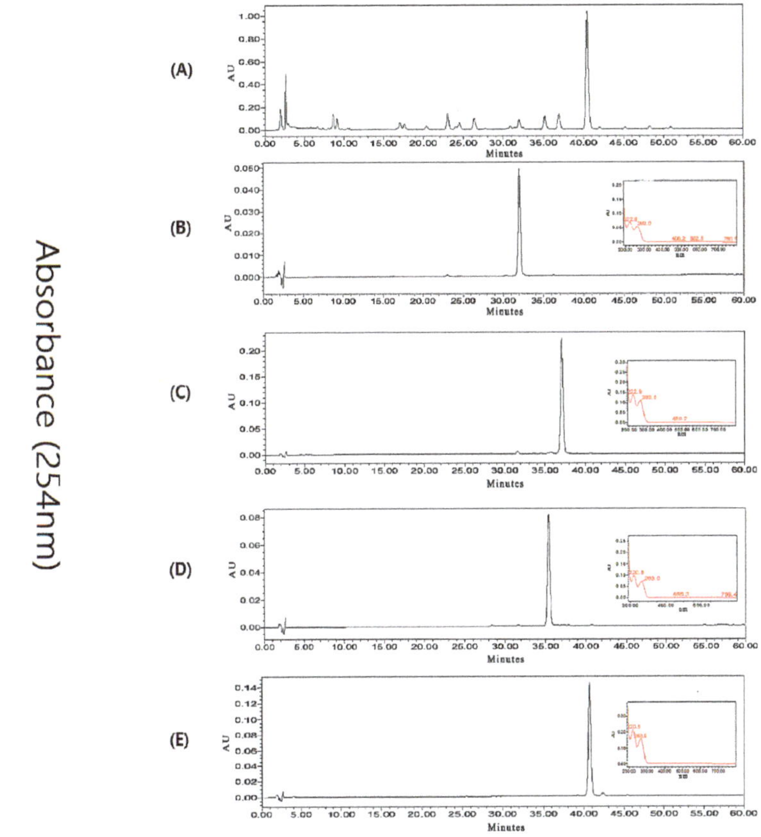

Figure 2. Representative analytical HPLC chromatograms. (**A**) Crude extract of *Fusarium* sp; (**B**) refined peak 1 from HSCCC, corresponding to compound **1**; (**C**) refined peak 2 from HSCCC, corresponding to compound **3**; (**D**) refined peak 3 from HSCCC, corresponding to compound **2**; (**E**) refined peak 4 from HSCCC, corresponding to compound **4**. For B–D, UV profiles of the major peak are inset at 254 nm.

2.2. Optimization of Suitable HSCCC Solvent System

In order to efficiently separate and purify target compounds, the selection of an optimal biphasic solvent system is critical for preparative HSCCC. According to the "golden rules of HSCCC", satisfactory partition coefficient K_D values should meet some basic requirements: (1) the target compounds should each be in the range of $0.5 \leq K_D \leq 2.0$; (2) each set of two target compounds should have the separation factor $\alpha > 1.5$, where α is the ratio of the two K_D values ($\alpha = K_D^1/K_D^2$, for $K_D^1 > K_D^2$); and (3) higher retention of the stationary phase will provide better peak resolution [22]. Thus, preliminary studies were carried out to examine the K_D values of the trichothecene mycotoxins **1–4** in different hexanes–EtOAc–CH_3OH–H_2O solvent systems of different volume ratios by liquid-liquid partitioning and HPLC analysis. The K_D values for **1–4** in the various solvent systems tested are shown in Table 1.

Table 1. Partition coefficients (K_D) of compounds **1–4** in several hexanes–EtOAc–CH_3OH–H_2O solvent systems tested for high-speed countercurrent chromatography (HSCCC) separation.

Solvent System (*v*/*v*) Hexanes–EtOAc–CH_3OH–H_2O	K_D			
	Compound 1	Compound 2	Compound 3	Compound 4
1:1:1:1	2.08	2.61	2.33	10.58
5.5:4.5:5:5	0.93	2.25	2.14	4.73
6:4:5:5	0.61	1.83	1.26	3.32
6.5:3.5:5:5	0.37	1.43	1.12	2.58
7:3:5:5	0.45	1.25	0.80	3.21
7.5:2.5:5:5	0.36	1.10	0.68	2.73
8:2:5:5	0.19	0.58	0.54	1.87
8.5:1.5:5:5	0.11	0.37	0.32	1.12
9:1:5:5	0.10	0.30	0.25	0.83

No single suitable biphasic solvent system was found that had K_D values between 0.5 and 2 for each of compounds **1–4** at the same time. To overcome this challenge, a stepwise HSCCC elution mode was chosen in order to separate compounds with significantly different K_D values in a single run. This technique had been successfully applied previously by some research groups [23,24].

The use of the "HeMWat", or hexanes–EtOAc–CH_3OH–H_2O, solvent system at volumetric ratios of 1:1:1:1 and 5.5:4.5:5:5 both afforded larger K_D values unsuitable for the separation of the trichothecene mycotoxins investigated. However, the biphasic solvent system of hexanes–EtOAc–CH_3OH–H_2O at a volumetric ratio of 6.5:3.5:5:5 yielded acceptable K_D values of compounds **1–3** between 0.5 and 2, although compounds **2** and **3** had an unsuitable separation factor $\alpha < 1.5$. However, the biphasic hexanes–EtOAc–CH_3OH–H_2O solvent system at a volume ratio of 6:4:5:5 led to the observation of the K_D values between 0.5 and 2 for compounds **1**, **2**, and **3**, and each pair had a separation factor $\alpha > 1.5$. Nevertheless, this solvent system offered an unsuitable K_D value (2.58) for compound **4**. To overcome this problem, the hexanes–EtOAc–CH_3OH–H_2O 8.5:1.5:5:5 solvent system was selected for the second part of the HSCCC run, since it produced a suitable K_D value of 1.12 for compound **4**, and it would only be used in stepwise mode after the elution of **1–3**.

2.3. Stepwise HSCCC Separation

The optimized stepwise elution method was applied for the direct preparative HSCCC separation of 200 mg of crude *Fusarium* extract in a single run. As shown in Figure 3, the separation initiated with the solvent system of hexanes–EtOAc–CH_3OH–H_2O 6:4:5:5, and the upper phase was used as the stationary phase while the lower phase was used as the mobile phase in the head-to-tail elution mode. Retention of the stationary phase was 63%, and after peaks 1–3 eluted at 102, 180, and 205 min, respectively, the mobile phase was switched to the lower phase of the solvent system (8.5:1.5:5:5) at 250 min. Peak 4 was well resolved, and eluted at 350 min. Timewise fractions were collected from the HSCCC separation and pooled after evaluation by HPLC, to yield compound **1** (11.3 mg), compound **2** (7.7 mg), compound **3** (4.7 mg), and compound **4** (21.3 mg). Each compound isolated had a purity of >98% based on UV peak integrations (Figure 2, Panels B–E). The chromatogram of HSCCC separation is shown in Figure 3.

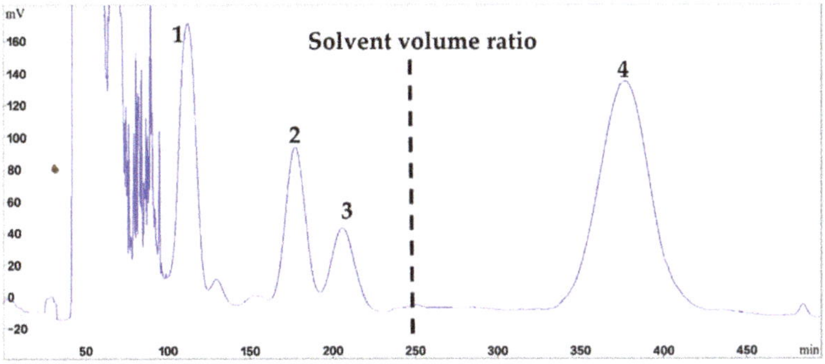

Figure 3. HSCCC chromatogram of the crude extract from *Fusarium* sp. LS68 using stepwise elution with solvent systems A and B. The dotted line represents the time at which the solvent system was switched from A to B. Solvent system A: hexanes–EtOAc–CH_3OH–H_2O (6:4:5:5, *v*/*v*/*v*/*v*), solvent system B: hexanes–EtOAc–CH_3OH–H_2O (8.5:1.5:5:5, *v*/*v*/*v*/*v*); stationary phase: upper phase of solvent system A; mobile phase: lower aqueous phase of solvent system A and B; column capacity, 350 mL; rotation speed, 800 rpm; column temperature, 25 °C; flow rate, 2.0 mL/min; detection, 254 nm; sample injected, 200 mg in 6 mL biphasic solution; retention of the stationary phase, 63%; peak identification: roridin E (**1**), roridin E acetate (**2**), verrucarin L acetate (**3**), verrucarin J (**4**).

2.4. Structural Identification

The structural identification of **1–4** was conducted by HRESI-MS, ^1H and ^{13}C NMR analyses, as well as specific rotation data, and these were compared with literature values. Accordingly, the molecules isolated were identified as roridin E (**1**) [25], roridin E acetate (**2**) [26], verrucarin L acetate (**3**) [27], and verrucarin J (**4**) [27] (see Supplementary Materials).

3. Materials and Methods

3.1. Reagents and Materials

All solvents used for HSCCC were of analytical grade (Huadong Chemicals, Hangzhou, China). Reverse osmosis Milli-Q water (18 M) (Millipore, Bedford, MA, USA) was used for all solutions and dilutions. Methanol used for HPLC analyses was of chromatographic grade and purchased from Anpel Laboratory Technologies (Shanghai, China). The $CDCl_3$ used for NMR analyses was purchased from Tenglong Weibo Technology (Qingdao, China).

3.2. Fungal Material

The marine fungi *Fusarium* sp. LS68, was isolated and cultured from a *Halicloma* sp. sponge collected from Linshui, Hainan Province, China. It was identified as *Fusarium* sp. according to the morphological and molecular (ITS rDNA sequence) analyses (GenBank accession number EU860057, 99% similarity). A voucher specimen was deposited at the School of Marine Sciences, Ningbo University (Ningbo, China).

3.3. Apparatus

HSCCC was carried out using a model TBE-300C high-speed countercurrent chromatograph (Tauto Biotech Co. Ltd., Shanghai, China), containing a self-balancing three-coil centrifuge rotor equipped with three preparative multilayer coils and a total capacity of 320 mL. The internal diameter of PTFE (Polytetrafluoroethylene) tubing was 1.9 mm. The apparatus maximum rotational speed is 1000 rpm and has a 20 mL manual sample loop. The revolution radius was 5 cm and the β value of the multilayer coil varied from 0.5 at the internal terminal to 0.8 at the external terminal.

An integrated TBP 5002 (Tauto Biotech Co. Ltd.) was used to pump the two-phase HSCCC solvent system, and the UV absorbance of the effluent was measured at 254 nm by a UV 1001 detector (Shanghai Sanotac Scientific Instruments Co. Ltd., Shanghai, China). A DC-0506 constant temperature regulator (Tauto Biotech Co. Ltd.) was used to control the temperature during HSCCC. An N2000 data analysis system (Institute of Automation Engineering, Zhejiang University, Hangzhou, China) was employed for HSCCC data collection and analysis. The analytical HPLC equipment was an Alliance 2695 equipped with a model 2998 diode array detector and Empower System (Waters Co., Milford, MA, USA). NMR experiments were carried out using a DirectDrive2 600 MHz NMR spectrometer (Agilent, Santa Clara, CA, USA) at 25 °C and Auto Triple Resonance (Agilent, Santa Clara, CA, USA). HRESIMS data were measured using a Waters Q-TOF Premier LC/MS spectrometer (Waters Co., Milford, MA, USA). Column chromatography was conducted with silica gel (200–300 mesh, Qingdao Marine Chemical Inc. Qingdao, China). The UV spectra were recorded on an NADE Evolution 201 spectrophotometer (Waters Co., Milford, CT, USA). Optical rotations were measured on an Autopol VI (Rudolph Research Analytical, Hackettstown, NJ, USA).

3.4. Culturing and Extraction

The fungus *Fusarium* sp. LS68 was cultivated in a seawater-based potato dextrose broth (PDB) medium and incubated on a rotary shaker at 150 rpm and 25 °C for 14 days. The fermentation broth (30 L) was extracted with EtOAc (3 × 30 L). The organic solvent partitions were combined and evaporated under reduced pressure at 40 °C to yield a crude extract (30 g). This sample was stored in a refrigerator at 4 °C until the subsequent HSCCC separation.

3.5. Determination of Partition Coefficients (K_D)

In order to determine the appropriate solvent systems for optimal partition coefficients (K_D), various solvent combinations of hexanes–EtOAc–CH_3OH–H_2O were attempted. A 2-mg sample of crude extract was added to a 10 mL test tube along with 8 mL of an experimental biphasic solvent system. The test tube was then capped and shaken vigorously for 3 min, to allow the distribution of the extract between the two phases. After reaching equilibration, equal aliquots of each phase (10 μL) were analyzed by HPLC-DAD to determine the partition coefficient (K_D) of each target compound. The K_D values were defined as the integrated peak area of each target compound in the upper phase divided by that in the lower phase, as observed at 254 nm.

3.6. HSCCC Separation

The biphasic solvent systems of hexanes–EtOAc–CH_3OH–H_2O (6:4:5:5 and 8.5:1.5:5:5) were selected for the HSCCC separation. A 200 mg sample of crude extract was dissolved in 6 mL of each phase of a solvent mixture consisting of equal volumes of both upper and lower phases for preparative HSCCC separation. In the single run, the upper (stationary) phase was pumped into and filled the coil column of TBE-300C (320 mL, Tauto Biotech Co. Ltd., Shanghai, China) by a constant flow at 10.0 mL/min. The column was then rotated at a speed of 800 rpm, and the lower (mobile) phase was pumped into the column in the "head to tail" elution mode at 2.0 mL/min. When the mobile phase began to elute at the tail outlet, the hydrodynamic equilibrium state of the two phases was established. Subsequently, the sample solution (6 mL) containing 200 mg of crude extract was injected through the sample port. After 250 min, the pump was stopped and then the lower phase of hexanes–EtOAc–CH_3OH–H_2O (8.5:1.5:5:5) was pumped into the column as the new mobile phase at 2.0 mL/min. The separation temperature was controlled at 25 °C. The effluent was continuously monitored with a UV detector (Shanghai Sanotac Scientific Instruments Co. Ltd., Shanghai, China) at 254 nm. After the separation procedure, the solvents in the column were completely eluted and collected. Fractions were collected near 110 min, 180 min, 210 min, and 380 min, respectively, and analyzed by HPLC to allow for fraction pooling.

3.7. HPLC Analysis and Identification of the Peaks

Each fraction generated by preparative HSCCC was evaluated by HPLC, using a 150 mm × 4.6 mm i.d., 5 μm, YMC-Pack ODS-A column (Waters Co., Milford, CT, USA) that was maintained at 25 °C. The samples were separated with a CH_3CN/H_2O gradient (flow rate 0.8 mL/min, 25–75% CH_3CN from 0–60 min). The effluent was continuously monitored by a UV detector at 220 nm and 254 nm. Fractions that showed only one peak in the chromatogram were respectively pooled together to yield compounds **1** (11.3 mg, the t_R(HPLC) 32 min, t_R(HSCCC) 102–120 min), **2** (7.7 mg, t_R(HPLC) 37 min, t_R(HSCCC) 180–195 min), **3** (4.7 mg, t_R(HPLC) 35 min, t_R(HSCCC) 205–220 min), and **4** (21.3 mg, t_R(HPLC) 40 min, t_R(HSCCC) 350–400 min). Compounds **1–4** were identified as roridin E (**1**) [25], roridin E acetate (**2**) [26], verrucarin L acetate (**3**) [27], and verrucarin J (**4**) [27] by comparison of their UV, ^1H and ^{13}C NMR, and specific rotation data with literature values. The purity levels of these samples were determined by peak area percentage after the automated integration of each chromatogram.

4. Conclusions

Trichothecenes are worldwide plant toxins that cause enormous yield losses in major economic crops. Some researchers have highlighted the need to decontaminate mycotoxins in foods and feeds [28]. However, investigations of trichothecene phytotoxicity are limited due to the difficulty and expense of obtaining trichothecene mycotoxins in high purity and sufficient quantity. In this study, the first efficient preparative separation of four trichothecene mycotoxins from the marine fungi *Fusarium* sp. LS68 by a stepwise HSCCC elution method was developed. The purities of the trichothecene mycotoxins isolated, **1–4**, were >98%. Therefore, the stepwise HSCCC method is an efficient technique for the isolation of high purity trichothecene mycotoxins. This method is industrially scalable with the size of the HSCCC instrumentation, and may provide a means to obtain pure trichothecene mycotoxins in the quantities needed for broader biological examinations and the generation of analytical standards for the agricultural food, supplement, and feedstock industries.

Supplementary Materials: The following are available online at www.mdpi.com/1660-3397/16/2/73/s1, Figure S1a, ^1H NMR spectrum of compound **1** ($CDCl_3$, 600 MHz); Figure S1b, ^{13}C NMR spectrum of compound **1** ($CDCl_3$, 150 MHz); Figure S1c, HRESIMS spectrum of compound **1**; Figure S1d, UV spectrum of compound **1**; Figure S2a, ^1H NMR spectrum of compound **2** ($CDCl_3$, 600 MHz); Figure S2b, ^{13}C NMR spectrum of compound **2** ($CDCl_3$, 150 MHz); Figure S2c, HRESIMS spectrum of compound **2**; Figure S2d, UV spectrum of compound **2**; Figure S3a, ^1H NMR spectrum of compound **3** ($CDCl_3$, 600 MHz); Figure S3b, ^{13}CNMR spectrum of compound **3** ($CDCl_3$, 150 MHz); Figure S3c, HRESIMS spectrum of compound **3**; Figure S3d, UV spectrum of compound **3**; Figure S4a, ^1H NMR spectrum of compound **4** ($CDCl_3$, 600 MHz); Figure S4b, ^{13}CNMR spectrum of compound **4** ($CDCl_3$, 150 MHz); Figure S4c, HRESIMS spectrum of compound **4**; Figure S4d, UV spectrum of compound **4**; Table S1, NMR data of compound **1** in $CDCl_3$; Table S2, NMR data of compound **2** in $CDCl_3$; Table S3, NMR data of compound **3** in $CDCl_3$; Table S4, NMR data of compound **4** in $CDCl_3$; Table S5, Specific rotation values of compounds **1–4**; Table S6, UV values of compounds **1–4**.

Acknowledgments: This study was supported by the National Natural Science Foundation of China (41776168, 41706167), the Natural Science Foundation of Zhejiang Province (LY15C200004), Scientific Research Fund of Zhejiang Provincial Education Department (Y201737271), Ningbo Sci. & Tech. Projects for Common Wealth (2015C10026, 2017C10016), the National 111 Project of China, the Li Dak Sum Yip Yio Chin Kenneth Li Marine Biopharmaceutical Development Fund, and the K.C. Wong Magna Fund in Ningbo University.

Author Contributions: Conceived and designed the experiments: Lijian Ding, Shan He. Collect the samples: Shan He, Yong Liu, Yanbin Lu. Performed the experiments: Yong Liu, Xuezhen Zhou. Analyzed the data: Yong Liu, Lijian Ding. Wrote the paper: Yong Liu, C. Benjamin Naman, Lijian Ding.

Conflicts of Interest: The authors declare no conflict of interest.

References

1. Cast, I. *Mycotoxins: Risks in Plant, Animal, And Human Systems*; Task Force Report No. 139; Council for Agriculture Science and Technology: Ames, IA, USA, 2003.

2. Berthiller, F.; Crews, C.; Dall'Asta, C.; Saeger, S.D.; Haesaert, G.; Karlovsky, P.; Oswald, I.P.; Seefelder, W.; Speijers, G.; Stroka, J. Masked mycotoxins: A review. *Mol. Nutr. Food Res.* **2013**, *57*, 165–186. [CrossRef] [PubMed]
3. McMullen, M.; Jones, R.; Gallenberg, D. Scab of wheat and barley: A re-emerging disease of devastating impact. *Plant Dis.* **1997**, *81*, 1340–1348. [CrossRef]
4. Goswami, R.S.; Kistler, H.C. Heading for disaster: *Fusarium graminearum* on cereal crops. *Mol. Plant Pathol.* **2004**, *5*, 515–525. [CrossRef] [PubMed]
5. Starkey, D.E.; Ward, T.J.; Aoki, T.; Gale, L.R.; Kistler, H.C.; Geiser, D.M.; Suga, H.; Tóth, B.; Varga, J.; O'Donnell, K. Global molecular surveillance reveals novel fusarium head blight species and trichothecene toxin diversity. *Fungal Genet. Biol.* **2007**, *44*, 1191–1204. [CrossRef] [PubMed]
6. Kazan, K.; Gardiner, D.M.; Manners, J.M. On the trail of a cereal killer: Recent advances in *Fusarium graminearum* pathogenomics and host resistance. *Mol. Plant Pathol.* **2012**, *13*, 399–413. [CrossRef] [PubMed]
7. Grove, J.F. Macrocyclic trichothecenes. *Nat. Prod. Rep.* **1993**, *10*, 429–448. [CrossRef]
8. Grove, J.F. The trichothecenes and their biosynthesis. *Prog. Chem. Org. Nat. Prod.* **2007**, *38*, 63–130. [CrossRef]
9. Wilkins, K.; Nielsen, K.F.; Din, S.U. Patterns of volatile metabolites and nonvolatile trichothecenes produced by isolates of *Stachybotrys, Fusarium, Trichoderma, Trichothecium* and *Memnoniella*. *Environ. Sci. Pollut. Res.* **2003**, *10*, 162–166. [CrossRef]
10. Trapp, S.; Hohn, T.; McCormick, S.; Jarvis, B. Characterization of the gene cluster for biosynthesis of macrocyclic trichothecenes in *Myrothecium roridum*. *Mol. Gen. Genet.* **1998**, *257*, 421–432. [CrossRef] [PubMed]
11. Jarvis, B.B.; Mazzola, E.P. Macrocyclic and other novel trichothecenes: Their structure, synthesis, and biological significance. *Acc. Chem. Res.* **1982**, *15*, 388–395. [CrossRef]
12. Desjardins, A.E.; Mccormick, S.P.; Appell, M. Structure-activity relationships of trichothecene toxins in an *Arabidopsis thaliana* leaf assay. *J. Agric. Food Chem.* **2007**, *55*, 6487–6492. [CrossRef] [PubMed]
13. Alexander, N.J.; McCormick, S.P.; Ziegenhorn, S.L. Phytotoxicity of selected trichothecenes using *Chlamydomonas reinhardtii* as a model system. *Nat. Toxins* **1999**, *7*, 265–269. [CrossRef]
14. Eudes, F.; Comeau, A.; Rioux, S.; Collin, J. Phytotoxicité de huit mycotoxines associées à la fusariose de l'épi chez le blé. *Can. J. Plant Pathol.* **2000**, *22*, 286–292. [CrossRef]
15. Veprikova, Z.; Zachariasova, M.; Dzuman, Z.; Zachariasova, A.; Fenclova, M.; Slavikova, P.; Vaclavikova, M.; Mastovska, K.; Hengst, D.; Hajslova, J. Mycotoxins in plant-based dietary supplements: Hidden health risk for consumers. *J. Agric. Food Chem.* **2015**, *63*, 6633–6643. [CrossRef] [PubMed]
16. Cutler, H.G.; Jarvis, B.B. Preliminary observations on the effects of macrocyclic trichothecenes on plant growth. *Environ. Exp. Bot.* **1985**, *25*, 115–128. [CrossRef]
17. Ryu, S.M.; Lee, H.M.; Song, E.G.; Seo, Y.H.; Lee, J.; Guo, Y.Q.; Kim, B.S.; Kim, J.J.; Jin, S.H.; Ryu, K.H. Antiviral activities of trichothecenes isolated from *Trichoderma albolutescens* against pepper mottle virus. *J. Agric. Food Chem.* **2017**, *65*, 4273–4279. [CrossRef] [PubMed]
18. Yang, Y.; Zhao, Y.; Gu, D.; Ayupbek, A.; Huang, Y.; Dou, J.; Ito, Y.; Zhang, T.; Aisa, H.A. Separation of the minor flavonols from flos gossypii by high-speed countercurrent chromatography. *J. Liq. Chromatogr. Relat. Technol.* **2010**, *33*, 1502–1515. [CrossRef] [PubMed]
19. Sutherland, I.A.; Fisher, D. Role of counter-current chromatography in the modernisation of chinese herbal medicines. *J. Chromatogr. A* **2009**, *1216*, 740–753. [CrossRef] [PubMed]
20. Sticher, O. Natural product isolation. *Nat. Prod. Rep.* **2008**, *25*, 517–554. [CrossRef] [PubMed]
21. Oka, F.; Oka, H.; Ito, Y. Systematic search for suitable two-phase solvent systems for high-speed counter-current chromatography. *J. Chromatogr. A* **1991**, *538*, 99–108. [CrossRef]
22. Ito, Y. Golden rules and pitfalls in selecting optimum conditions for high-speed counter-current chromatography. *J. Chromatogr. A* **2005**, *1065*, 145–168. [CrossRef] [PubMed]
23. He, S.; Wang, H.; Yan, X.; Zhu, P.; Chen, J.; Yang, R. Preparative isolation and purification of macrolactin antibiotics from marine bacterium *Bacillus amyloliquefaciens* using high-speed counter-current chromatography in stepwise elution mode. *J. Chromatogr. A* **2013**, *1272*, 15–19. [CrossRef] [PubMed]
24. Huang, X.Y.; Ignatova, S.; Hewitson, P.; Di, D.L. An overview of recent progress in elution mode of counter current chromatography. *Trac-Trend Anal. Chem.* **2016**, *77*, 214–225. [CrossRef]
25. Ridge, C.D.; Mazzola, E.P.; Colesb, M.P.; Hinkley, S.F.R. Isolation and characterization of roridin E. *Magn. Reson. Chem.* **2016**, *55*, 337–340. [CrossRef] [PubMed]

26. Isaka, M.; Punya, J.; Lertwerawat, Y.; Tanticharoen, M.; Thebtaranonth, Y. Antimalarial activity of macrocyclic trichothecenes isolated from the fungus *Myrothecium verrucaria*. *J. Nat. Prod.* **1999**, *62*, 329–331. [CrossRef] [PubMed]
27. Namikoshi, M.; Kobayashi, H.; Yoshimoto, T.; Meguro, S.; Akano, K. Isolation and characterization of bioactive metabolites from marine-derived filamentous fungi collected from tropical and sub-tropical coral reefs. *Chem. Pharm. Bull.* **2000**, *48*, 1452–1457. [CrossRef] [PubMed]
28. Temba, B.A.; Sultanbawa, Y.; Kriticos, D.J.; Fox, G.P.; Harvey, J.J.; Fletcher, M.T. Tools for defusing a major global food and feed safety risk: Nonbiological postharvest procedures to decontaminate mycotoxins in foods and feeds. *J. Agric. Food Chem.* **2016**, *64*, 8959–8972. [CrossRef] [PubMed]

© 2018 by the authors. Licensee MDPI, Basel, Switzerland. This article is an open access article distributed under the terms and conditions of the Creative Commons Attribution (CC BY) license (http://creativecommons.org/licenses/by/4.0/).

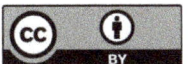

marine drugs MDPI

Article

A Dereplication and Bioguided Discovery Approach to Reveal New Compounds from a Marine-Derived Fungus *Stilbella fimetaria*

Sara Kildgaard [1], Karolina Subko [1], Emma Phillips [2], Violaine Goidts [2], Mercedes de la Cruz [3], Caridad Díaz [3], Charlotte H. Gotfredsen [4], Birgitte Andersen [1], Jens C. Frisvad [1], Kristian F. Nielsen [1] and Thomas O. Larsen [1,*]

1 DTU Bioengineering, Technical University of Denmark, Søltofts Plads 221, DK-2800 Kgs. Lyngby, Denmark; sarki@bio.dtu.dk (S.K.); karosu@dtu.dk (K.S.); ba@bio.dtu.dk (B.A.); jcf@bio.dtu.dk (J.C.F.); kfn@bio.dtu.dk (K.F.N.)
2 German Cancer Research Center, Brain Tumor Translational Targets, Im Neuenheimer Feld 580, D-69120 Heidelberg, Germany; e.phillips@dkfz-heidelberg.de (E.P.); v.goidts@dkfz-heidelberg.de (V.G.)
3 Fundación MEDINA, Av del Conocimiento, 34, 18100 Armilla, Granada, Spain; mercedes.delacruz@medinaandalucia.es (M.d.l.C.); caridad.diaz@medinaandalucia.es (C.D.)
4 Department of Chemistry, Technical University of Denmark, Kemitorvet, Building 207, DK-2800 Kgs. Lyngby, Denmark; chg@kemi.dtu.dk
* Correspondence: tol@bio.dtu.dk; Tel.: +45-4525-2632

Received: 4 July 2017; Accepted: 31 July 2017; Published: 13 August 2017

Abstract: A marine-derived *Stilbella fimetaria* fungal strain was screened for new bioactive compounds based on two different approaches: (i) bio-guided approach using cytotoxicity and antimicrobial bioassays; and (ii) dereplication based approach using liquid chromatography with both diode array detection and high resolution mass spectrometry. This led to the discovery of several bioactive compound families with different biosynthetic origins, including pimarane-type diterpenoids and hybrid polyketide-non ribosomal peptide derived compounds. Prefractionation before bioassay screening proved to be a great aid in the dereplication process, since separate fractions displaying different bioactivities allowed a quick tentative identification of known antimicrobial compounds and of potential new analogues. A new pimarane-type diterpene, myrocin F, was discovered in trace amounts and displayed cytotoxicity towards various cancer cell lines. Further media optimization led to increased production followed by the purification and bioactivity screening of several new and known pimarane-type diterpenoids. A known broad-spectrum antifungal compound, ilicicolin H, was purified along with two new analogues, hydroxyl-ilicicolin H and ilicicolin I, and their antifungal activity was evaluated.

Keywords: bioguided-discovery; dereplication; cytotoxicity; antifungal; MS/HRMS; marine-derived; pimarane-type diterpenoids; ilicicolin H

---

1. Introduction

With the ocean covering almost two thirds of the Earth's surface area, the marine environment offers a great diversity of microorganisms and thereby a promising potential for new bioactive natural products displaying unique chemical scaffolds [1–3]. Fungal strains isolated from the marine environment have attracted increased attention due to the discovery of several secondary metabolites rich in biological activity [1–4]. The majority of fungal strains have been isolated from sources such as algae, sponges, and mangrove habitats [1] with deep sea sediments emerging as a new niche of potentially interesting compounds [1,5]. It is under much debate, however, what the real origin of these fungal strains is; being true marine or opportunistic strains adapted to the marine environment [4].

This is due to the fact that many fungal strains are isolated from intertidal zones and mangrove habitats and thereby not likely true marine habitats [4,6–8]. The most common secondary metabolite producing species come from *Aspergillus* and *Penicillium*, with only few belonging to the well-documented lineage of marine fungi [4,6–8]. That said, the origin of these marine-derived fungal strains, whether true marine or opportunistic, may not be as critical when it comes to drug discovery if the opportunistic strains produce new bioactive compounds not found in their terrestrial counterparts.

Dereplication is an essential step in natural product (NP) discovery to prevent re-isolation and re-characterization of known bioactive compounds. It is especially important in primary bioactivity screening, where the target is often non-selective and there is a high chance of rediscovering general cytotoxic compounds. This is due to a great number of highly bioactive compounds being observed across the fungal kingdom of which several are found in multiple fungal species [9–11]. One dereplication approach is based on ultra-high performance liquid chromatography-diode array detection-quadrupole time of flight mass spectrometry (UHPLC-DAD-QTOFMS) and database searching [10,12,13]. This can be combined with auto tandem high resolution mass spectrometry (MS/HRMS) and use of a MS/HRMS library, which has been shown to be a robust and effective way of tentatively identifying known bioactive compounds on a given instrument [9,11]. The MS/HRMS library may serve as a database of compounds for targeted dereplication, matching peaks in the unknown spectrum against the library spectrum and vice versa, or to identify compounds sharing similar fragment ions, but that do not share the same molecular formula [11]. Another dereplication strategy based on MS/MS involves molecular networking proposed by the Dorrestein/Bandeira labs [14–16], where a pairwise comparison of MS/MS spectra results in clustered networks of structurally related compounds. Early integration of the MS/MS networking approach and bioassay data has been shown to enable the targeted discovery of new bioactive compounds [17]. However, a limiting factor is the lack of back-integration of raw data to find the corresponding full scan data and retention times resulting in detailed analysis being time consuming.

Pre-fractionation serves as another highly valuable step in NP discovery for the success of both the initial dereplication and bioactivity screening. This is because metabolites present in minor amounts may go undetected, their activity being masked or interfered with by major components in a complex crude extract [18–20]. Wyeth [19] and Appleton et al. [18] reported that primary bioactivity screening of pre-fractionated crude samples showed that the bioactivity was masked in up to 80% of the cases with no activity being observed for the original crude extracts, but only for the fractions. Meanwhile, up to 13% of the crude samples lost their activity upon fractionation [18,19], meaning that it can be advantageous to screen both the crude extract and fractions in the primary assay. In addition to using traditional reversed phase (RP) chromatography for pre-fractionation, orthogonal purification strategies such as Explorative Solid-Phase Extraction (E-SPE) can be used to facilitate the removal or reduction of co-eluting interferences [21]. Pre-fractionation can aid the discovery of new compounds or activities which would have otherwise been missed either due to: (1) the crude extract containing more than one compound responsible for the observed activity; (2) a single compound displaying multiple activities, or (3) several compounds displaying various activities.

In this paper, we describe a combined bioassay-guided and dereplication based discovery approach for a marine-derived fungus *Stilbella fimetaria* IBT 28361 using cytotoxicity and antimicrobial screening assays and UHPLC-DAD-QTOFMS with MS/HRMS in combination with our in-house MS/HRMS library [9]. This method led to the discovery of different bioactive compound families in *Stilbella fimetaria,* including pimarane-type diterpenoids and hybrid polyketide-non ribosomal peptides belonging to the ilicicolin H family. To the best of our knowledge, the latter has not previously been obtained from the genus *Stilbella*. New and known compounds of both families were isolated and elucidated by nuclear magnetic resonance (NMR) spectroscopy and their cytotoxicity and antimicrobial activities evaluated. The outcome of the primary bioassay screening on both the crude extracts and their fractions assisted in the dereplication of the crude extract allowing for a quick tentative identification of known antimicrobial compounds and potential new bioactive analogues.

2. Results and Discussion

Bioactivity-guided purification was performed using cytotoxicity and antimicrobial bioassays on the marine-derived fungus *Stilbella fimetaria* IBT 28361 isolated from a seawater sample off the coast of the island Fanoe, Western part of Denmark. The fungus was cultivated in small cultivation on yeast extract sucrose agar (YES) and czapek yeast extract agar (CYA) plates. The YES and CYA plates were combined and extracted together with EtOAc containing 1% formic acid (FA). An EtOAC extract of plates from both YES and CYA media were chosen in order to increase the spectrum of compounds produced by the fungus. The EtOAc crude extract was fractionated by RP flash chromatography with a gradient of acetonitrile (MeCN) and water going from 15% to 100% MeCN into six fractions and both the crude extract and the six fractions were subsequently evaluated for their cytotoxicity and antimicrobial activity. No activity was observed for the screening of the crude extract on its own, whereas the fourth, fifth, and sixth flash fractions (ranging from 40% to 100% organic) displayed cytotoxic, antibacterial, and antifungal activities, respectively (Figure 1). Dereplication of the separate bioactive fractions using UHPLC-DAD-QTOFMS allowed a quick tentative identification of several bioactive compound families likely responsible for the observed activities (Figure 1).

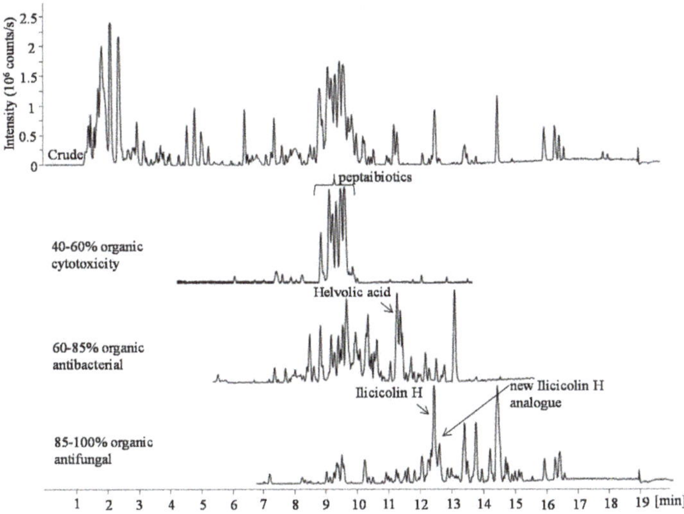

Figure 1. Base peak chromatograms (BPC) of the EtOAc crude extract and three bioactive fractions (ranging from 40% to 100% organic) in positive electrospray ionization (ESI) mode. The fractions were obtained by RP flash chromatography with a gradient of MeCN and water going from 15% to 100% MeCN. In the bioactive fractions the marked peaks indicate the tentatively identified peptaiboitics, helvolic acid, ilicicolin H, and a potential new ilicicolin H analogue.

Different further fungal cultivations (1–3, see below) were prepared in order to purify potential new compounds and confirm the bioactivity of the known compounds in the applied bioassays. The identity of the cytotoxic compounds and their analogues were obtained using bio-guided isolation on large scale cultivation YES media (Cultivation 1). YES media was chosen as it displayed weak activity when crude extracts for one YES and one CYA plate were tested separately. Further media optimization was performed to find the optimal growth conditions for potential cytotoxic compounds otherwise only present in trace amounts on YES media and in order to circumvent a group of co-eluting peptaibiotics (Cultivation 2, rice media incubated for 10 days at 25 °C in the dark) [Section 2.1]. The known antibacterial nortriterpenoid, helvolic acid [22–24] was identified as one of the main components in the fraction displaying antibacterial activity against methicillin-resistant

Staphylococcus aureus (MRSA) reported by Kildgaard et al. [11]. This was done using an in-house MS/HRMS library and comparison of its retention time to a standard from our compound library and suggested to be the compound exhibiting the observed activity. In this study, the activity of the pure compound against MRSA was confirmed, MIC_{90} < 0.25 μg/mL (1D NMR data shown in Figures S9–S11). The compound responsible for the antifungal activity was tentatively identified as the broad-spectrum antifungal metabolite, ilicicolin H [25–28]. Due to the tentative identification of new ilicicolin H analogues with similar retention times to ilicicolin H, it was isolated along with two new analogues on large cultivation rice media incubated for 21 days at 25 °C in the dark (Cultivation 3) [Section 2.2].

2.1. Pimarane-Type Diterpenoids Exhibiting Cytotoxicity

From cultivation 1, the RP flash chromatography fractions (40–60% organic) displayed cytotoxicity against patient derived glioblastoma stem-like cells (GSCs). The observed cytotoxicity was comparable to that of the fraction from the original small scale EtOAc crude extract of the YES and CYA plates combined and extracted together. GSCs were chosen for the study as there is an acute need for novel therapeutics targeting this tumor subpopulation as they exhibit resistance to the current standard therapy for glioblastoma [29]. UHPLC-DAD-QTOFMS-MS/HRMS and use of an in-house MS/HRMS library [11] and The Comprehensive Peptaibiotics Database [30] tentatively identified the major components of the active fractions to be peptaibiotics belonging to the antiamebins family. Antiamebin I [31] was tentatively identified by comparison to its reference standard in the MS/HRMS library reported by Kildgaard et al. [11]. Furthermore, *Stilbella fimetaria* (syn. *S. erythrocephala*) is well-known for its production of antiamebins [32,33]. At a glance, the antiamebins might be suspected as responsible for the observed bioactivity, but a second fractionation revealed the active component to be the compound obscured by the group of co-eluting antiamebins and present only in trace amount in the first fractionation. The molecular formula for the compound was established to be $C_{20}H_{22}O_4$ based on the pseudomolecular ion, $[M + H]^+$ of m/z 329.1745 with an accuracy of 0.6 ppm (HRESITOFMS) and the ultraviolet (UV) spectrum displayed absorption bands at λ_{max} 215 and 270 nm. A NMR spectroscopic analysis of the isolated compound and comparison to the data reported for myrocins A-E [34–37] allowed for the structural elucidation of a new pimarane-type diterpene, myrocin F (**1**) (Figure 2). ^1H, ^{13}C, HMBC and NOESY data is shown in Table 1.

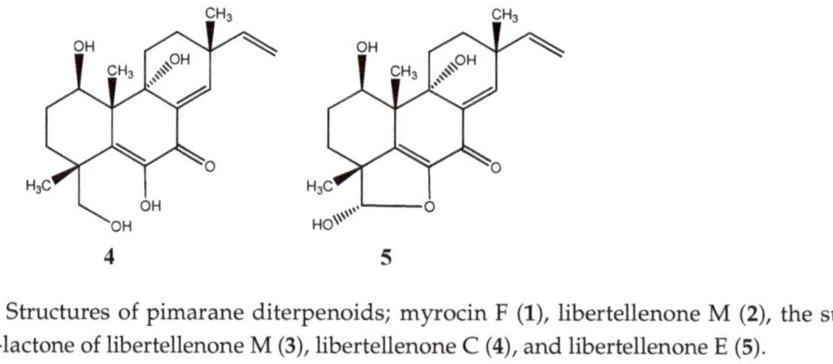

Figure 2. Structures of pimarane diterpenoids; myrocin F (**1**), libertellenone M (**2**), the suggested opened γ-lactone of libertellenone M (**3**), libertellenone C (**4**), and libertellenone E (**5**).

Table 1. NMR spectroscopic data (400 MHz, MeOD, δ in ppm, *J* in Hz) for myrocin F (**1**).

Position	$\delta^{13}C$	$\delta^{1}H$ (Mult, *J*)	HMBC	NOESY
1	14.0	1.63 m	3	2b,5,11,20b
2a	19.8	1.78 m	3,4	3a,20a
2b		1.81 m	3,4	1,5,18
3a	28.8	1.44 m	1,4,5,19	2a,20a
3b		1.74 m	4,19	18
4	42.8	-		
5	52.5	2.11 s	4,6,9,10,18–20	1,2b,7,16a,18
6	107.6	-		
7	77.4	4.24 s	5,6,8,9,14	5,14
8	135.5	-		
9	138.6	-		
10	20.5	-		
11	114.6	5.24 t(4.5)	8,10,12–14	1,12,20b
12	37.0	2.19 m	9,11,13–15,17	11,15,17
13	38.9	-		
14	135.8	5.56 s	7,9,11–13,15,17	7,16a,17
15	144.0	5.67 dd(17.4/10.4)	13,14,17	12,16a/b,17
16a	112.3	5.03 dd (17.4/1.5)	13	5,14,15,17
16b		4.89 dd(10.4/1.5)	13	15
17	28.0	1.15 s	12–15	12,14,15,16a
18	29.6	1.42 s	3–5,19	2b,3b,5
19	185.6	-		
20a	17.1	0.85 t(5.2)	1,5,9	2a,3a
20b		0.25 dd(8.2/5.7)	2,9	1,11

^{1}H-NMR spectrum revealed the presence of six methines (including one oxygenated and three olefinic), five methylenes (including one cyclopropylic and one olefinic), and two singlet methyl groups. The ^{13}C-NMR spectrum identified one ester carbonyl group and six quaternary carbon signals (including one oxygenated and two olefinic). The DQF-COSY spectrum defined three spin systems besides the two singlet methyl signals at δ_H 1.15 (CH_3-17) and δ_H 1.42 (CH_3-18). One spin system included the terminal vinyl group with protons at δ_H 5.67 (1H, dd, *J* = 17.4, 10.4, H-15), δ_H 5.03 (1H, dd, *J* = 17.4, 1.5, H-16a), and δ_H 4.89 (1H, dd, *J* = 10.4, 1.5, H-16b). The second spin system included the olefinc methine at δ_H 5.24 (CH-11) and the enantiotopic methylene at δ_H 2.19 (CH_2-12). The third spin system included the diastereotropic methylenes at δ_H 1.74/1.44 (CH_2-3) and δ_H 1.81/1.78 (CH_2-2) and cyclopropylic protons (as indicated by the characteristic upfield chemical shift and coupling pattern of H-20) at δ_H 1.63 (H-1), δ_H 0.85 (1H, t, *J* = 5.2, H-20a), and δ_H 0.25 (1H, dd, *J* = 8.2, 5.7, H-20b). The connection of these COSY spin systems and assignment of remaining signals and quaternary carbons was done by analysis of the HMBC spectrum obtaining the long range H-C correlations. The important HMBC correlations from H-16 to C-13, H-17 to C-12, C-13, C-14, and C-15, H-11 to C-8, C-10, and C-13, H-14 to C-7, C-9, C-12, C-13, and C-17, H-7 to C-5, C-6, C-8, and C-9, H-5 to C-4, C-6, C-9, C-10, and C-18, H-2 and H-3 to C-4 confirmed the presence of the pimarane-type diterpene structure [36]. The fusion of the lactone ring through C-4 and C-6 and the cyclopropyl ring (C-1-C-20-C-10) to the pimarane skeleton was supported by the important HMBC correlations from H-5, H-3, and H-18 to the ester carbonyl signal at δ_H 185.6 (C-19) and from H-20a to C-1, C-5, and C-9 and H-20b to C-2 and C-9 (See Figure 3 for important HMBC correlations). The relative configuration of myrocin F is based on an analysis of the NOESY spectrum with key NOE correlations from H-1 to H-2b and H-5, from H-5 to H-2b, CH_3-18, H-7, and H-16a, and from CH_3-18 to H-2b, H-5, and H-3b. Further key NOEs from H-20a to H-2a and H-3a and between the latter two and from H-20b to H-1 and H-11 and between the latter two suggested the cyclopropyl group with the cyclopropylic protons H-20a/H-20b in each direction, CH_3-17 and the hydroxyl group at C-7 to be on the same face of the molecule and CH_3-18, H-5, and the vinyl group on the opposite face. The hydroxyl group at C-6 is suggested to be positioned to the latter face based on observed strong NOE correlation between

H-7 and H-14 and no correlation between H-7 and CH_3-18 (See Figure 3). The relative configuration of myrocin F is in agreement with that of previously reported myrocin A-C [34,35] with absolute configuration reported by X-ray diffraction analysis of myrocin C monoacetate [38].

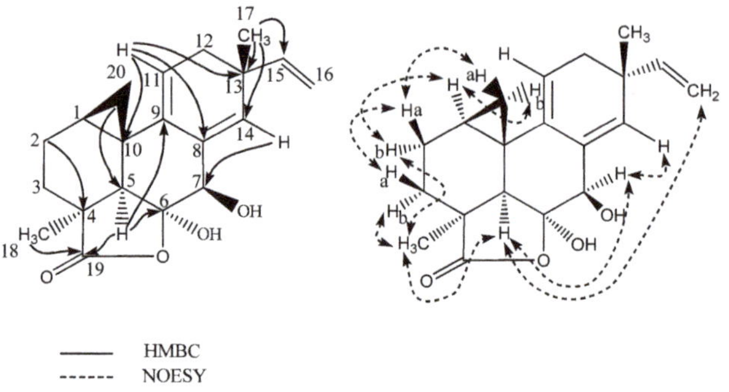

Figure 3. Selected key HMBC and NOESY correlations for myrocin F (**1**).

Optimization of media and growth conditions led to the discovery of a highly enriched profile of the pimarane-type diterpenoids when *Stilbella fimetaria* IBT 28361 was grown on rice media for 10 days at 25 °C in the dark (Cultivation 2). This enabled the purification of two new libertellenones obtained from the same fraction, libertellenone M (**2**) and what we propose to be the opened γ-lactone ring of libertellenone M (**3**) that were both present as trace amounts in cultivation 1 (Figure 2). The two known compounds, libertellenone C (**4**) [39] and libertellenone E (**5**) [36] (Figures 2 and S31 and Table 2 with NMR Spectroscopic Data, Supplementary information) were isolated from the same extract and identified based on their spectroscopic profiles (1D and 2D NMR, HRMS, MS/HRMS, UV, $[\alpha]_D^{20}$). Both compounds have been reported with their absolute configurations, determined by X-ray diffraction analysis for libertellenone E [36]. The BPC of the crude rice extract with extracted ion chromatogram (EIC) identifying the libertellenones is shown in Figure S4, Supplementary information.

Table 2. NMR spectroscopic data (800 MHz CD_3CN, δ in ppm, *J* in Hz) for libertellenone M (**2**) and (800 MHz MeOD, δ in ppm, *J* in Hz) for the suggested opened γ-lactam libertellenone M (**3**).

	Libertellenone M (2)			**Opened γ-lactam libertellenone M (3)**		
Position	$\delta^{13}C$	$\delta^{1}H$ **(Mult, *J*)**	**HMBC**	$\delta^{13}C$	$\delta^{1}H$ **(Mult, *J*)**	**HMBC**
1	130.7	5.78 dd(9.9,3.0)	3,5,6,10,20	130.7	5.94 m	3,10
2	127.4	5.91 m	3,4,10	126.7	5.98 m	3,10
3a	34.3	2.36 dt(16.5,2.5)	1,2,4,5,18	36.2	2.16 m	-
3b		2.43 dd(16.5,5.9)	1,2,4,18,19		2.64 m	1,2
4	46.2	-		46.8	-	-
5	146.9	-		137.0	-	-
6	143.1	-		*	-	-
7	177.3	-		183.6	-	-
8	137.6	-		*	-	-
9	76.6	-		76.0	-	-
10	45.5	-		46.6	-	-
11a	27.5	2.24 m	9,10,12,13	27.4	2.16 m	-
11b		1.72 ddd(14.0,5.0,3.5)	8–10,12,13		1.93 m	-
12a	30.9	1.59 m	9,11,14,17	30.6	1.60 m	-
12b		1.78 td(13.0,3.5)	9,11,13–15,17		1.92 m	17
13	39.8	-		40.0	-	-
14	148.8	6.90 s	7–9,12,13,15,17	148.8	6.98 s	7,9,12,15
15	147.0	5.93 m	12–14,17	147.0	5.92 m	-

Table 2. *Cont.*

	Libertellenone M (2)			Opened γ-lactam libertellenone M (3)		
Position	δ^{13}C	δ^{1}H (Mult, *J*)	**HMBC**	δ^{13}C	δ^{1}H (Mult, *J*)	**HMBC**
16a	113.5	5.09 d(17.5)	13,15	113.0	5.12 d(17.2)	13
16b		5.07 d(10.5)	13,15		5.06 d(10.5)	13
17	24.8	1.17 s	12–15	23.8	1.16 s	12–15
18	23.4	1.48 s	3–5,19	24.1	1.55 s	3–5,19
19	181.2	-		181.1	-	
20	24.1	1.29 s	1,5,9,10	28.3	1.23 s	1,5,9,10

* ^{13}C chemical shift not observed.

Libertellenone M (**2**) possessed the molecular formula $C_{20}H_{22}O_4$ based on the pseudomolecular ion, $[M + H]^+$ of m/z 327.1592 (accuracy −0.27 ppm). The ^{1}H and ^{13}C NMR spectra were similar to those of libertellenone C with the exception of the C-1/C-2 double bond with the downfield carbon shifts of δ_C 130.7 (C-1) and δ_C 127.4 (C-2) compared to δ_C 70.1 (C-1) and δ_C 29.3 (C-2) and replacement of the ketone at δ_C 181.2 (C-19) with the hydroxyl methylene group at δ_C 70.2 (opened γ-lactam ring). The planar structure of libertellenone M is the same as that reported for libertellenone G [40] with a different relative configuration suggested based on the NOESY spectra (Figure 4). Key NOEs of compound (**2**) were observed from CH_3-17 to H-11a and H-12a, from H-11a to H-12a, CH_3-20 and a weak NOE to CH_3-18, from CH_3-20 to H-12a and CH_3-18, and from H-11b to H-12b and H-1 placing all the methyl groups (CH_3-17, CH_3-20, and CH_3-18) on the same face of the molecule (Figure 4). The position of the hydroxyl group at C-9 was assigned to the opposite face of the methyl groups based upon strong NOE correlations observed between CH_3-20 and H-11a. Furthermore, libertellenone M showed a similar relative configuration to those of the closely structurally related known compounds (**4**) and (**5**) supporting the assignment (Figure 2).

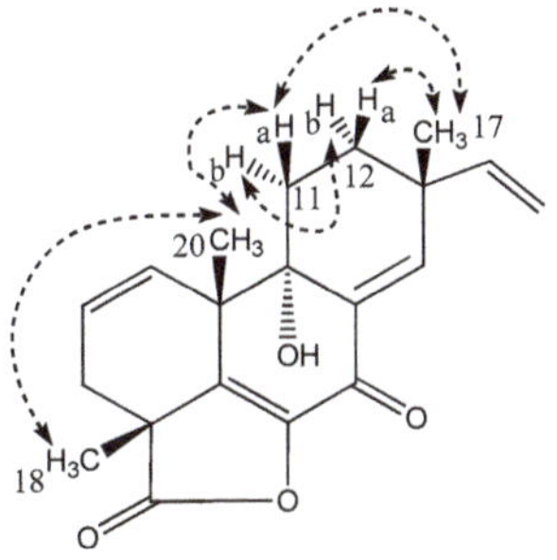

Figure 4. Selected key NOESY correlations for libertellenone M (**2**).

HRESITOFMS showed a 18.01 Da mass difference between compounds (**3**) ($[M + H]^+$ m/z 345.1692, accuracy −0.76 ppm) and (**2**) suggesting the latter to be a dehydrated analogue of the former. Compound (**3**) degenerated gradually during the NMR run, complicating the interpretation of the NMR data and preventing further analysis and bioactivity studies of the compound. With this in regard, ^{1}H, DQF-COSY and HSQC spectra of compounds (**3**) and (**2**) were highly similar, suggesting compound (**3**) to be the opened γ-lactone ring of libertellenone M (**2**) formed through hydrolysis of the ester. Further in the HMBC experiment, key correlations were observed resembling those exhibited by compound (**2**) and with the most notable difference in the carbon chemical shift seen at C-5 that shifted upfield to δ_C 137.0 ppm compared to 146.9 ppm for compound (**2**) (a similar upfield shift was observed for libertellenone C (**4**) in comparison to compound (**2**)). A table with NMR spectroscopic data is shown for both compounds (**2**) and (**3**) in Table 2. Analysis of the MS/HRMS data assisted in the confirmation of the structure of compound (**3**) to be the opened γ-lactone ring of libertellenone

M (**2**). The major degeneration product of compound (**3**) was observed at m/z 299.1644 [M + H]$^+$ (also present as a fragment ion in the MS/HRMS spectra of both compounds (**2**) and (**3**)) indicating the loss of HCO_2H (Δ 46.0048 between fragment ion and [M + H]$^+$, calcd. 46.0054). The three compounds displayed highly similar fragmentation patterns with similarity scores $\geq$84% (compound (**3**)) and $\geq$88% (m/z 299.1644) for all MS/HRMS spectra (10, 20 and 40 eV) compared to libertellenone M (**2**). These were observed searching the MS/HRMS spectra of both analogues against our MS/HRMS library spectra (libertellenone M included) by similarity scoring as in Kildgaard et al. [11], identifying compounds that share the same fragment ions but have different molecular masses. MS/HRMS spectra are shown for compounds (**2**) and (**3**) in Figures S2 and S3, Supplementary information. In addition compound (**2**) was observed as a minor degeneration product of compound (**3**), suggesting the relative configuration of both to be the same.

Myrocin F (**1**), libertellenone M (**2**), libertellenone C (**4**) and libertellenone E (**5**) were all evaluated for their activity towards GSCs and compounds (**1**), (**2**), and (**4**) were shown to display IC_{50} values of 40, 18, and 40 μM, respectively. The cytotoxicity of the diterpenoids was also evaluated towards the following cancer cell lines: A549 (lung carcinoma), MCF7 (breast carcinoma), SW480 (colorectal adenocarcinoma), and DU145 (prostate carcinoma). Myrocin F (**1**) showed the strongest effect with IC_{50} values between 20–50 μM, whereas compounds (**2**) and (**4**) proved to be much less cytotoxic towards these cell lines (See Figures S46 and S47 for data). Libertellenone E (**5**) did not display any activity towards any of the cell lines at the tested concentrations (IC_{50} > 300 μM). The higher cytotoxicity displayed against all cancer cell lines for myrocin F could indicate the cyclopropane ring's influence on the bioactivity, in agreement with previous reports for other pimarane diterpenoids [38].

As far as antibacterial (*Escherichia coli* and methicillin-sensitive *S. aureus* (MSSA)) and antifungal activity (*Aspergillus fumigatus* and *Candida albicans*) was concerned, none of the compounds were active at the concentrations tested (MIC_{90} > 64 μg/mL).

2.2. *Ilicicolin H, A Broad-Spectrum Antifungal, and New Analogues*

From the original small scale cultivation (eight plates) combined YES and CYA extract, the sixth flash fraction (ranging from 85% to 100% organic) displayed antifungal activity against *A. fumigatus*. UHPLC-DAD-QTOFMS revealed the molecular formula $C_{27}H_{31}NO_4$ (0.7 ppm accuracy) for one of the major compounds in the fraction. AntiBase 2012 [41] suggested the broad spectrum antifungal compound, ilicicolin H (Figure 5, (**7**)) as a candidate, consistent with UV data [25] and the biological activity of the fraction [27,28]. Ilicicolin H is a hybrid polyketide—non-ribosomal peptide derived fungal metabolite that was originally isolated in 1971 from the 'imperfect fungus' *Cylindrocladium ilicicola* [42], with its structure elucidation described in 1976 [25], biosynthesis in 1983 [26], and total synthesis of racemic ilicicolin H in 1985 [43]. The production of this compound was highly increased when incubation time on rice media was extended from 10 days (as was optimal for the pimarane diterpenoids) to three weeks at 25 °C in the dark (Cultivation 3). This led to isolation of the compound in high amounts (>50 mg) and 1D and 2D NMR confirmation (See Table 3) of the structure to be ilicicolin H, confirmed by comparing ^{1}H- and ^{13}C- chemical shifts to that of published data [25,26].

Table 3. NMR spectroscopic data (500 MHz and 800 MHz, MeCN-d3, δ in ppm, *J* in Hz) for hydroxyl-ilicicolin H (**6**), ilicicolin H (**7**), and ilicicolin I (**8**).

	Hydroxyl-ilicicolin H (6)		**Ilicicolin H (7)**		**Ilicicolin I (8)**	
Position	δ^{13}C	δ^1H (Mult, *J*)	δ^{13}C	δ^1H (Mult, *J*)	δ^{13}C	δ^1H (Mult, *J*)
1′	125.9	-	125.8	-	126.0	-
3′5′	116.4	6.83 d(8.6)	116.6	6.83 d(8.6)	116.4	6.84 d(8.6)
2′6′	131.8	7.27 d(8.6)	131.7	7.26 d(8.6)	131.8	7.29 d(8.6)
4′	157.8	-	157.8	-	157.9	-
4′OH	-	16.7 br.s.	-	17.6 br.s.	-	-
1NH	-	9.46 br.s.	-	9.56 br.s.	-	9.44 br.s.

Table 3. *Cont.*

Position	Hydroxyl-ilicicolin H (6) δ^{13}C	δ^{1}H (Mult, *J*)	Ilicicolin H (7) δ^{13}C	δ^{1}H (Mult, *J*)	Ilicicolin I (8) δ^{13}C	δ^{1}H (Mult, *J*)
2	163.0	-	162.9	-	163.3	-
3	108.7*	-	108.1	-	107.5	-
4	178.2	-	178.0	-	179.5	-
5	114.9	-	114.8	-	115.1	-
6	141.3	7.40 s	141.4	7.40 s	141.2	7.42 s
7	210.8	-	211.0	-	195.7	-
8	54.1	4.98 m	54.1	4.97 m	127.5	7.98 d(16.0)
9	45.7	2.56 q(10.4)	46.2	2.48 q(10.4)	160.2	7.26 d(16.0)
10	44.5	1.28 m	44.5	1.23 m	42.6	-
11a	40.6	0.61 q(11.8)	40.6	0.58 q(11.8)	43.2	1.41 m
11b		1.78 m		1.77 m		
12a	33.8	1.40 m	33.8	1.38 m	28.5	1.07 dq(12.4,3.4)
12b						1.40 m
13a	36.6	0.97 m	36.6	0.97 m	36.8	1.73 m
13b		1.76 m		1.77 m		1.00 dq(12.5,3.4)
14a	31.0	2.07 m	31.0	2.04 m	34.3	1.47 m
14b		0.99 m		0.99 m		
15a	45.6	1.70 m	45.4	1.68 m	43.1	1.80 m
15b						0.80 q(12.5)
16	139.5	-	139.5	-	39.3	1.81 m
17	121.0	5.22 s	120.9	5.21 m	131.1	5.41 d(10.0)
18	21.4	1.65 s	21.5	1.63 s	132.5	5.58 ddd(10.0,4.7,2.6)
19	23.3	0.90 d(6.5)	23.4	0.89 d(6.5)	44.5	1.91 m
20	134.1	5.41 dd(15.5,8.2)	134.8	5.21 m	23.2	0.90 d(6.5)
21	132.6	5.47 dt(15.5,5.1)	127.3	5.32 m	18.6	0.98 d(7.0)
22	63.5	3.85 d(4.8)	18.5	1.53 d(6.5)	18.5	1.10 s

* very weak carbon chemical shift.

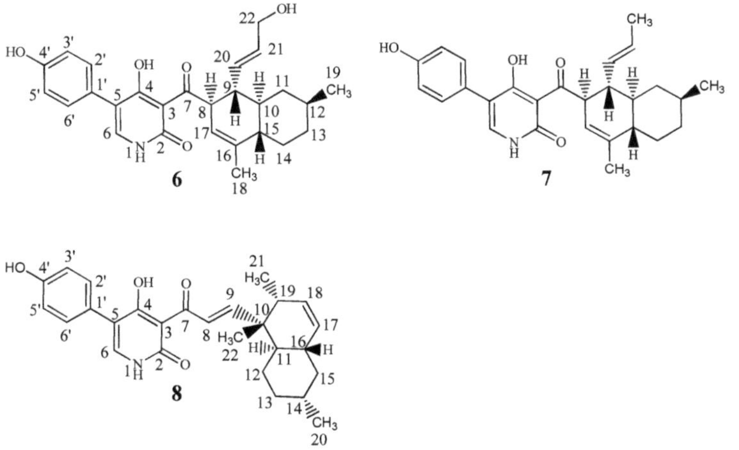

Figure 5. Structures of hydroxyl-ilicicolin H (**6**), ilicicolin H (**7**), ilicicolin I (**8**).

HRMS and MS/HRMS of a group of peaks eluting in close proximity to ilicicolin H in cultivation 3 showed the presence of several ilicicolin H analogues in searching their MS/HRMS spectra against our MS/HRMS library spectra (ilicicolin H included) by similarity scoring as in Kildgaard et al. [11]. Ilicicolin H and the tentatively identified analogues all shared the dominant fragment ion at m/z 230.0451 that corresponds to the left hand part of the molecule (Figure 5) with incorporation of phenylalanine, $[C_{12}H_8NO_4]^+$ formed from cleavage of the C-7/C-8 bond. See Figure S5, Supplementary information for BPC of the crude rice extract with EIC from MS/HRMS showing the fragment ion m/z 230.0451 and EIC from MS displaying ilicicolin H (434.2323 calculated for $[C_{27}H_{31}NO_4 + H]^+$) and the tentatively identified analogues and their position in the chromatogram. Two new analogues, hydroxyl-ilicicolin H (**6**) and ilicicolin I (**8**) (See Figure 5) were isolated from the crude rice extract and their structures elucidated by NMR spectroscopy (See Table 3). The first new analogue (**6**) was purified in low amounts (0.4 mg), eluting slightly earlier than ilicicolin H in the ESI$^+$ chromatogram. The ESI$^+$ HRMS spectrum displayed the pseudomolecular ion, $[M + H]^+$ with m/z 450.2278, from which the molecular formula could be deduced as $C_{27}H_{31}NO_5$ (accuracy −1.23 ppm), indicating the addition of an oxygen atom. In relation to ilicicolin H, a similarity score of 90% was observed by comparing the MS/HRMS spectra at 40 eV and the same absorptions maxima at 250 nm, 295 nm, and 350 nm were displayed in the UV spectra. The structure of hydroxyl-ilicicolin H (**6**) was proposed from 1D and 2D NMR spectroscopic analysis (See Table 3 for ^{1}H and ^{13}C chemical shifts). The NMR data for the phenyl-pyridone moiety were comparable to those of ilicicolin H elucidated in the same solvent. For the decalin moiety, the ^{1}H-NMR spectrum exhibited eight methines (including three vinylic), four methylenes (including three diastereotopic), and two methyl groups (including one singlet). This indicated the difference of an oxidation of the methyl group at δ_H 1.53 (CH_3-22) in ilicicolin H to the enantiotopic methylene at δ_H 3.85 (CH_2-22) in hydroxyl-ilicicolin H, with the observed downfield chemical shift of the methylene supporting the presence of the hydroxyl group at C-22. The position of the CH_2-22 was confirmed by identification of observed vicinal couplings in the COSY spectrum between δ_H 5.47 (CH-21) and δ_H 3.85 (CH_2-22) belonging to the spin system including CH-8 to CH-15, CH-17, CH_3-19 and CH-20 to CH_2-22. Furthermore, HMBC correlations were observed from the vinylic protons at δ_H 5.41 (CH-20) and δ_H 5.47 (CH-21) to the methylene carbon at δ_C 63.5 (C-22) (See Figure 6). The relative configuration of hydroxyl-ilicicolin H (**6**) was suggested to be the same as ilicicolin H (**7**), based on the inspection of coupling constants and observed NOEs in the NOESY spectra (See Figure 6) together with the close structural similarity of compounds (**6**) and (**7**). A trans diaxial relationship was suggested for the protons at H-8 and H-9 and H-9 and H-10, as H-9 was observed as a quartet in the ^{1}H-NMR spectrum with a coupling constant J = 10.4 Hz. Furthermore, the proton at δ_H 0.61 (H-11a) also appeared in the ^{1}H-NMR spectrum as a quartet with a coupling constant J = 11.8 Hz, indicating a trans diaxial relationship between the protons H-10 and H-11a and H-11a and H-12. This was supported by observed NOEs of H-10 with H-8, H-11b and H-14b, and of H-11b with H-12 that placed these protons on the same face of the molecule, whereas NOEs of H-11a with H-9, H-15, CH_3-19 and H-13a and of H-15 with H-9, H-13a and H-14a placed these protons on the opposite face of the molecule. The size of the vicinal coupling constants for H-20/H-21 of J = 15.5 Hz suggested trans stereochemistry and NOEs were observed of H-20 with H-11b and of H-21 with H-9.

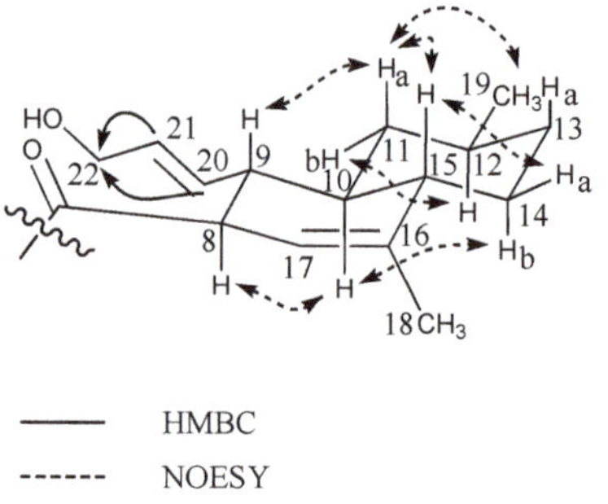

Figure 6. Selected important HMBC correlations (^{1}H-^{13}C) to C-22 and NOESY correlations for the decalin moiety of hydroxyl-ilicicolin H (**6**).

The second new analogue (**8**) was observed eluting as a small peak at almost the same retention time as ilicicolin H in the ESI$^+$ chromatogram and it was deduced to possess the same molecular formula of $C_{27}H_{31}NO_4$ ($[M + H]^+$ with *m*/*z* 434.2325, −0.20 ppm accuracy), indicating the presence of an ilicicolin H isomer. The compound showed a similarity score of 92% (MS/HRMS spectra, 40 eV) and the UV spectrum displayed a slight bathochromic shift to longer wavelength with absorption maxima at 254 nm, 308 nm, and 365 nm to that of ilicicolin H. The structure of ilicicolin I (**8**) was elucidated by 1D and 2D NMR spectroscopic analysis (See Table 3). The NMR data for the phenyl-pyridone moiety were comparable to those of ilicicolin H, whereas observed changes to the decalin moiety revealed the compound to be a structural isomer. The ^{1}H-NMR spectrum for the decalin moiety displayed eight methines (including four vinylic), three methylenes (all diastereotopic), and three methyl groups (including one singlet). The DQF-COSY spectrum defined two spin systems besides the singlet methyl group at δ_H 1.10 (CH_3-22). One spin system consisted of the two vinylic protons at δ_H 7.98 (CH-8) and δ_H 7.26 (CH-9) with the size of the coupling constant of J_{89} = 16.0 Hz, indicating trans stereochemistry. The second spin system consisted of the two vinylic methines at δ_H 5.41 (CH-17) and δ_H 5.58 (CH-18), four methines at δ_H 1.41 (CH-11), δ_H 1.47 (CH-14), δ_H 1.81 (CH-16) and δ_H 1.91 (CH-19), three diastereotopic methylenes at δ_H 1.40/1.07 (CH_2-12), δ_H 1.73/1.00 (CH_2-13), and δ_H 1.80/0.80 (CH_2-15) and two methyl groups at δ_H 0.90 (CH_3-20) and δ_H 0.98 (CH_3-21). The linking between these two COSY spin systems and the phenyl-pyridone moiety together with the assignment of the singlet methyl group at CH_3-22 and quaternary carbons was accomplished by analysis of the HMBC spectrum (See Figure 7). Important HMBC correlations from the vinylic protons H-8 and H-9 to the ketone at δ_C 195.7 (C-7) assisted in the connection of this spin system to the phenyl-pyridone moiety. The upfield shift observed for the ketone at C-7 (decreasing from 211.0 to 195.7 ppm) in comparison to ilicicolin H and the downfield shift of the β carbon at δ_C 160.2 (C-9) supports that the C-8/C-9 double bond is in conjugation with the ketone at C-7. HMBC correlations from H-8 and H-9 to δ_C 42.6 (C-10), H-9 to δ_C 18.5 (C-22), H-12, H-18, H-21, and H-22 to C-10 and H-11 and H-19 to C-22 linked the spin system of CH-8 and CH-9 to the remaining spin system of the polyketide chain (including CH-11 to CH-21) via the quaternary carbon at C-10 and singlet methyl group at C-22. Further key HMBC correlations from H-12 and H-18 to δ_C 39.3 (C-16) and from H-15 and H-17 to δ_C 43.2 (C-11) assisted in the assembly of the decalin ring system. The relative stereochemistry of ilicicolin I was proposed based on coupling constants and observed NOEs in the NOESY experiments (See Figure 7). A trans diaxial relationship was suggested for the protons H-16 and H-15b and H-15b and H-14 based on the observation that H-15b appears as a quartet in the ^{1}H-NMR spectrum with a coupling constant of J = 12.5 Hz. Furthermore, a trans diaxial relationship was also assumed for the protons H-14 and H-13b, H-13b, and H-12a and H-12a and H-11 based on H-13b and H-12a appearing in the ^{1}H-NMR spectrum as double quartets with coupling constants of J = 12.4 and 3.4 Hz. This was supported by observed NOEs of H-8 with CH_3-22, CH_3-22 with H-16 and H-19, H-16 with H-14 and H-15a, H-14 with H-12a and H-13a placing these protons on the same side of the plane, whereas correlations of H-9 with CH_3-21, H-11, and H-12b, H-11 with H-15b and CH_3-21, and of H-12b with H-13b placed these protons on the opposite side of the plane.

Based on the structural similarities between ilicicolin I and ilicicolin H, we hypothesize that the decalin moiety for ilicicolin I is biosynthesized by the fungus via cyclization between C-10 and C-19 and between C-11 and C-16 through an intermolecular Diels-Alder reaction of the reduced octaketide chain instead of cyclization between C-8 and C-9 and C-10 and C-15 as in ilicicolin H [26].

Two other ilicicolin H analogues with the pseudomolecular ions, $[M + H]^+$ *m*/*z* 452.2436 ($C_{27}H_{33}NO_5$, accuracy −1.26 ppm) and *m*/*z* 420.2126 ($C_{26}H_{29}NO_4$, accuracy −0.87 ppm) were tentatively identified by HRMS and MS/HRMS to also elute in close proximity to ilicicolin H. This suggested the new structures with the possible addition of H_2O for the former and one less methyl group (difference of a CH_2 unit) for the latter compound compared to ilicicolin H. The two compounds shared the dominant fragment ion at *m*/*z* 230.0451 and showed similarity scores of 80% and 92% to that of ilicicolin H for their 40 eV MS/HRMS spectra, respectively (See Figures S5 and S6, Supplementary information for MS/HRMS spectra). Only trace amounts insufficient for purification were present of these two possibly new analogues in the crude extract.

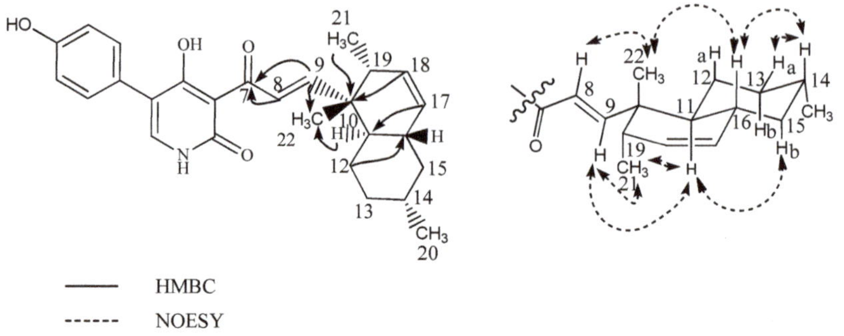

Figure 7. Selected important HMBC correlations (^{1}H-^{13}C) and NOESY correlations for the decalin moeity of ilicicolin I (**8**).

Hydroxyl-ilicicolin H (**6**) and ilicicolin I (**8**) were evaluated together with ilicicolin H (**7**) for their antifungal activity against *A. fumigatus*, *C. albicans*, *Candida parapsilosis*, and *Candida tropicalis*. Compounds (**6**) and (**8**) did not show any activity at the tested concentrations (MIC_{90} > 128 µg/mL). In contrast, ilicicolin H (**7**) exhibited strong activities against *A. fumigatus* (MIC_{90} 0.5–1 µg/mL), *C. albicans* (MIC_{90} < 0.25 µg/mL), and *C. parapsilosis* (MIC_{90} 0.5 µg/mL) to confirm the observed activity of the antifungal fraction. Structure–activity relationship (SAR) studies have previously been performed during structural modifications (chemical, biotransformation, and enzymatic) to ilicicolin H [27,28,44]. As shown here, a series of semisynthetic analogues produced by biotransformation of ilicicolin H generally showed a significant loss of activity when oxidized [44]. The importance of the β-diketone feature (C-4-C-3-C-7) has been indicated in the antifungal activity and in general a significant reduction or loss of activity has been seen for compounds with modification around the β-diketone and hindrance of an established bioactive conformation with a perpendicular orientation between the left hand phenyl-pyridone side and right hand decalin side [27,28]. The loss of activity seen for ilicicolin I may be due to the hindrance of this structural isomer to take up the right bioactive conformation.

3. Materials and Methods

3.1. General Experimental Procedures

UHPLC-DAD-QTOFMS was performed on an Agilent Infinity 1290 UHPLC system (Agilent Technologies, Santa Clara, CA, USA) equipped with a DAD. Separation was achieved on an Agilent Poroshell 120 phenyl-hexyl column (2.1 × 150 mm, 2.7 µm) with a flow rate of 0.35 mL/min at 60 °C using a linear gradient of 10% acetonitrile (MeCN) in Milli-Q water buffered with 20 mM formic acid (FA) increased to 100% in 15 min staying there for 2 min, returned to 10% in 0.1 min and kept there for 3 min before the following run. MeCN was LC-MS grade. MS detection was done on an Agilent 6545 QTOF MS equipped with Agilent Dual Jet Stream electrospray ion source with a drying gas temperature of 160 °C, a gas flow of 13 L/min, and a sheath gas temperature of 300 °C and flow of 16 L/min. Capillary voltage was set to 4000 V and a nozzle voltage to 500 V. Other MS parameters including description of the automated data-dependent MS/HRMS (at 10, 20, and 40 eV) can be found in Kildgaard et al. 2014 [11]. The MS data were analyzed in three different ways. First, full scan HRMS data were data mined (aggressive dereplication) for $[M + H]^+$, $[M + Na]^+$, $[M - H]^-$, and $[M + HCOO]^-$ adducts of all known elemental compositions described from *Stilbella* and related genera [11], here the mass accuracy, isotopic ratios, and isotopic spacing [45] were added into a combined score (0–100%), where only hits above 70% were considered. Secondly, the MS/HRMS spectra were searched against the in-house library using the Agilent MassHunter PCDL manager (Agilent Technologies), with 20 ppm accuracy on the parent ion and 30 ppm on the fragment ions, giving a score of 0–100%. Finally, the elemental composition of peaks not identified in the previous two steps, were identified based on the mass accuracy, isotopic ratios, and isotopic spacing (sometimes providing several candidates above 70%). Then similarity search (>50% of 100%) was used for matching peaks in the library spectrum against the unknown spectrum (independent on parent mass) [11] to pinpoint related pimarane diterpenoids and hybrid polyketide-non ribosomal peptides, since both had groups displaying unique and very different fragment ions (Supplementary information). Pre-fractionation was performed using flash chromatography of the crude extract with an Isolera One automated flash system (Biotage, Uppsala, Sweden). Purification of compounds was conducted using a Waters 600 Controller (Milford, MA, USA) coupled to a Waters 996 Photodiode Array Detector. One and two dimensional NMR experiments were acquired using standard pulse sequences on a 400 MHz Bruker Ascend spectrometer with a Prodigy cryoprobe, 600 MHz Bruker Ascend with a SmartProbe (BBO) and a 800 MHz Bruker Avance spectrometer with a 5 mm TCI cryoprobe, alternatively on a 500 MHz Bruker Avance with a 1.7 mm cryoprobe at Fundación Medina, Spain. Optical rotations were measured on a Perkin Elmer 341 polarimeter (Perkin Elmer, Waltham, MA, USA).

3.2. Fungal Strain and Identification

The filamentous fungus was isolated from a sea water sample off the coast of the Danish island Fanoe. The fungus was 3-point inoculated on CYA, OAT, PDA, and V8 agar plates [46] and incubated at 25 °C in the dark. After 11 days of growth on V8, microscope slides were made and a morphological examination identified the fungus as *Stilbella fimetaria* (Pers.) Lindau. Molecular sequencing of the ITS region confirmed the morphological identification. The fungus (IBT 28361) is stored in the IBT culture collection at DTU Bioengineering, Technical University of Denmark.

3.3. Cultivation

Original small scale cultivation: the marine-derived fungus was 3-point inoculated on ten agar plates (five CYA and five YES) and incubated for 9 days in the dark at 25 °C [46]. Cultivation 1: the fungus was 3-point inoculated on 200 YES plates and incubated for 9 days in the dark at 25 °C. Cultivation 2: the fungus was inoculated into 6 × 1.8 L conical culture flasks with organic grain rice (150 g per flask) and Milli-Q water (150 g per flask) and incubated at 25 °C in the dark for 10 days. Cultivation 3: the fungus was inoculated into 15 small conical flasks 0.5 L with organic grain rice (50 g per flask) and Milli-Q water (50 g per flask) and incubated for 21 days at 25°C in the dark.

3.4. Extraction and Isolation

Original small scale cultivation: Extraction of the eight plates (four CYA and four YES) was achieved with 150 mL EtOAc containing 1% FA. The crude extract was then fractionated on a RP C_{18} flash column (Sepra ZT, Isolute, 10 g) using the Isolera One automated flash system. The gradient used was MeCN and water buffered with 20 mM FA going from 15% to 100% MeCN over 28 min (12 mL/min). Six flash fractions were automatically collected based on UV signal (210 nm and 254 nm). MeCN was of HPLC grade and water was purified and deionized by a Millipore system with a 0.22 μm membrane filter (Milli-Q water). For one CYA plate and one YES plate 4 plugs were taken from one colony with a 6-mm plug drill, covering the diameter of the colony and extracted with 1 mL EtOAc containing 1% FA and otherwise prepared in accordance with the micro-scale extraction method described by Smedsgaard [47].

Cultivation 1: Extraction was achieved with 150 mL EtOAc with 1% FA for every 10 plates. Liquid-liquid extraction was performed with 1:9 Milli-Q water:methanol (MeOH) and 1:1 heptane, resulting in two phases, the Milli-Q water/MeOH phase was added Milli-Q water to a ratio 1:1, and metabolites were extracted with dichloromethane (DCM). This was done to remove unwanted carbohydrates from the media as well as fatty acids. The crude extract from the DCM phase was fractionated on a RP C_{18} flash column (Sepra ZT, Isolute, 25 g) using the Isolera One automated flash system. The gradient used was 15–100% MeCN buffered with 20 mM FA over 28 min (25 mL/min). Fractions were automatically collected based on UV signal (210 nm and 254 nm). The bioactive fraction (going from 40–50% MeCN) was further fractionated on the Isolera system using a diol flash column (Diol, 25 g, 33 mL) and fractions were eluted with two column volumes (2 col. vols.) per fraction with DCM, DCM/EtOAc, EtOAc, EtOAc/MeOH, and MeOH with a flow rate of 25 mL/min. The bioactive fractions going from 50% to 60% and 60% to 85% MeCN were fractionated further on the Isolera system using a RP C_{18} flash column (10 g/15 mL). The gradient was 5% stepwise (13 col. vols.) from 35% to 100% MeOH buffered with 20 mM FA with a flow rate of 15 mL/min. Fractions were collected manually for every 5%. Myrocin F and helvolic acid were purified on the Waters 600 semi-preparative HPLC. Myrocin F separation was achieved on a Luna II C_{18}, 5 μm, 250 × 10 mm column (Phenomenex, Torrance, CA, USA) with a flow rate of 5 mL/min using a linear gradient of 45% MeCN in Milli-Q water with 20 mM FA going to 75% MeCN in 20 min. Helvolic acid separation was achieved on a Luna II C_{18}, 5 μm, 250 × 10 mm column (Phenomenex, Torrance, CA, USA) with a flow rate of 4 mL/min using a linear gradient 60% MeCN in Milli-Q water going to 100% MeCN in 20 min.

Cultivation 2: Extraction was achieved using 600 mL per flask of EtOAc with 1% FA. Liquid-liquid extraction was performed with 1:9 Milli-Q water:MeOH and 1:1 heptane, the Milli-Q water/MeOH phase was added Milli-Q water to a ratio 1:1, and metabolites were extracted with DCM, leaving the crude extract from the DCM phase. The crude extract was fractionated on a diol flash column (Diol, 25 g, 33 mL) and compounds were eluted with 2 col. vols. per fraction: heptane, heptane/DCM, DCM, DCM 3: 1 EtOAc, DCM/EtOAc, EtOAc, EtOAc 3:1 MeOH, EtOAc/MeOH, and MeOH. Fractions DCM 3: 1 EtOAc and DCM/EtOAc were further fractionated on a RP C_{18} column (15 μm/100 Å, 10 g/15 mL) using the Isolera One automated flash system. The gradient was 5% stepwise (13 col. vols.) from 35% to 100% MeOH buffered with 20 mM FA with a flow rate of 15 mL/min. Fractions were collected manually for every 5%. Libertellenone M, the suggested opened γ-lactone of libertellenone M and libertellenone C were purified on the Waters 600 semi-preparative HPLC. Libertellenone M and the opened γ-lactone of libertellenone M separation was achieved on a Gemini C_6-Phenyl, 5 μm, 250 × 10 mm column (Phenomenex, Torrance, CA, USA) with a flow rate of 4 mL/min using a linear gradient 40% MeCN in Milli-Q water with 20 mM FA going to 100% MeCN in 28 min. Further libertellenone M separation was done on a Luna II C_{18}, 5 μm, 250 × 10 mm column (Phenomenex, Torrance, CA, USA) with a flow rate of 4 mL/min isocratic 55% MeCN in Milli-Q water with 20 mM FA in 20 min and a Kinetex Biphenyl, 5 μm 250 × 10 mm column (Phenomenex, Torrance, CA, USA) with a flow rate of 4 mL/min using a linear gradient 30% MeCN in Milli-Q water with 20 mM FA going to 100% MeCN in 25 min. Libertellenone C separation was achieved on a Luna II C_{18}, 5 μm, 250 × 10 mm column (Phenomenex, Torrance, CA, USA) with a flow rate of 5 mL/min using a linear gradient of 30% MeCN in Milli-Q water with 20 mM FA going to 70% MeCN in 30 min. Libertellenone E was purified from the EtOAc 3:1 MeOH fraction on the Waters 600 semipreparative HPLC. Separation was achieved on a Luna II C_{18}, 5 μm, 250 × 10 mm column (Phenomenex, Torrance, CA, USA) with a flow rate of 5 mL/min using a linear gradient of 30% MeCN in Milli-Q water with 20 mM FA going to 70% MeCN in 20 min and a Kinetex Biphenyl, 5 μm 250 × 10 mm column (Phenomenex, Torrance, CA, USA) with a flow rate of 4 mL/min using a linear gradient of 30% MeCN in Milli-Q water with 20 mM FA going to 100% MeCN in 25 min.

Cultivation 3: Extraction was achieved using 150 mL EtOAc per flask. Liquid-liquid extraction was performed with 1:9 Milli-Q water:MeOH and 1:1 heptane, the Milli-Q water/MeOH phase was added Milli-Q water to a ratio 1:1, and metabolites were extracted with DCM, leaving the crude extract from the DCM phase. The crude extract was pre-fractionated on a diol flash column (Diol, 25 g, 33 mL) and compounds were eluted with 2 col. vols. per fraction: heptane, heptane/DCM, DCM, DCM 3:1 EtOAc, DCM/EtOAc, EtOAc, EtOAc 3:1 MeOH, EtOAc/MeOH, and MeOH. Interesting fractions were further fractionated on a RP C_{18} column (15 µm/100 Å, 10 g/15 mL) using the Isolera One automated flash system. The gradient was 5% stepwise (13 col. vols.) from 35% to 100% MeOH buffered with 20 mM FA with a flow rate of 15 mL/min. Fractions were collected manually for every 5%. Ilicicolin H and hydroxy-ilicicolin H purification was achieved from the 80% MeOH and 50% MeOH fractions, respectively, on a Gemini C_6-Phenyl, 5 µm, 250 × 10 mm column (Phenomenex, Torrance, CA, USA) with a flow rate of 4 mL/min using a linear gradient from 80% MeCN in Milli-Q water with 20 mM FA going to 100% MeCN in 15 min for ilicicolin H and from 50% MeCN in Milli-Q water with 20 mM FA going to 90% MeCN in 20 min for hydroxy-ilicicolin H. Ilicicolin I was purified from the 60% MeOH fraction on a Kinetex Biphenyl, 5 µm 250 × 10 mm column (Phenomenex, Torrance, CA, USA) with a flow rate of 4 mL/min using an isocratic gradient at 75% MeCN in Milli-Q water with 20 mM FA for 20 min.

Helvolic acid: white solid; UV (MeCN) λ_{max}: 234 nm; ^{13}C NMR see Figure S12 and Table 1; HRESIMS m/z 591.2932 ($[M + Na]^+$ calculated for $C_{33}H_{44}O_8Na$, m/z 591.2922)

Myrocin F: white solid; UV (MeCN) λ_{max}: 215 nm, 270 nm; ^{13}C- and ^{1}H-NMR see Table 1; HRESIMS m/z 329.1745 ($[M + H]^+$ calculated for $C_{20}H_{25}O_4$, m/z 329.1746)

Libertellenone M: white solid; $[\alpha]_D^{20}$ −81° (c 0.10, MeOH); UV (MeCN) λ_{max}: 220 sh nm, 270 sh nm, 290 nm; ^{13}C- and ^{1}H-NMR see Table 2; HRESIMS m/z 327.1592 ($[M + H]^+$ calculated for $C_{20}H_{23}O_4$, m/z 327.1590)

Opened γ-lactone ring of libertellenone M: white solid; UV (MeCN) λ_{max}: 220 sh nm, 270 nm, 315 nm; ^{13}C- and ^{1}H-NMR see Table 2; HRESIMS m/z 345.1692 ($[M + H]^+$ calculated for $C_{20}H_{25}O_5$, m/z 345.1695)

Libertellenone C: white solid; $[\alpha]_D^{20}$ −98° (c 0.11, MeOH); UV (MeCN) λ_{max}: 218 nm, 270 nm, 325 nm; ^{13}C- and ^{1}H-NMR see Figure S31 and Table 2; HRESIMS m/z 349.2012 ($[M + H]^+$ calculated for $C_{20}H_{29}O_5$, m/z 349.2007)

Libertellenone E: white solid; $[\alpha]_D^{20}$ +24.6° (c 0.13, MeOH); UV (MeCN) λ_{max}: 214 nm, 268 nm, 314 nm; ^{13}C- and ^{1}H-NMR see Figure S31 and Table 2; HRESIMS m/z 347.1858 ($[M + H]^+$ calculated for $C_{20}H_{27}O_5$, m/z 347.1851)

Ilicicolin H: yellow solid; $[\alpha]_D^{20}$ −159° (c 0.11, MeOH); UV (MeCN) λ_{max}: 250 nm, 295 nm, 350 nm; ^{13}C- and ^{1}H-NMR see Table 3; HRESIMS m/z 434.2325 ($[M + H]^+$ calculated for $C_{27}H_{32}NO_4$, m/z 434.2323)

Hydroxyl-ilicicolin H: yellow solid; UV (MeCN) λ_{max}: 250 nm, 295 nm, 350 nm; ^{13}C- and ^{1}H-NMR see Table 3; HRESIMS m/z 450.2278 ($[M + H]^+$ calculated for $C_{27}H_{32}NO_5$, m/z 450.2272)

Ilicicolin I: yellow solid; UV (MeCN) λ_{max}: 254 nm, 308 nm, 365 nm; ^{13}C- and ^{1}H-NMR see Table 3; HRESIMS m/z 434.2325 ($[M + H]^+$ calculated for $C_{27}H_{32}NO_4$, m/z 434.2323

3.5. Cytotoxicity Assay

NCH421k GSCs were derived from primary GBM patients who underwent surgical resection according to the research proposals approved by the Institutional Review Board at the Medical Faculty of Heidelberg. Tissues were enzymatically dissociated and cells were cultivated as floating neurospheres under standard conditions (37 °C, 95% humidity, and 5% CO_2) in serum-free stem cell medium (DMEM/F-12 medium, 20% (v/v) BIT-admixture and 20 ng/mL each of basal fibroblast growth factor (bFGF) and epidermal growth factor (EGF)). Cells were generally cultivated in 75 cm^2 untreated cell culture flasks (Sarstedt, Newton, MA, USA). When spheres reached around 150–300 µm in diameter, cells were passaged into new medium. Spheres were separated from debris and dead cells by gravity sedimentation, before suspension in 1 mL accutase and shaking at 1100 rpm at 37 °C. Accutase was removed after centrifugation at 900 g for 4 min and cells resuspended in 1 mL stem cell medium. Cells were passaged at 1:5–1:10 into 13 mL fresh stem cell medium, depending on the density of the previous culture. Malignant cell lines A549 (lung carcinoma), MCF7 (breast adenocarcinoma), SW480 (colorectal adenocarcinoma) and DU 145 (prostate carcinoma) were cultivated adherently in DMEM supplemented with 10% FCS and 1% (*v*/*v*) penicillin/streptomycin. *Stilbella fimetaria* extracts were initially tested for anticancer activity in NCH421k cells. To this end, cells were seeded in 96-well plates (Greiner, Munich, Germany) at a density of 20,000 cells per well in 100 μL medium. Dried fractionated fungal extracts were dissolved in DMSO and 10, 2, 0.4, 0.1, and 0.025 μg/well was applied to the cells. 48 h after incubation under standard cell culture conditions, cell viability was assessed using the CellTiter-Glo® luminescent cell viability assay (Promega, Madison, WI, USA). Cells incubated with DMSO only were used as a control. In order to determine IC_{50} values for the pure diterpenoids, cells were seeded in 96-well plates (Greiner, Munich, Germany) at a density of 5000 cells per well for adherent cells and 8500 cells per well for NCH421k cells. Adherent cells were seeded 24 h in advance to allow the cells to attach. Compound was dissolved to 30 mM in 100% DMSO and three-fold serial dilutions were performed in cell culture medium. The compound containing medium was then applied with a dilution factor of ten, contributing to eight concentrations, starting at 300 μM for all the assays. Cell viability was assessed by the CellTiter-Glo® (Promega, Madison, WI, USA) luminescent cell viability assay after 48 h incubation with the compound. Data were normalised to the DMSO control. Viability curves were plotted using Excel and IC_{50} values estimated from the curves. The assay was performed in biological triplicate.

3.6. *Antibacterial and Antifungal Assays*

Previously described methods were used for evaluating antibacterial and antifungal properties of extracts/compounds [48,49]. The pimarane diterpenoids were tested for their ability to inhibit the growth of Gram-negative and Gram-positive bacteria (*E. coli* ATCC25922 and MSSA MB2865), fungi (*A. fumigatus* ATCC46645) and yeast (*C. albicans* ATCC64124). Ilicicolin H and analogues were tested for their ability to inhibit the growth of *A. fumigatus* ATCC46645 and yeast (*C. albicans* ATCC64124, *C. parapsilosis* ATCC22019, and *C. tropicalis* ATCC750). Helvolic acid was tested for its ability to inhibit the growth of MRSA MB5393. Briefly, each compound was 3-fold serially diluted in DMSO with a dilution factor of 2 to provide 10 concentrations starting at 128 μg/mL for all the assays (for the pimarane diterpenoids only nine concentrations were used starting at 64 μg/mL). The MIC was defined as the lowest concentration of an antibacterial or antifungal compound that inhibited $\geq$90% of the growth of a microorganism after overnight incubation. The Genedata Screener software (Genedata, Inc., Basel, Switzerland) was used to process and analyse the data and also to calculate the RZ′ factor which predicts the robustness of an assay [50]. In all experiments performed in this work the RZ′ factor obtained was between 0.87 and 0.98.

4. Conclusions

In this study, our combined bio-guided and dereplication-based discovery approach of cytotoxicity and antimicrobial assays, UHPLC-DAD-QTOFMS-MS/HRMS using an in-house MS/HRMS library and pre-bioassay fractionation of a marine-derived fungus *Stilbella fimetaria* proved to be quick and effective in the identification of new and known bioactive natural products. There was no observed bioactivity for the *Stilbella fimetaria* crude extract on its own, whereas pre-fractionation allowed the observation of cytotoxicity, and antibacterial and antifungal activity, respectively, in three different fractions. This led to the discovery of several cytotoxic pimarane-type diterpenoids, including the two new diterpenes, myrocin F and libertellenone M, with IC_{50} values of 40 an 18 μM, respectively, towards patient derived glioblastoma stem-like cells. Myrocin F exhibited general cytotoxicity towards various cancer cell lines with IC_{50} values between 20 to 50 μM. The known broad-spectrum antifungal compound, ilicicolin H was revealed as the active compound contributing to the observed antifungal activity and MS/HRMS was applied to tentatively identify several new ilicicolin H analogues, including the two purified compounds, hydroxyl-ilicicolin H and ilicicolin I. Optimization on rice media allowed for the purification of compounds in the required amount for structure elucidation and bioassay analysis, with the production being optimal at around one week for the pimarane-type ditepenoids and three weeks for the ilicicolin H analogues.

Supplementary Materials: The following are available online at www.mdpi.com/1660-3397/15/8/253/s1, HRESITOFMS, MS/HRMS, UV and 1D and 2D NMR data of all new compounds are provided.

Acknowledgments: Funding is acknowledged from PharmaSea (Grant Agreement No 312184). Thanks to Lisette Knoth-Nielsen for assistance with media and crude extracts. We thank the NMR center • DTU and the Villum foundation for 800 MHz NMR time. We are grateful to Agilent Technologies for the Thought Leader Donation of the UHPLC-QTOF system.

Author Contributions: Sara Kildgaard and Karolina Subko performed the purifications and structural elucidations. Emma Phillips, Violaine Goidts, Mercedes de la Cruz, Caridad Díaz and Sara Kildgaard performed the bioassay analyses and wrote the experimental bioassay sections. Birgitte Andersen and Jens C. Frisvad provided and identified the strain and together with Charlotte H. Gotfredsen, Kristian F. Nielsen and Thomas O. Larsen assisted in compound identification. Sara Kildgaard wrote the paper. All authors read and corrected the paper.

Conflicts of Interest: The authors declare no conflict of interest.

References

1. Rateb, M.E.; Ebel, R. Secondary metabolites of fungi from marine habitats. *Nat. Prod. Rep.* **2011**, *28*, 290–344. [CrossRef] [PubMed]
2. Debbab, A.; Aly, A.H.; Lin, W.H.; Proksch, P. Bioactive compounds from marine bacteria and fungi. *Microb. Biotechnol.* **2010**, *3*, 544–563. [CrossRef] [PubMed]
3. Duarte, K.; Rocha-Santos, T.A.P.; Freitas, A.C.; Duarte, A.C. Analytical techniques for discovery of bioactive compounds from marine fungi. *Trends Anal. Chem.* **2012**, *34*, 97–109. [CrossRef]
4. Overy, D.P.; Bayman, P.; Kerr, R.G.; Bills, G.F. An assessment of natural product discovery from marine (*sensu strictu*) and marine-derived fungi. *Mycology* **2014**, *5*, 145–167. [CrossRef] [PubMed]
5. Burgaud, G.; Le Calvez, T.; Arzur, D.; Vadenkoornhuyse, P.; Barbier, G. Diversity of culturable marine filamentous fungi from deep-sea hydrothermal vents. *Environ. Microbiol.* **2009**, *11*, 1588–1600. [CrossRef] [PubMed]
6. Jones, E. Are there more marine fungi to be described? *Bot. Mar.* **2011**, *54*, 343–354. [CrossRef]
7. Jones, E. Fifty years of marine mycology. *Fungal Divers.* **2011**, *50*, 73–112. [CrossRef]
8. Richards, T.A.; Jones, M.D.M.; Leonard, G.; Bass, D. Marine fungi: Their ecology and molecular diversity. *Annu. Rev. Mar. Sci.* **2012**, *4*, 495–522. [CrossRef] [PubMed]
9. El-Elimat, T.; Figueroa, M.; Ehrmann, B.M.; Cech, N.B.; Pearce, C.J.; Oberlies, N.H. High-resolution MS, MS/MS, and UV database of fungal secondary metabolites as a dereplication protocol for bioactive natural products. *J. Nat. Prod.* **2013**, *76*, 1709–1716. [CrossRef] [PubMed]
10. Bladt, T.B.; Dürr, C.; Knudsen, P.B.; Kildgaard, S.; Frisvad, J.C.; Gotfredsen, C.H.; Seiffert, M.; Larsen, T.O. Bio-activity and dereplication-based discovery of ophiobolins and other fungal secondary metabolites targeting leukemia cells. *Molecules* **2013**, *18*, 14629–14650. [CrossRef] [PubMed]
11. Kildgaard, S.; Mansson, M.; Dosen, I.; Klitgaard, A.; Frisvad, J.C.; Larsen, T.O.; Nielsen, K.F. Accurate dereplication of bioactive secondary metabolites from marine-derived fungi by UHPLC-DAD-QTOFMS and a MS/HRMS library. *Mar. Drugs* **2014**, *12*, 3681–3705. [CrossRef] [PubMed]
12. Nielsen, K.F.; Månsson, M.; Rank, C.; Frisvad, J.C.; Larsen, T.O. Dereplication of microbial natural products by LC-DAD-TOFMS. *J. Nat. Prod.* **2011**, *74*, 2338–2348. [CrossRef] [PubMed]
13. Klitgaard, A.; Iversen, A.; Andersen, M.R.; Larsen, T.O.; Frisvad, J.C.; Nielsen, K.F. Aggressive dereplication using UHPLC-DAD-QTOF—Screening extracts for up to 3000 fungal secondary metabolites. *Anal. Bioanal. Chem.* **2014**, *406*, 1933–1943. [CrossRef] [PubMed]
14. Guthals, A.; Watrous, J.D.; Dorrestein, P.C.; Bandeira, N. The spectral networks paradigm in high throughput mass spectrometry. *Mol. BioSyst.* **2012**, *8*, 2535–2544. [CrossRef] [PubMed]
15. Yang, J.Y.; Sanchez, L.M.; Rath, C.M.; Liu, X.; Boudreau, P.D.; Bruns, N.; Glukhov, E.; Wodtke, A.; de Felicio, R.; Fenner, A.; et al. Molecular networking as a dereplication strategy. *J. Nat. Prod.* **2013**, *76*, 1686–1699. [CrossRef] [PubMed]

16. Watrous, J.; Roach, P.; Alexandrov, T.; Heath, B.S.; Yang, J.Y.; Kersten, R.D.; van der Voort, M.; Pogliano, K.; Gross, H.; Raaijmakers, J.M.; et al. Mass spectral molecular networking of living microbial colonies. *Proc. Natl. Acad. Sci. USA* **2012**, *109*, E1743–E1752. [CrossRef] [PubMed]
17. Naman, C.B.; Rattan, R.; Nikoulina, S.E.; Lee, J.; Miller, B.W.; Moss, N.A.; Armstrong, L.; Boudreau, P.D.; Debonsi, H.M.; Valeriote, F.A.; et al. Integrating molecular networking and biological assays to target the isolation of a cytotoxic cyclic octapeptide, samoamide A, from an American Samoan marine cyanobacterium. *J. Nat. Prod.* **2017**, *80*, 625–633. [CrossRef] [PubMed]
18. Appleton, D.R.; Buss, A.D.; Butler, M.S. A simple method for high-throughput extract prefractionation for biological screening. *Chimia* **2007**, *61*, 327–331. [CrossRef]
19. Wagenaar, M.M. Pre-fractionated microbial samples—The second generation natural products library at Wyeth. *Molecules* **2008**, *13*, 1406–1426. [CrossRef] [PubMed]
20. Butler, M.S.; Fontaine, F.; Cooper, M.A. Natural product libraries: Assembly, maintenance, and screening. *Planta Med.* **2014**, *80*, 1161–1170. [CrossRef] [PubMed]
21. Månsson, M.; Phipps, R.K.; Gram, L.; Munro, M.H.G.; Larsen, T.O.; Nielsen, K.F. Explorative solid-phase extraction (E-SPE) for accelerated microbial natural product discovery, dereplication, and purification. *J. Nat. Prod.* **2010**, *73*, 1126–1132. [CrossRef] [PubMed]
22. Ratnaweera, P.B.; Williams, D.E.; de Silva, E.D.; Wijesundera, R.L.C.; Dalisay, D.S.; Andersen, R.J. Helvolic acid, an antibacterial nortriterpenoid from a fungal endophyte, *Xylaria* sp. of orchid *Anoectochilus setaceus* endemic to Sri Lanka. *Mycology* **2014**, *5*, 23–28. [CrossRef] [PubMed]
23. Qin, L.; Li, B.; Guan, J.; Zhang, G. In vitro synergistic antibacterial activities of helvolic acid on multi-drug resistant *Staphylococcus aureus*. *Nat. Prod. Res.* **2009**, *23*, 309–318. [CrossRef] [PubMed]
24. Fujimoto, H.; Negishi, E.; Yamaguchi, K.; Nishi, N.; Yamazaki, M. Isolation of new tremorgenic metabolites from an Ascomycete, *Corynascus setosus*. *Chem. Pharm. Bull.* **1996**, *44*, 1843–1848. [CrossRef]
25. Matsumoto, M.; Minato, H. Structure of ilicicolin H, an antifungal. *Tetrahedron Lett.* **1976**, *42*, 3827–3838. [CrossRef]
26. Tanaba, M.; Uranot, S. Biosynthetic studies with 13C the antifungal antibiotic ilicicolin H. *Tetrahedron* **1983**, *39*, 3569–3574. [CrossRef]
27. Singh, B.S.; Liu, W.; Li, X.; Chen, T.; Shafiee, A.; Card, D.; Abruzzo, G.; Flattery, A.; Gill, C.; Thompson, J.R.; et al. Antifungal spectrum, *in vivo* efficacy, and structure-activity relationship of ilicicolin H. *ACS Med. Chem. Lett.* **2012**, *3*, 814–817. [CrossRef] [PubMed]
28. Singh, S.B.; Liu, W.; Li, X.; Chen, T.; Shafiee, A.; Dreikorn, S.; Hornak, V.; Meinz, M.; Onishi, J.C. Structure—activity relationship of cytochrome bc1 reductase inhibitor broad spectrum antifungal ilicicolin H. *Bioorg. Med. Chem. Let.* **2013**, *23*, 3018–3022. [CrossRef] [PubMed]
29. Shervington, A.; Lu, C. Expression of multidrug resistance genes in normal and cancer stem cells. *Cancer Investig.* **2008**, *26*, 535–542. [CrossRef] [PubMed]
30. Stoppacher, N.; Neumann, N.K.N.; Burgstaller, L.; Zeilinger, S.; Degenkolb, T.; Bruckner, H.; Schuhmacher, R. The Comprehensive Peptaibiotics Database. *Chem. Biodivers.* **2013**, *10*, 734–743. [CrossRef] [PubMed]
31. Thirumalachar, M.J. Antiamoebin anti parasit a new anti protozoal anti helminthic antibiotic I production and biological studies *Emericellopsis-Poonensis Emericellopsis-Synnematicola Cephalosporium-Pimprina*. *Hindustan Antibiot. Bull.* **1968**, *10*, 287–289. [PubMed]
32. Lehr, N.-A.; Meffert, A.; Antelo, L.; Sterner, O.; Anke, H.; Weber, R.W.S. Antiamoebins, myrocin B and the basis of antifungal antibiosis in the coprophilous fungus *Stilbella erythrocephala* (syn. *S. fimetaria*). *FEMS Microbiol. Ecol.* **2006**, *55*, 105–112. [CrossRef] [PubMed]
33. Jaworski, A.; Bruckner, H. New sequences and new fungal producers of peptaibol antibiotics antiamoebins. *Pept. Sci.* **2000**, *6*, 149–167. [CrossRef]
34. Klemke, C.; Kehraus, S.; Wright, A.D.; König, G.M. New secondary metabolites from the marine endophytic fungus *Apiospora montagnei*. *J. Nat. Prod.* **2004**, *67*, 1058–1063. [CrossRef] [PubMed]
35. Hsu, Y.-H.; Nakagawa, M.; Hirota, A.; Shima, S.; Nakayama, M. Structure of myrocin B, a new diterpene antibiotic produced by *Myrothecium verrucaria*. *Agric. Biol. Chem.* **1988**, *52*, 1305–1307. [CrossRef]
36. Tsukada, M.; Fukai, M.; Miki, K.; Shiraishi, T.; Suzuki, T.; Nishio, K.; Sugita, T.; Ishino, M.; Kinoshita, K.; Takahashi, K.; et al. Chemical constituents of a marine fungus, *Arthrinium sacchari*. *J. Nat. Prod.* **2011**, *74*, 1645–1649. [CrossRef] [PubMed]

37. Shiono, Y.; Matsui, N.; Imaizumi, T.; Koseki, T.; Murayama, T.; Kwon, E.; Abe, T.; Kimura, K.-I. An unusual spirocyclic isopimarane diterpenoid and other isopimarane diterpenoids from fruiting bodies of *Xylaria polymorpha*. *Phytochem. Lett.* **2013**, *6*, 439–443. [CrossRef]
38. Hsu, Y.-H.; Hirota, A.; Shima, S.; Nakagawa, M.; Adachi, T.; Nozaki, H.; Nakayama, M. Myrocin C, a new diterpene antitumor antibiotic from *Myrothecium verrucaria*. *J. Antibiot.* **1989**, *42*, 223–229. [CrossRef] [PubMed]
39. Oh, D.-C.; Jensen, P.R.; Kauffman, C.A.; Fenical, W. Libertellenones A–D: Induction of cytotoxic diterpenoid biosynthesis by marine microbial competition. *Bioorg. Med. Chem.* **2005**, *13*, 5267–5273. [CrossRef] [PubMed]
40. Tan, R.; Wei, W.; Jiang, R.; Zhao, G. Yi Zhong Er Tie Libertellenone G Ji Qi Zhi Bei Fang Fa Yu Yong Tu. CN Patent 103073527 A, 1 May 2013.
41. Laatsch, H. *AntiBase 2012*; Wiley-VCH: Weinheim, Germany, 2012. Available online: http://www.wileyvch.de/stmdata/antibase.php (accessed on 1 July 2017).
42. Hayakawa, S.; Minato, H.; Katagiri, K. The ilicicolins, antibiotics from *Cylindrocladium ilicicola*. *J. Antibiot.* **1971**, *24*, 653–654. [CrossRef] [PubMed]
43. Williams, D.R.; Bremmer, M.L.; Brown, D.L.; D'Antuono, J. Total Synthesis of (f)-Ilicicolin H. *J. Org. Chem.* **1985**, *50*, 2807–2809. [CrossRef]
44. Singh, S.B.; Li, X.; Chen, T. Biotransformation of antifungal ilicicolin H. *Tetrahedron Lett.* **2011**, *52*, 6190–6191. [CrossRef]
45. Andersen, A.J.C.; Hansen, P.J.; Jørgensen, K.; Nielsen, K.F. Dynamic cluster analysis: An unbiased method for identifying A + 2 element containing compounds in liquid chromatographic high-resolution time of flight mass spectrometric data. *Anal. Chem.* **2016**, *88*, 12461–12469. [CrossRef] [PubMed]
46. Samson, R.A.; Houbraken, J.; Thrane, U.; Frisvad, J.C.; Andersen, B. *Food and Indoor Fungi*; CBS-KNAW Fungal Biodiversity Centre: Utrecht, The Netherlands, 2010.
47. Smedsgaard, J. Micro-Scale extraction procedure for standardized screening of fungal metabolite production in cultures. *J. Chromatogr. A* **1997**, *760*, 264–270. [CrossRef]
48. Audoin, C.; Bonhomme, D.; Ivanisevic, J.; de la Cruz, M.; Cautain, B.; Monteiro, M.C.; Reyes, F.; Rios, L.; Perez, T.; Thomas, O.P. Balibalosides, an original family of glucosylated sesterterpenes produced by the Mediterranean sponge *Oscarella balibaloi*. *Mar. Drugs* **2013**, *11*, 1477–1489. [CrossRef] [PubMed]
49. Monteiro, M.C.; de la Cruz, M.; Cantizani, J.; Moreno, C.; Tormo, J.R.; Mellado, E.; De Lucas, J.R.; Asensio, F.; Valiante, V.; Brakhage, A.A.; et al. A new approach to drug discovery: High-throughput screening of microbial natural extracts against *Aspergillus fumigatus* using resazurin. *J. Biomol. Screen.* **2012**, *17*, 542–549. [CrossRef] [PubMed]
50. Zhang, J.H.; Chung, T.D.; Oldenburg, K.R. A simple statistical parameter for use in evaluation and validation of high throughput screening assays. *J. Biomol. Screen.* **1999**, *4*, 67–73. [CrossRef] [PubMed]

© 2017 by the authors. Licensee MDPI, Basel, Switzerland. This article is an open access article distributed under the terms and conditions of the Creative Commons Attribution (CC BY) license (http://creativecommons.org/licenses/by/4.0/).

marine drugs

MDPI

Article

Isolation and Tissue Distribution of an Insulin-Like Androgenic Gland Hormone (IAG) of the Male Red Deep-Sea Crab, *Chaceon quinquedens*

Amanda Lawrence, Shadaesha Green and Jum Sook Chung *

Institute of Marine and Environmental Technology, University of Maryland Center for Environmental Science, 701 E. Pratt Street Columbus Center, Baltimore, MD 21202, USA; alawrence@umces.edu (A.L.); sgreen@umces.edu (S.G.)

* Correspondence: chung@umces.edu; Tel.: +1-410-234-8841

Received: 14 July 2017; Accepted: 29 July 2017; Published: 1 August 2017

Abstract: The insulin-like androgenic gland hormone (IAG) found in decapod crustaceans is known to regulate sexual development in males. IAG is produced in the male-specific endocrine tissue, the androgenic gland (AG); however, IAG expression has been also observed in other tissues of decapod crustacean species including *Callinectes sapidus* and *Scylla paramamosain*. This study aimed to isolate the full-length cDNA sequence of IAG from the AG of male red deep-sea crabs, *Chaceon quinquedens* (*ChqIAG*), and to examine its tissue distribution. To this end, we employed polymerase chain reaction cloning with degenerate primers and 5′ and 3′ rapid amplification of cDNA ends (RACE). The full-length *ChqIAG* cDNA sequence (1555 nt) includes a 366 nt 5′ untranslated region a 453 nt open reading frame encoding 151 amino acids, and a relatively long 3′ UTR of 733 nt. The ORF consists of a 19 aa signal peptide, 32 aa B chain, 56 aa C chain, and 44 aa A chain. The putative ChqIAG amino acid sequence is most similar to those found in other crab species, including *C. sapidus* and *S. paramamosain*, which are clustered together phylogenetically.

Keywords: *Chaceon quinquedens*; cold water species; red deep-sea crab; insulin-like androgenic gland hormone (IAG); androgenic gland

1. Introduction

Insulin-like androgenic gland hormone (IAG) is produced by the male endocrine organ referred to as the androgenic gland (AG) and is unique to male crustaceans. This gland, first described in the blue crab, *Callinectes sapidus*, is located near the sub-terminal region of the vas deferens, surrounded by muscles of the coxopodite of the last thoracic leg [1]. Following its discovery in *C. sapidus*, AG has been found to be present in other crustacean species including an amphipod species, *Orchestia gammarella* [2].

Androgenic gland hormone (AGH) produced by the AG is known to be involved in male sexual differentiation. The presence of AGH has been supported initially by experiments involving AG manipulations in crustaceans [3]. AG implantation into a female isopod, *Armadillidium vulgae*, resulted in the development of male sexual traits [4]. In female *Cherax quadricarinatus*, AG implantation caused the development of male secondary sexual characteristics including red patching on the propodus and the inhibition of vitellogenesis [5]. With clear evidence of the presence of AGH in crustaceans, its structural elucidation was reported first in the isopod *A. vulgare* [6,7]. The structure of IAGs (=AGHs) share six conserved cysteine residues with that of vertebrate insulin, whereas the rest of the primary sequences show much less similarity [6–11].

IAG, being involved in male sexual development, is thought to be exclusively found in male crustaceans. However, it has been reported that IAG has been expressed in tissues aside from the AG. Females of two decapod crab species (*C. sapidus* and *S. paramamosain*) express IAG in both the hepatopancreas and ovary, and male *C. sapidus* show a similar IAG expression in the hepatopancreas [9,10]. In shrimp, IAG expression is reported in the hepatopancreas and nerve cord of *Fenneropenaeus chinensis* in both sexes and the hepatopancreas of *M. nipponense* males [12,13]. Interestingly, in *C. sapidus*, IAG cDNA found in different tissues encode the same putative IAG sequence, while 5′ and 3′ UTR sequences differ [10,14,15]. These findings imply that IAG may be a multifunctional hormone, the function is reported as tissue-specific [14].

The red deep-sea crab, *Chaceon quinquedens*, is an important commercial species in the northeastern United States, where its fishery is federally managed. The *C. quinquedens* fishery is based on the harvesting of males with carapace width exceeding 114 mm as these animals are considered to be adults. *C. quinquedens* are distributed along the continental shelf and slope from Nova Scotia and into the Gulf of Mexico, inhabiting depths from 200 to 1800 m. Compared to warm water crustacean species, much remains unknown about their biology and physiology, including size-related sexual maturity. Like most decapod crustacean species, *C. quinquedens* are sexually dimorphic, females upon maturity exhibit specific morphological features specifically at pubertal molt, such as gonopore formation, ovigerous hair development, etc. [16]. Adult males on the other hand, show no clear external morphological feature(s) distinguishing them from juveniles. With the lack of available knowledge on when and at what size male *C. quinquedens* become sexually mature [17], it is important to garner information on size-related sexual maturity to provide more appropriate regulatory guidelines for male-oriented fisheries.

In this study, we aimed to develop a molecular tool, which can be used for determining the sexual maturity of male *C. quinquedens*. To this end, we isolated the full-length cDNA sequence of male *ChqIAG* from the AG using polymerase chain reaction (PCR) with the degenerate primers, and 5′ and 3′ rapid amplification of cDNA ends (RACE) and examined its tissue distribution in adult male and female *C. quinquedens*.

2. Results

2.1. cDNA Sequence Analysis

The full-length cDNA of *ChqIAG* (GenBank accession number KY497474) was isolated from the AG of an adult male, *C. quinquedens* (Figure 1). The *ChqIAG* cDNA sequence (1555 nt) contains a 366 nt 5′ UTR, a 453 nt ORF encoding 151 amino acids, and a relatively long 3′ UTR of 733 nt. The signal peptide (19 aa): MFLPVIILLMLLTATQTKA was identified (p = 0.879) using SignalP (http://www.cbs.dtu.dk/services/SignalP/).

Similar to vertebrate insulin, the putative ChqIAG sequence predicts B and A chains, with six conserved cysteine residues likely involved in three disulfide bridges (two interchains: C_{B9} and C_{A12} and C_{B20} and C_{A28}, and one intrachain: C_{A11} and C_{A19}). The ChqIAG sequence seen in Figure 1, contains a 19 aa signal peptide, followed by a B chain of 33 aa (underlined), a C chain of 55 aa (in bold and italicized), and an A chain of 44 aa (double underlined). Two cleavage sites, RHKR and RFRR, are located at the end of the B chain and C chain, respectively (boxed). The presence of a putative *N*-glycosylation site at N_{A18} (marked with a triangle) was found in the A chain.

```
>ChqIAG (KY497474)
     GGGGGAGGATAGGGGTGAAAATTGTAAGGATGTGAA                         36
     GTGACCTTTTGTTAACATGATCCTAATCTATCCTAGCACACCCCAAAAAATAGCTAGGGT 96
     GGCGAGTCTTCATGTGATAATTTTTTGAGACTCCTATCGCTGCGGTGCACCATCAGGAGC 156
     TGCTCCCGGCACTTAGCACTTCAGCACACCACCCGCCACGTCCTTCTTCCACCACCTCTT 216
     CACTTTCCTCCCAAGTCACCAGTAACTGTGTCTATTCCTCTCCTTCGCTTTCCTCCTAAG 276
     ACTAACCTCGACGCGTCCTCCTCCGTTTCTGTTCCTCCAGCTTAGGTCTTCCTCATCTA 336
     ACTCTCAAGCCGCGCACGGTACTCTCAAGAATGTTCCTGCCCGTGATTATACTACTGATG 396
10                                    M  F  L  P  V  I  I  L  L  M
     CTGCTGACGGCGACGCAGACGAAGGCGGACGCTAACAACTTCTCTGTGGACTGTGCTAAC 456
30   L  L  T  A  T  Q  T  K  A  D  A  N  N  F  S  V  D  C  A  N
     CTACCAAGAACCTTATCTCTGTATGCCTGACCTACAAACAACCTCCCAACAACAGACAT 516
50   L  P  R  T  L  S  S  V  C  L  T  Y  K  Q  P  P  N  N  R  H
     AAACGAGACACCGAGTCACAGGGCGCTGACACCCCTGATGATACCAACCCTGCCTTCCGC 576
70   K  R  D  T  E  S  Q  G  A  D  T  P  D  D  T  N  P  A  F  R
     CCCCGCCCACCTCACGCAGTCCCCATGATAACAGACGACGGCCCGATACTGTCCCCGGAG 636
90   P  R  P  P  H  A  V  P  M  I  T  D  D  G  P  I  L  S  P  E
     CTCGCCTTCCAGCTTGTCAAGACACAATGGACAGGGGGAAGGTTCCGCAGGTCTCAGCGG 696
110  L  A  F  Q  L  V  K  T  Q  W  T  G  G  R  F  R  R  S  Q  R
     TCTGTCAACGCCTATGACGAGTGCTGCCCTCAGTCCACCAAGAACTGCACCGTGTATGAG 756
130  S  V  N  A  Y  D  E  C  C  P  Q  S  T  K  N  C  T  V  Y  E
     GTAGCGGGGTACTGCGCTACTCTCAGGTCGCCCTACAGGGAAATTATAGCAGCTCAGAAT 816
150  V  A  G  Y  C  A  T  L  R  S  P  Y  R  E  I  I  A  A  Q  N
     CAGTAGGAAGATGAGGACGACGCGGCCCCAGCAGCTCCGAACACCCCAGCGATAGGAGTC 876
151  Q  *
     TCAAAAAATTATCATATGAAGACTCGCCACCCTAGCTATTTTTGGGGTGTGCTAGGATA 936
     GATTAGGATCATGTTAACAAAAGGTCACTTCACATCCTTACAATTTTCACCCCTATCCTC 996
     CCCAGAAAAGGTACTGAGGCTCATGTTAACAAAATGCTCACTTCAAAATCTTACAAGTTT 1056
     CATCCCTACCTCCGCAAAAAAGGTACCTAAGGCTCATGTTAACAAAAGATTACTTCAAAA 1116
     CCTTACAATTTTCATCCCTATCCTCCCCAAAACAGGTACTAAGGCTCATGTTAACAAATG 1176
     CTCACTTCAAAACCTTACAATTTTCACCCCTATCCCCCCATAAAGGTACTCAAGACTCCT 1236
     GTTAACAAATTGACCACTTCACAACCTTAGAAGTTTCACCCCACAGATCTCTCATTCACT 1296
     TAAACCAGTATGAAGGTGTGTGCACTGTGCATACACCAACATACACACAGGAAAACGCAA 1356
     ATTCCTTAAGATCCCCCATGTCTGTTTCACACCTGCCTACCGCTCAGCTTCCCCACGCAC 1416
     CTGTTGAGGAAGGTAACAACTATCTAACCCTCCCCATAGTAGTGCCTCGATGCCCCAAAT 1476
     TACCTTGTTCCCATCCTATGATTAGCGACGCGTAAGCAAATAAAGGTTTCAATATGATGC 1536
     GAGAGGAAAAAAAAAAAAA                                          1555
```

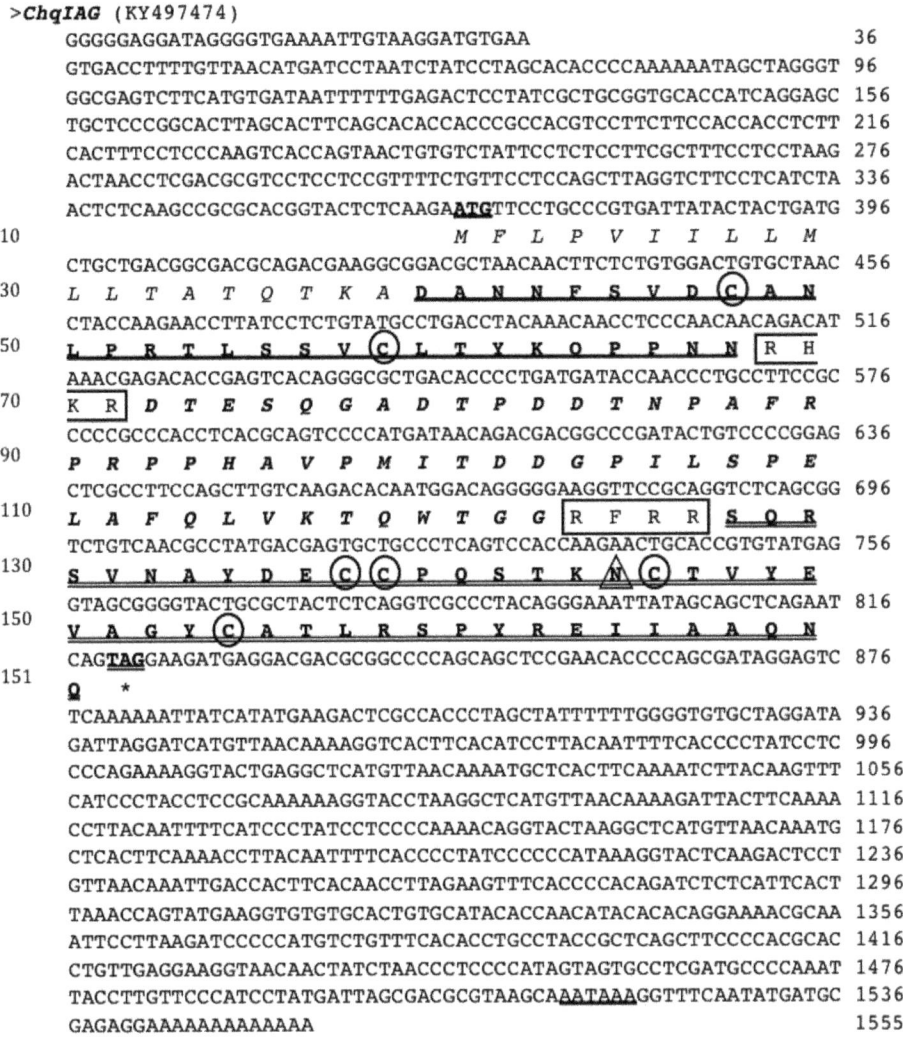

Figure 1. The full-length cDNA and deduced amino acid sequence of ChqIAG isolated from the androgenic gland (AG) of male *C. quinquedens* (GenBank Accession No. KY497474). Predicted signal peptide is italicized. The predicted start codon (ATG) is bolded and underlined, and the stop codon (TAG) is bolded, double underlined and marked with "*". The nucleotide number is on the right and the amino acid number is on the left hand side of the figure. Two predicted cleavage sites (RHKR/RFRR) are boxed and a polyadenylation signal (AATAAA) is underlined in the 3′ untranslated region (UTR). The six conserved cysteine residues are circled. The B chain is bold and underlined, the C chain is bold and italicized and the A chain is bold and double underlined. The predicted *N*-glycosylation site is noted with a triangle.

2.2. Phylogenetic Tree Analysis

A phylogenetic tree of the ORFs of decapod IAGs and AGH found in isopods was generated using neighbor-adjoining methods, as shown (Figure 2). The phylogenetic tree clusters crustacean

IAGs in relative correspondence to their taxonomy. Figure 2 contains two main branches clustering one group including the IAGs of the crayfish, lobsters, and the majority of prawn species, *Jasus edwardsii*, *Sagmariasus verreaux*, *C. destructor*, *P. clarkii*, *C. quadricarinatus*, *P. monodon*, *F. chinensis* and a crab species *Portunus pelagicus*. The other main branch groups crab species; *S. paramamosain*, *C. quinquedens*, *C. sapidus* and *Eriocheir sinensis* with a prawn species *M. rosenbergii* and all but one shrimp species *M. japonicas*. *Armadillidium vulgare* as an isopod outgroup clusters away from all malacostraca crustacean species.

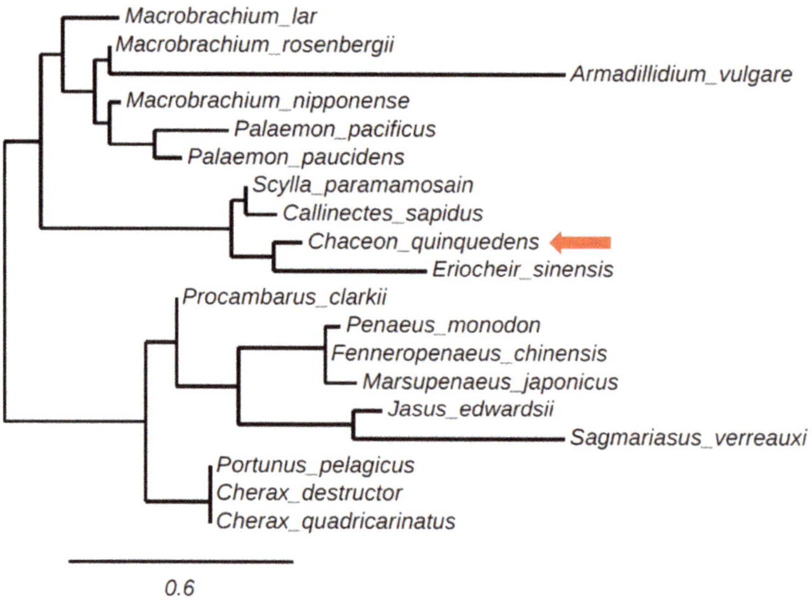

Figure 2. Maximum likelihood tree (using phylogeny.fr) of the open reading frame (ORF) sequence of crustacean insulin-like androgenic gland hormones (IAGs) and androgenic gland hormones (AGHs) obtained from the following species: *C. quinquedens*, KY497474; *M. rosenbergii*, ACJ38227.1; *P. pelagicus*, HM459854; *E. sinensis*, KU724192; *S. paramamosain*, JQ681748.1; *Jasus edwardsii*, KF908794; *Macrobrachium lar*, AB579012.1; *Callinectes sapidus*, KF792074.1; *M. nipponense*, KC460325; *Sagmariasus verreauxi*, KF220491; *Cherax destructor*, ACD91988; *Palaemon pacificus*, AB588014.1; *Procambarus clarkii*, KT343750. *Armadillidium vulgare*, BAA86893.1. *Cherax quadricarinatus*, DQ851163.1; *F. chinensis*, JQ388277.1; *P. monodon*, GU208677.1; *P. paucidens*, AB588013.1; *M. japonicus*, AB598415.1. The scale bar indicates the number of amino acid sequence substitutions per site. Distance represents neighbor-adjoining bootstrap values.

2.3. *Tissue Distribution of ChqIAG*

The spatial distribution of *ChqIAG* expression was examined in various tissues that were dissected from an adult male and female *C. quinquedens* using an end-point reverse-transcriptase polymerase chain reaction (RT-PCR) assay (Promega, Madison, WI, USA). The primers *ChqIAG*-start and -end were used to amplify the entire ORF region of *ChqIAG* (Table 1) (Figure 3a,b, respectively). The AG is the only tissue that expresses *ChqIAG* (Figure 3a, lane 13 boxed). The expression of arginine kinase (AK) as a reference gene is common in all the same tissue cDNA examined. There was no amplification noted by the no template control (lane 14). In contrast to earlier findings in other species, *ChqIAG* expression is absent in the male and female hepatopancreas (Figure 3a, lane 11) as well as the ovary (Figure 3b, Lane 11 and 12, respectively).

Table 1. Primer sequences used for the isolation of the full-length cDNA of *ChqIAG* from the AG of *C. quinquedens* (d = degenerate).

Primer Name	Primer Sequences (5′ → 3′)
dF1	GAYTTYGAYTGYGGNSAYYT
dR2	ACTGCGGCSACMTSGSCGACA
ChqIAG-3F1	ACCAAGAACCTTATCCTCTGTATGCCTGACC
ChqIAG-3F2	GCCCCCGCCCACCTCACGCAGTCCCCATGA
ChqIAG-3F3	AGCGGTCTGTCAACGTGCACGACGAGTGCTGC
ChqIAG-5R1	GCAGCACTCGTCGTGCACGTTGACAGACCGC
ChqIAG-5R2	TGTCCATTGTGTCTTGACAAGCTGGAAGGCGA
ChqIAG-5R3	ATCATCAGGGGTGTCAGCGCCCTGTGACTCGG
ChqIAG-st	ATGTTCCTGCCCGTGATTATACTACTGAT
ChqIAG-end	TACTGATTCTGAGCTGCTATAATTTCCCT
ChqAK-QF	CTGGGCCAGGTATACCGCCGCCTTGTCAGC
ChqAK-QR	GGGGAGCTTGATGTGGACGGAGGCACGCAC

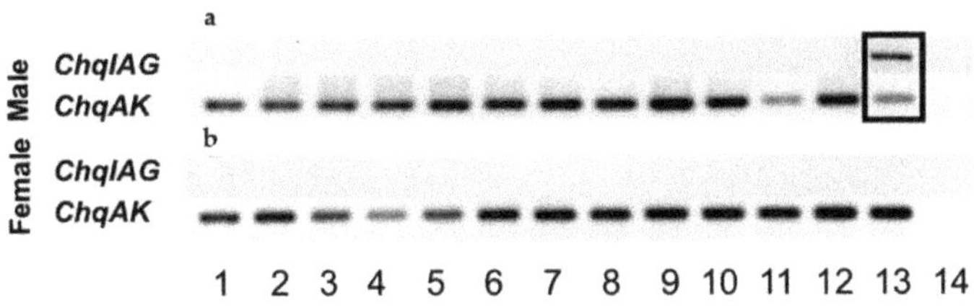

Figure 3. Spatial expression analysis of *ChqIAG* in adult male (**a**) and female (**b**) tissues 1: eyestalk ganglia; 2: thoracic ganglia complex; 3: brain; 4: hypodermis; 5: muscle; 6: gill; 7: midgut; 8: hindgut; 9: heart; 10: hemocytes; 11: hepatopancreas; 12: testis/ovary; 13: androgenic gland/spermatheca; 14: no template control. Arginine kinase (*ChqAK*) was used as a reference gene for amplification.

2.4. Translational Regulatory Sites in ChqIAG cDNA Sequence

Several decapod IAG sequences including that of *C. quinquedens* have been analyzed for putative translational regulatory sites present in 5′ and 3′ UTR using the RegRNA finder (Table 2). *C. quinquedens* share several of these sites with those of other decapod species IAG sequences. Terminal oligopyrimidine tract (TOP) motifs were found in the 5′ and in the 3′ UTRs of the *ChqIAG* sequence. An internal ribosome entry site (IRES) and upstream open reading frame (uORF) were present in both the 5′ and 3′ UTRs. A K-Box and Brd-Box were present only in the 5′ UTR of *ChqIAG*. A gamma interferon inhibitor of translation (GAIT element) located in the 3′ UTR of the ceruloplasmin mRNA is only found in the 3′ UTR.

Table 2. Putative translational regulatory sites * present in the 5′ (top of the table) and 3′ (bottom of the table) UTRs of decapod crustacean *IAG cDNA* sequences.

	TOP	IRES	uORF	GAIT Element	SECIS	ADH_DRE	KB	CPE	GY	Brd	BRE
Species:											
C. quinquedens	5	1	1				1			1	
M. nipponense	6										
P. pelagicus											
M. rosenbergii	9				1						
E. sinensis	7								1		
P. pacificus	3			3							
C. destructor											
S. verreauxi	9								1		
S. paramamosain	6	1									
M. japonicus	4										
M. lar	6										
C. quadricarinatus	4				2						
C. sapidus	3										
F. chinensis	5										
P. paucidens	2			1							
P. clarkii	3										

Table 2. *Cont.*

	TOP	IRES	uORF	GAIT Element	SECIS	ADH_DRE	KB	CPE	GY	Brd	BRE
C. quinquedens	5	4	3	1							
M. nipponense	24	2	4	1					1	3	
P. pelagicus	5	1	2	2					1		
M. rosenbergii	31		3	1				1	1	3	
E. sinensis	7	3	2	2	1			1			
P. pacificus	23		3	1	1					8	
C. destructor	3	1	1	2					1		
S. verreauxi	9	2	4	6	2						
S. paramamosain	2	3	2	6	1					1	
M. japonicus	2									1	
M. lar	24	2	3	4	1	1		1	1	1	
C. quadricarinatus	2	1	2					1		1	
C. sapidus	3	2	2	1	1				1		
F. chinensis	12	4	2								1
P. paucidens	8		2	1							
P. clarkii	1										
motif distribution	233	27	36	32	10	1	1	4	8	19	1
motif frequency	0.63	0.07	0.1	0.09	0.03	0.003	0.003	0.01	0.02	0.05	0.003

* Regulatory sites were analyzed using regrna.mbc.nctu.edutw/html/prediction.html: Terminal oligopyrimidine tract (TOP), internal ribosome entry site (IRES), upstream open reading frame (uORF), gamma interferon activated inhibitor of ceruloplasmin mRNA translation (GAIT element), selenocysteine insertion sequence (SECIS), alcohol dehydrogenase 3′ UTR down regulation control element (ADH_DRE), K-box (KB)/cytoplasmic polyadenylation response element (CPE), GY-box (GY), and Brd-box (BRD), Bruno 3′ UTR responsive element (BRE). Motif distribution row represents the number of sequences containing that particular motif (n = 16). Motif frequency row represents the frequency of that motif as a percentage of all motifs (n = 372). *A. vulagre, J. edwardsii* and *P. monodon* are excluded from this figure because only the coding region, not the full-length cDNA sequence of IAGs including 5′ and 3′ UTRs are available in National Center for Biotechnology Information (NCBI).

3. Discussion

In this study, we isolated the full-length *ChqIAG* cDNA sequence from the androgenic gland of a male red deep-sea crab, *C. quinquedens,* and determined the spatial distribution of its expression in male and female tissues. To examine translational control of IAG, we also analyzed putative translational motifs of IAG sequences in 15 other crustacean species listed from GenBank together with *ChqIAG*.

ChqIAG differentiates itself from other crustacean IAG sequences by exhibiting a 733 nt long 3′ UTR, implicating that this region may contain putative translation regulatory sites. The crab species as a group, including *C. sapidus, S. paramamosain, E. sinensis,* and *C. quinquedens,* have longer 3′ UTRs (~500–830 nt) followed by *P. pelagicus* with a 377 nt 3′ UTR and the lobster, prawn and crayfish species having the smallest 3′ UTR < 300 nt [7]. It is reported that the IAG sequence is possibly encoded by four or more exons separated by three introns: the first one located within the signal peptide, and both the second and third located inside the C peptide [9,18]. The length of the 3′ UTR that is encoded in exon four differs by species. The 3′ UTR length is known to reflect translational efficiency [19], suggesting that *C. quinquedens'* lengthy 3′ UTR may involve a more proficient translation process.

ChqIAG is clustered with three other crab species *S. paramamosain, C. sapidus,* and *E. sinensis*. This grouping reflects sequence similarities of the ORFs. The six conserved cysteines within the A and B chains allow for the formation of the intra- and inter-disulfide bonds. The putative amino acid sequence of ChqIAG is most similar to that of *S. paramamosain* and *C. sapidus,* showing 63.6% and 62.9% sequence identity, respectively. *E. sinensis* shares the least sequence identity within the crab cluster at 40.9%. Oddly, the *C. destructor* sequence shows greater similarity to another crab species, *P. pelagicus* than a crayfish belonging to the same genus, *C. quadricarinatus.* The least similar clusters are the prawn/shrimp species cluster and the lobster species cluster at less than ~25% sequence similarity. Overall, IAG sequences isolated from all crab species except for *P. pelagicus* are more similar to each other than those of crayfish or prawn.

IAG is expressed exclusively in the AG of male *C. quinquedens.* It is expected that *ChqIAG* would show a similar expression pattern as that of *C. sapidus* and *S. paramamosain.* However, the exclusive expression of *ChqIAG* expression in the AG is similar to other crustacean species [8] but differs from that of *C. sapidus. S. paramamosain, F. chinensis,* and *M. nipponense* where IAG has been expressed in both male and female tissues [12,14]. To date, it is still not known if these additional tissues of *S. paramamosain*, *F. chinensis*, and *M. nipponense* contain the same IAG as in the AG as in *C. sapidus* [10]. It is proposed that *C. quinquedens* may have different forms of IAG in these tissues. Hence, they might not have been amplified with the pair of primers used in this study.

The analysis of putative translation regulatory sites in the IAG cDNA sequences shows that *ChqIAG* contains five different motifs: five TOPs, one IRES, one uORF, one K-box and one Brd-box. The presence of IRES in the 5′ UTR of the IAG sequence is unique to *C. quinquedens* and *S. paramamosain*. As another unique feature, *ChqIAG* 5′ UTR also lists a Brd-box which is typically found in the 3′ UTR. The Brd-box found in 3′ UTR is known to down-regulate transcription and subsequently leads to a reduction in protein levels [20]. Having two translational regulatory sites in the 5′ UTR of *ChqIAG* suggests that the translation of IAG levels in AG may be regulated tightly.

Although the ChqIAG cDNA sequence is the only IAG sequence obtained from cold-water species to date, we propose that IRES and Brd-box may be related to ChqIAG translation and may be associated with water temperature. IRES presence is usually associated with the mRNA of growth regulatory genes, which are known to respond to and during environmental stressors [21]. The *ChqIAG* sequence displays the IRES motif more frequently than IAG sequences of any other species in the analysis. Both IRES and box motifs are present among other growth hormone mRNA in cold-water species including *C. japonicus* and *C. opilio* crustacean hyperglycemic hormones [22]. It appears that crustacean species inhabiting colder water are more sensitive to temperature changes than those living in warmer water and may depend on tighter translational control of these neuropeptide hormones than those living in warmer water.

Four different translational regulatory sites are predicted within the *ChqIAG* 3′ UTR, including five TOPs, one uORF, one GAIT, and one IRES. These motifs are most commonly found in the 3′ UTRs of all species in Table 2. The presence of at least three out of four of these regulatory sites present in 14 out of 16 crustaceans in the analysis suggests a more conserved 3′ UTR among IAGs.

There are in general difficulties in distinguishing the sexual maturity of male crustaceans. Unlike adult females, adult males do not exhibit externally visible morphological features. Attempts have been made to determine a relationship between the size and onset of sexual maturity in other deep-sea cold water crustaceans such as the Alaskan tanner crab, *Chionoecetes bairdi*, using chela allometry (using chela height/length, and carapace length/width). However, a clear relationship between size and maturity has not been found yet either in *C. bairdi* [23] or in *C. quinquedens* [17]. Hence it is proposed that establishing a relationship between the size and the levels of crustacean male hormone, IAG, can be used as a tool to define the maturity of male crustaceans.

IAG is known to regulate male sexual development, specifically secondary sexual features and spermatogenesis, suggesting that the levels of IAG expression in the AG and of the hemolymph IAG titers may be closely associated with male sexual maturity. It is reported that IAG requires a binding partner, an insulin-like binding protein, or an insulin-like binding protein like peptide [24]. The exact mode of the IAG mechanism by which it regulates such processes still remains to be studied. With the isolation of the *ChqIAG* cDNA sequence, it will be examined if there is a relationship between the levels of IAGs and the size at sexual maturity of *C. quinquedens* males. This information would provide management agencies guidance for male-driven fisheries that are currently regulated only based on the size, not maturity.

4. Materials and Methods

4.1. Animal Collection and Maintenance

Adult *C. quinquedens* were collected along the continental shelf off the coast of Virginia in June of 2016 (The Atlantic Red Crab Co., New Bedford, MA, USA). Crabs were captured using baited crab pots and stored in a refrigerated cooling tank onboard the fishing vessel. Adult males and females were then transported in coolers from Newport News, VA to the Institute of Marine and

Environmental Technology (IMET, Baltimore, MD, USA). The crabs were kept for three days in a dark, climate-controlled room at 4 °C in 30 ppt artificial seawater. Crabs were chilled on ice prior to dissection. AGs were collected and immediately placed on dry ice. These samples were kept at −80 °C until further processing.

4.2. Isolation of the Full-Length ChqIAG cDNA Using PCR with Degenerate Primers

The degenerate primers in Table 1 were based on conserved amino acid sequences of crustacean IAGs [10]. The total RNA was isolated from the AGs of an adult male using the QIAzol lysis reagent (Qiagen, Santa Ana, CA, USA), following the manufacturer's protocol. The total RNA was quantified using a NanoDrop Lite Spectrophotometer (Thermo Scientific, Waltham, MA, USA). The total RNA (~1–1.5 µg) was subjected to 5′ and 3′ RACE cDNA syntheses using the Switching Mechanism at 5′ End of RNA Template (SMART) cDNA synthesis kit (BD Biosciences, San Jose, CA, USA) following the manufacturer's protocol. A two-step PCR method was employed as reported [10]. Briefly, the first touch-down polymerase chain reaction (TD-PCR) (BD Biosciences, San Jose, CA, USA) reaction used the degenerate primer dF1 with a universal primer (BD Biosciences) with the following conditions: 94 °C for 2.5 min; eight cycles at 94 °C for 30 s; decreasing annealing temperatures 2 °C/cycle from 42 °C to 39 °C for 30 s; 68 °C for 1.5 min; 27 cycles at 94 °C for 30 s; 43 °C for 30 s; 68 °C for 1.5 min; and the final extension at 68 °C for 7 min. The TD-PCR products served as the template for the semi-nested PCR where dF1 and dR2 primers were used with the following PCR conditions: 94 °C for 2.5 min; 40 cycles at 94 °C for 30 s; 40 °C for 30 s; 72 °C for 1.5 min; followed by a final extension of 72 °C for 7 min. Products from the semi-nested PCR reaction were analyzed on a 1.5% agarose gel. A band of the expected size ~280 bp was excised for DNA extraction. Cloning and sequencing procedures were conducted as described in [13]. From the initially acquired sequencing results of *ChqIAG*, gene-specific primers were generated (see Table 1) for further isolation of the full-length cDNA sequence encoding *ChqIAG*.

4.3. 5′ and 3′ RACE of ChqIAG

The initial TD-PCRs for 5′ and 3′ RACE were carried out as described above; however, the gene specific primers *ChqIAG*-5R1 and *ChqIAG*-3F1 were utilized to obtain 5′ and 3′ RACE sequences, respectively. Both 5′ and 3′ RACE TD-PCRs were conducted using the following conditions: 94 °C for 2.5 min; annealing temperatures decreasing 2 °C/cycle from 57 °C to 53 °C for 9 cycles; followed by 27 cycles at 94 °C for 30 s; 58 °C for 30 s; 68 °C for 1.5 min; and the final extension at 68 °C for 7 min. One microliter of the initial TD-PCR product served as the template for the semi-nested PCR and was amplified using nested universal primer (BD Biosciences) and *ChqIAG*-5R2 for 5′ RACE and *ChqIAG*-3F2 for 3′ RACE. Bands with the expected size of ~450–550 bp were excised for DNA extraction (Qiagen), followed by subsequent cloning and sequencing as described in [10].

4.4. Sequence Analyses

The ORF finder was used for finding the ORF (www.ncbi.nlm.nih.gov/orffinder/). The putative amino acid ChqIAG was examined for the presence of a signal peptide using Signal P (http://www.cbs.dtu.dk/services/SignalP/). The transcriptional regulatory sites present in the *ChqIAG* sequence were analyzed using RegRNA2.0 (http://regrna2.mbc.nctu.edu.tw/ [25]. The *N*-glycosylation site was determined using (http://www.cbs.dtu.dk/services/NetNGlyc/). A phylogenetic tree was constructed using phylogeny.fr.

4.5. Tissue Distribution of ChqIAG Expression

Total RNA was extracted as described above from various tissues from an adult males and females including eyestalk ganglia, thoracic ganglia complex, brain, hypodermis, abdominal muscle, gill, midgut, hindgut, heart, hemocytes, hepatopancreas, testis, ovary, androgenic gland, and spermatheca. One-2 µg of the total RNA of each tissue sample was subjected to the first strand cDNA synthesis using the PrimeScript™ Reverse transcriptase reagent kit with a gDNA eraser (TaKaRa, Mountain View, CA, USA). The *ChqIAG* spatial distribution was determined using an end-point PCR assay. Each tissue's cDNA (12.5 ng of total RNA equivalent) was amplified with *ChqIAG*-start and end primers (Table 1) under the following PCR conditions: 94 °C for 2.5 min, followed by 30 cycles of 94 °C for 30 s, 60 °C for 30 s, and 72 °C for 1 min, and the final extension at 72 °C for 5 min. As a reference gene, arginine kinase (*ChqAK*) was amplified in the same cDNA samples using *ChqAK*-QF and *ChqAK*-QR primers.

Acknowledgments: We thank Jon Williams and Bruce Medeiros of the Atlantic Red Crab Company for obtaining red deep-sea crabs for this research and Stephanie Martinez at University of Maryland Eastern Shore for arranging deliveries and collection of the animals. The work was supported by a National Science Foundation program grant to JSC (1146774). AL internship was supported by the NOAA Living Marine Resources Cooperative Science Center (NOAA Award No. NA11SEC4810002). This article is contribution No. 5390 of the University of Maryland Center for Environmental Science and contribution No. 17-211 of the Institute of Marine and Environmental Technology.

Author Contributions: Jum Sook Chung conceived and designed the experiments; Amanda Lawrence performed experiments; Shadaesha Green contributed reagents and materials; Amanda Lawrence and Jum Sook Chung analyzed the data; Amanda Lawrence and Jum Sook Chung wrote the paper.

Conflicts of Interest: The authors declare no conflict of interest.

References

1. Cronin, L.E. Anatomy and histology of the male reproductive system of *Callinectes sapidus* Rathbun. *J. Morphol.* **1947**, *81*, 209–239. [CrossRef] [PubMed]
2. Charniaux-Cotton, H. Decouverte chez un crustace amphipode (*Orchestia gammarella*) d'une glande endocrine responsable de la differentiation de caracteres sexuels primaires et secondaires males. *C. R. Acad. Sci. Paris* **1954**, *239*, 780–782. [PubMed]
3. Charniaux-Cotton, H. Androgenic gland of crustaceans. *Gen. Comp. Endocrinol.* **1962**, *1*, 241–247. [CrossRef]
4. Suzuki, S.; Yamasaki, K. Sex reversal by implantations of ethanol-treated androgenic glands of female isopods, *Armadillidium vulgare* (Malacostraca, crustacea). *Gen. Comp. Endocrinol.* **1998**, *111*, 367–375. [CrossRef] [PubMed]
5. Manor, R.; Aflalo, E.D.; Segall, C.; Weil, S.; Azulay, D.; Ventura, T.; Sagi, A. Androgenic gland implantation promotes growth and inhibits vitellogenesis in *Cherax quadricarinatus* females held in individual compartments. *Invertebr. Reprod. Dev.* **2004**, *45*, 151–159. [CrossRef]
6. Martin, G.; Sorokine, O.; Moniatte, M.; Bulet, P.; Hetru, C.; Van Dorsselaer, A. The structure of a glycosylated protein hormone responsible for sex determination in the isopod, *Armadillidium vulgare*. *Eur. J. Biochem.* **1999**, *262*, 727–736. [CrossRef] [PubMed]
7. Okuno, A.; Hasegawa, Y.; Ohira, T.; Katakura, Y.; Nagasawa, H. Characterization and cDNA cloning of androgenic gland hormone of the terrestrial isopod *Armadillidium vulgare*. *Biochem. Biophys. Res. Commun.* **1999**, *264*, 419–423. [CrossRef] [PubMed]
8. Ventura, T.; Manor, R.; Aflalo, E.D.; Weil, S.; Khalaila, I.; Rosen, O.; Sagi, A. Expression of an androgenic gland-specific insulin-like peptide during the course of prawn sexual and morphotypic differentiation. *ISRN Endocrinol.* **2011**, *2011*, 476283. [CrossRef] [PubMed]
9. Huang, X.; Ye, H.; Huang, H.; Yang, Y.; Gong, J. An insulin-like androgenic gland hormone gene in the mud crab, *Scylla paramamosain*, extensively expressed and involved in the processes of growth and female reproduction. *Gen. Comp. Endocrinol.* **2014**, *204*, 229–238. [CrossRef] [PubMed]
10. Chung, J.S.; Manor, R.; Sagi, A. Cloning of an insulin-like androgenic gland factor (IAG) from the blue crab, *Callinectes sapidus*: Implications for eyestalk regulation of IAG expression. *Gen. Comp. Endocrinol.* **2011**, *173*, 4–10. [CrossRef] [PubMed]
11. Ventura, T.; Fitzgibbon, Q.; Battaglene, S.; Sagi, A.; Elizur, A. Identification and characterization of androgenic gland specific insulin-like peptide-encoding transcripts in two spiny lobster species: *Sagmariasus verreauxi* and *Jasus edwardsii*. *Gen. Comp. Endocrinol.* **2015**, *214*, 126–133. [CrossRef] [PubMed]
12. Li, S.; Li, F.; Sun, Z.; Xiang, J. Two spliced variants of insulin-like androgenic gland hormone gene in the Chinese shrimp, *Fenneropenaeus chinensis*. *Gen. Comp. Endocrinol.* **2012**, *177*, 246–255. [CrossRef] [PubMed]

13. Li, F.; Bai, H.; Xiong, Y.; Fu, H.; Jiang, S.; Jiang, F.; Jin, S.; Sun, S.; Qiao, H.; Zhang, W. Molecular characterization of insulin-like androgenic gland hormone-binding protein gene from the oriental river prawn *Macrobrachium nipponense* and investigation of its transcriptional relationship with the insulin-like androgenic gland hormone gene. *Gen. Comp. Endocrinol.* **2015**, *216*, 152–160. [CrossRef] [PubMed]
14. Chung, J.S. An insulin-like growth factor found in hepatopancreas implicates carbohydrate metabolism of the blue crab *Callinectes sapidus*. *Gen. Comp. Endocrinol.* **2014**, *199*, 56–64. [CrossRef] [PubMed]
15. Chung, J.S.; Zmora, N. Functional studies of crustacean hyperglycemic hormones (CHHs) of the blue crab, *Callinectes sapidus*—The expression and release of CHH in eyestalk and pericardial organ in response to envir. *FEBS J.* **2008**, *275*, 693–704. [CrossRef] [PubMed]
16. Zmora, N.; Chung, J.S. A novel hormone is required for the development of reproductive phenotypes in adult female crabs. *Endocrinology* **2014**, *155*, 230–239. [CrossRef] [PubMed]
17. Stevens, B.G.; Guida, V. Depth and temperature distribution, morphometrics, and sex ratios of red deepsea crab (*Chaceon quinquedens*) at 4 sampling sites in the mid-atlantic bight. *Fish. Bull.* **2016**, *114*, 343–359. [CrossRef]
18. Zhang, Y.; Qiao, K.; Wang, S.; Peng, H.; Shan, Z.; Wang, K. Molecular identification of a new androgenic gland-specific insulin-like gene from the mud crab, *Scylla paramamosain*. *Aquaculture* **2014**, *433*, 325–334. [CrossRef]
19. Tanguay, R.L.; Gallie, D.R. Translational efficiency is regulated by the length of the 3′ untranslated region. *Mol. Cell. Biol.* **1996**, *16*, 146–156. [CrossRef] [PubMed]
20. Lai, E.C.; Posakony, J.W. The Bearded box, a novel 3′ UTR sequence motif, mediates negative post-transcriptional regulation of Bearded and Enhancer of split Complex gene expression. *Development* **1997**, *124*, 4847–4856. [PubMed]
21. Hellen, T.U.C.; Sarrow, P. Internal ribosome entry sites in eukaryotic mRNA molecules. *J. Virol.* **2001**, *85*, 49–63. [CrossRef] [PubMed]
22. Chung, J.S.; Ahn, I.S.; Yu, O.H.; Kim, D.S. Crustacean hyperglycemic hormones of two cold water crab species, *Chionoecetes opilio* and *C. japonicus*: Isolation of cDNA sequences and localization of CHH neuropeptide in eyestalk ganglia. *Gen. Comp. Endocrinol.* **2015**, *214*, 177–185. [CrossRef] [PubMed]
23. Brown, R.B.; Powell, G.C. Size at maturity in the male alaskan tanner crab, *Chionoecetes bairdi*, as determined by chela allometry, reproductive tract weights, and size of precopulatory males. *J. Fish. Res. Board Can.* **1972**, *29*, 423–427. [CrossRef]
24. Rosen, O.; Weil, S.; Manor, R.; Roth, Z.; Khalaila, I.; Sagi, A. A crayfish insulin-like-binding protein: Another piece in the androgenic gland insulin-like hormone puzzle is revealed. *J. Biol. Chem.* **2013**, *288*, 22289–22298. [CrossRef] [PubMed]
25. Huang, H.Y.; Chien, C.H.; Jen, K.H.; Huang, H.D. RegRNA: A regulatory RNA motifs and elements finder. *Nucleic Acids Res.* **2006**, *34*, W429–W434. [CrossRef] [PubMed]

© 2017 by the authors. Licensee MDPI, Basel, Switzerland. This article is an open access article distributed under the terms and conditions of the Creative Commons Attribution (CC BY) license (http://creativecommons.org/licenses/by/4.0/).

MDPI
St. Alban-Anlage 66
4052 Basel
Switzerland
Tel. +41 61 683 77 34
Fax +41 61 302 89 18
www.mdpi.com

Marine Drugs Editorial Office
E-mail: marinedrugs@mdpi.com
www.mdpi.com/journal/marinedrugs

www.ingramcontent.com/pod-product-compliance
Lightning Source LLC
LaVergne TN
LVHW070608100526
838202LV00012B/595